# THE HANDBOOK OF COMMUNITY MENTAL HEALTH NURSING

*The Handbook of Community Mental Health Nursing* brings together authoritative contributions from leading mental health researchers, educators and practitioners to provide a comprehensive text for community mental health nurses in training and practice. In thirty-three chapters it covers a wide range of topics, from the history of the profession to current approaches to specific client groups, organised around three linked themes:

- professional context
- practice issues
- education and research.

Each chapter includes a summary of key points and suggestions for further reading. The book also includes useful appendices listing key professional and voluntary organisations, journals, internet sites and mailing lists.

*The Handbook of Community Mental Health Nursing* reflects the diversity and scope of the role of the CMHN and recognises the multidisciplinary and service user context in which nurses work. An essential text for CMHNs and mental health nurse educators, it also offers a useful source of reference for allied professionals.

**Ben Hannigan** is a Lecturer in the School of Nursing and Midwifery Studies, University of Wales College of Medicine, Cardiff. **Michael Coffey** is a Lecturer in Community Mental Health Nursing at the School of Health Science, University of Wales, Swansea.

# THE HANDBOOK OF COMMUNITY MENTAL HEALTH NURSING

Edited by Ben Hannigan and
Michael Coffey

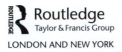
Routledge
Taylor & Francis Group

LONDON AND NEW YORK

First published 2003
by Routledge
11 New Fetter Lane, London EC4P 4EE

Simultaneously published in the USA and Canada
by Routledge
29 West 35th Street, New York, NY 10001

*Routledge is an imprint of the Taylor & Francis Group*

Designed and typeset in Sabon and Futura by
Keystroke, Jacaranda Lodge, Wolverhampton
Printed and bound in Great Britain by
TJ International Ltd, Padstow, Cornwall

*British Library Cataloguing in Publication Data*
A catalogue record for this book is available from the British Library

*Library of Congress Cataloging in Publication Data*
The handbook of community health nursing / edited by Ben Hannigan
and Michael Coffey.
p. ; cm.
Includes bibliographical references and index.
1. Psychiatric nursing–Handbooks, manuals, etc.  2. Community
mental health services–Handbooks, manuals, etc.
I. Hannigan, Ben, 1965–  II. Coffey, Michael, RMN.
[DNLM: 1. Community Health Nursing–methods. 2. Community Mental
Health Services. WY 106 H2355 2003]
RC440.H297 2003
610.73′68–dc21    20020037183

ISBN 0–415–28035–4 (hbk)
ISBN 0–415–28036–2 (pbk)

# CONTENTS

*List of tables, boxes and figures*  ix
*Notes on contributors*  xi
*Acknowledgements*  xv

Introduction  1
BEN HANNIGAN AND MICHAEL COFFEY

**PART 1**
**Context**  5

1  The history of community mental health nursing  7
   PETER NOLAN

2  The frontline workforce of community mental health care  19
   PAUL GODIN

3  The policy and legal context  30
   BEN HANNIGAN

4  Ethical issues  41
   CHRIS CHALONER

5  Social exclusion, discrimination and social isolation  54
   RACHEL PERKINS AND JULIE REPPER

6  Working in multidisciplinary community teams  67
   EDWARD PECK

7  Meeting mental health needs in primary care  78
   ELIZABETH ARMSTRONG

8  Collaborating with users of services  90
   PETER CAMPBELL

9 Gender issues     100
ANNE FOTHERGILL

10 Culture and ethnicity     111
SUMAN FERNANDO

11 Stress, burnout and coping     121
DEBORAH EDWARDS

12 Clinical supervision and reflective practice     132
JOHN CUTCLIFFE

PART 2
Practice     145

13 Promoting mental health     149
JUDY BOXER

14 Using evidence to inform practice     164
ROB NEWELL

15 Assessing needs in community mental health care     175
MIKE SLADE

16 Risk, decision-making and mental health     187
ANDY ALASZEWSKI

17 Preventing suicide     198
STEVE WOOD

18 Working with families I: systemic approaches     210
BILLY HARDY

19 Working with families II: psychosocial interventions     222
GEOFF BRENNAN

20 Cognitive behaviour therapy for psychosis     235
NORMAN YOUNG

21 Relapse prevention in psychosis     250
MICHAEL COFFEY

22 Case management and assertive outreach     261
STEVE MORGAN

23 Psychopharmacology and medication management     274
RICHARD GRAY, ELIZABETH BREWIN AND
DANIEL BRESSINGTON

24  Creativity and the therapeutic use of the creative arts        287
    TONY GILLAM

25  Working with mentally disordered offenders        299
    MICHAEL COFFEY

26  Working with people with coexisting mental health and
    substance misuse problems        310
    JEFF CHAMPNEY-SMITH

27  Working with people with dementia and their carers        319
    JOHN KEADY

28  Working with people with mental health problems and
    learning disabilities        331
    DAVE COYLE

29  Current approaches to working with children and adolescents        343
    RICHARD WILLIAMS AND FIONA GALE


PART 3
Education and research        357

30  Education and training for community mental health nurses        359
    MICHAEL COFFEY AND BEN HANNIGAN

31  Developing courses in psychosocial interventions        370
    NORMAN YOUNG AND IAN HULATT

32  The contribution of quantitative approaches to community
    mental health nursing research        385
    KEVIN GOURNAY

33  The contribution of qualitative approaches to community
    mental health nursing research        397
    IAN BEECH

    Conclusion        406
    BEN HANNIGAN AND MICHAEL COFFEY

Appendix I: Professional organisations        408
Appendix II: Voluntary organisations        410
Appendix III: Journals and magazines        414
Appendix IV: Internet sites and discussion lists        417

Index        418

# TABLES, BOXES AND FIGURES

## TABLES

1.1   Development of community psychiatric nursing at Moorhaven
      Hospital, Devon                                                    12
7.1   Diagnostic groups and ways of organising care                     81
7.2   An integrated approach to mental health care                      86
15.1  Psychometric properties of needs assessment measures             179
16.1  Definitions of risk                                              190
27.1  CPN and dementia care: selected overview of role attributes and
      practice domains                                                 324
30.1  'Specialist practice' courses for CMHNs: educational philosophies
      and aims                                                         363
30.2  'Specialist practice' courses for CMHNs: areas of content identified
      by course leaders related to the development of skills and
      knowledge associated with professional practice                  363
30.3  'Specialist practice' courses for CMHNs: areas of content identified
      by course leaders related to the preparation of nurses to work in
      contemporary community mental health settings                    363
31.1  Applying Rogers's model to the adoption of psychosocial
      interventions                                                    382

## BOXES

1.1   Greene's formulation of the role of the community psychiatric
      nurse in 1968                                                      13
1.2   Criticisms of CPN training in the early 1990s                     15
4.1   Two ethical theories                                              43
4.2   Ethical principles                                                44
4.3   Ethical reflection                                                45
4.4   Autonomy                                                          48
6.1   The CPNs' story                                                   74

| | | |
|---|---|---|
| 12.1 | Cutcliffe, Butterworth and Proctor's (2001) view of the central rudiments of clinical supervision | 134 |
| 12.2 | Ghaye and Lillyman's (2000) twelve key principles of reflective practice | 135 |
| 13.1 | Health for all | 151 |
| 13.2 | The concept of mental health promotion | 151 |
| 13.3 | Three levels of mental health promotion analysis | 152 |
| 13.4 | Anti-oppressive practice | 153 |
| 13.5 | Effective mental health promotion | 156 |
| 13.6 | Primary care trusts | 156 |
| 13.7 | An example of a user-focused monitoring project | 160 |
| 14.1 | Introducing an evidence-based care initiative | 166 |
| 19.1 | Caring about carers | 223 |
| 19.2 | A six-step problem-solving strategy | 227 |
| 19.3 | Case study | 229 |
| 20.1 | Changes in cognition in psychosis | 237 |
| 20.2 | Overview of CBT for psychosis | 239 |
| 20.3 | Overview of problem assessment | 241 |
| 20.4 | Ongoing monitoring | 243 |
| 20.5 | Vulnerability | 244 |
| 20.6 | Coping strategies for voices or paranoia | 246 |
| 21.1 | Five fundamental principles of relapse prevention | 255 |
| 21.2 | Strategies for helping manage illness | 257 |
| 23.1 | Medication management | 283 |
| 25.1 | Potential negative consequences of socially supportive relationships | 306 |
| 31.1 | General items required for a curriculum document | 377 |
| 31.2 | Thorn initiative evaluators' checklist | 380 |

## FIGURES

| | | |
|---|---|---|
| 20.1 | Stress vulnerability | 239 |
| 20.2 | The development of an ongoing formulation using Mind Maps® | 244 |
| 23.1 | Neurotransmission | 276 |
| 31.1 | Overview of course development | 372 |
| 31.2 | An example of a Gantt chart for a medication management module | 375 |
| 32.1 | A structural framework for development and evaluation of RCTs for complex interventions to improve health | 393 |

# NOTES ON CONTRIBUTORS

**Andy Alaszewski** is Professor in the Centre for Health Services Studies, University of Kent at Canterbury.

**Elizabeth Armstrong** is a Non-executive Director of Northampton Primary Care Trust.

**Ian Beech** is a Senior Lecturer in the School of Care Sciences, University of Glamorgan.

**Judy Boxer** is a Senior Lecturer in Social Work at Sheffield Hallam University.

**Geoff Brennan** is Head of Nursing Practice at Oxleas NHS Trust.

**Daniel Bressington** is a Tutor-Practitioner in Medication Management at the Institute of Psychiatry, King's College London/ South London and Maudsley NHS Trust.

**Elizabeth Brewin** is a Research Nurse at the Institute of Psychiatry, King's College London.

**Peter Campbell** is a mental health system survivor and writer.

**Chris Chaloner** is a Senior Lecturer in Ethics in the School of Health, Greenwich University.

**Jeff Champney-Smith** is a Lecturer/Practitioner in the School of Nursing and Midwifery Studies, University of Wales College of Medicine/Cardiff and Vale NHS Trust.

**Michael Coffey** is a Lecturer in Community Mental Health Nursing in the School of Health Science, University of Wales Swansea.

**Dave Coyle** is Director of Mental Health and Learning Disabilities Nursing in the School of Nursing and Midwifery Studies, University of Wales College of Medicine.

**John Cutcliffe** is Chair of Nursing, College of Arts and Social and Health Sciences, University of Northern British Columbia, Canada.

**Deborah Edwards** is a Researcher in the School of Nursing and Midwifery Studies, University of Wales College of Medicine.

**Suman Fernando** is an Honorary Senior Lecturer at The Tizard Centre, University of Kent.

**Anne Fothergill** is a Principal Lecturer in the School of Care Sciences, University of Glamorgan.

**Fiona Gale** is Joint Commissioning and Strategy Manager for Child and Adolescent Mental Health Services Leicester, Leicestershire and Rutland, Leicester City West Primary Care Trust.

**Tony Gillam** is a Project Worker with the Meriden Programme, Northern Birmingham Mental Health NHS Trust.

**Paul Godin** is a Lecturer in the Department of Applied Psychosocial Sciences, St Bartholomew School of Nursing, City University.

**Kevin Gournay** is Professor of Psychiatric Nursing at the Institute of Psychiatry, King's College London.

**Richard Gray** is an MRC Fellow in Health Services Research at the Institute of Psychiatry, King's College London.

**Ben Hannigan** is a Lecturer in the School of Nursing and Midwifery Studies, University of Wales College of Medicine.

**Billy Hardy** is a Senior Lecturer and Family Therapist at the School of Care Science, University of Glamorgan/Family Therapy Institute.

**Ian Hulatt** is a Lecturer in the School of Nursing and Midwifery Studies, University of Wales College of Medicine.

**John Keady** is a Senior Lecturer in the School of Nursing, Midwifery and Health Studies, University of Wales Bangor.

**Steve Morgan** works in 'Practice Based Evidence' (a Practice Development Consultancy for Mental Health), London.

**Rob Newell** is Professor of Nursing Research in the School of Health Studies, Bradford University.

**Peter Nolan** is Professor of Mental Health Nursing in the School of Health, Staffordshire University/South Staffordshire Healthcare NHS Trust.

**Edward Peck** is Professor in Healthcare Partnerships in the Health Services Management Centre, University of Birmingham.

**Rachel Perkins** is Clinical Director for General Adult Services at Springfield University Hospital, London.

**Julie Repper** is a Senior Research Fellow in the School of Health and Related Research, University of Sheffield and Lead Research Nurse for Community Health Sheffield.

**Mike Slade** is an MRC Clinician Scientist Fellow in the Health Services Research Department, Institute of Psychiatry, King's College London.

**Richard Williams** is Professor of Mental Health Strategy at the Welsh Institute for Health and Social Care Research, University of Glamorgan.

**Steve Wood** is a Lecturer/Practitioner in the School of Nursing and Midwifery Studies, University of Wales College of Medicine/Cardiff and Vale NHS Trust.

**Norman Young** is a Lecturer/Practitioner in the School of Nursing and Midwifery Studies, University of Wales College of Medicine/Cardiff and Vale NHS Trust.

# ACKNOWLEDGEMENTS

We are indebted to many people who, at some stage along the way, helped us see this book through to publication.

Our first expression of thanks goes to Philip Burnard. Phil made this project seem possible, and his unfailing encouragement and support made all the difference in the early stages.

Second, we are grateful to Edwina Welham and Michelle Bacca at Routledge, for their faith in this book and for their guidance.

Finally, and most importantly of all, we are grateful to our families for tolerating our absences. It is to them – Kara, Tom and Jack and Cathy, Milo and Eva – that this book is dedicated.

Ben Hannigan and Michael Coffey
October 2002

# INTRODUCTION

*Ben Hannigan and Michael Coffey*

The number of mental health nurses working in community settings in the UK has risen steadily since the appointment of the first 'outpatient nurses' in the mid-1950s. Data from the 1996 quinquennial survey of community mental health nurses (CMHNs) in England and Wales suggested that around 7,000 CMHNs were at that time working in these two countries (Brooker and White 1997). As mental health policy continues to promote the development of community, rather than institutional, care, the number of CMHNs working in the UK may continue expanding. As educators of community mental health nurses it struck us as somewhat odd, then, that there was no up-to-date dedicated text prepared specifically for this group of practitioners. True, there have been some very useful book contributions over the years, both nursing-oriented and addressing issues from a multidisciplinary perspective. However, as the largest group of health professionals providing specialist mental health services in the community, we felt that community mental health nurses deserved access to a single, comprehensive text that could be of use as a central resource. This edited book is the outcome of our deliberations.

Community mental health nursing in recent times has sometimes seemed like a ship at sea, in which the occupants continually fight over who should steer and in what direction. This ship has been subject to the vagaries of the political climate as well as the routes taken by other ships (professions). To stretch this analogy slightly further, we might imagine that the constant here is the service user and their families (the sea). Their needs remain, whatever the current emphasis in service provision. These debates and dilemmas over the direction of community mental health nursing have been felt in all arenas: in practice, education and research.

As the CMHN workforce has expanded, so too has the availability of education courses designed to prepare mental health nurses for practice in the community. Between thirty and forty UK universities were known to have offered degree-level (or higher) 'specialist practice' courses for CMHNs in the 1998–9 academic year (Hannigan *et al.* 2001). At pre-registration level, all students of mental health nursing are required to undertake periods of theory and practice relating to nursing in the community. In recent years there has also been more emphasis on providing education and training which equips nurses to address the needs of specific groups: for instance, those termed the 'seriously mentally ill'.

Education and other initiatives have, of course, been influenced by policy developments. Some of these have been driven by considered reviews of mental health care, others by cost-effective evidence-based practices, and others perhaps motivated by political and financial expediency. Community mental health nurses, like others working in the UK public services, are required to respond to policy and professional pressures, and they can be said to have done so with varying degrees of success. It seems to us that community mental health nurses often have an acute awareness of general mental health need amongst the community at large, but have struggled to reconcile this with the emphasis on providing services to priority groups to the exclusion of others. In attempting to provide services to those in mental distress, community mental health nurses, like their multidisciplinary colleagues, must be cognisant of the extent of mental health need encountered in the communities in which they work. They must also possess the breadth of knowledge, skill and creativity which will enable them to provide the type of responses that, ultimately, service users find useful.

Critically, community mental health nurses must accommodate the demands and pressures of their professional colleagues, policy-makers and the wider public whilst preserving the relationships they have with the users of their services. This relationship is fundamental, and despite the apparent allure of increased profes-sional status promised by legislative developments we would do well to remember that common humanity unites us all. As Peter Campbell reminds us in his chapter, mental health nurses have not always matched with action the rhetoric of the therapeutic relationship. Service users, those who experience mental ill health, can instruct us in developing our profession so that it does what it sets out to do and actually provides help.

This edited book brings together contributions from leading mental health researchers, educators and practitioners. The handbook aims to be a comprehen-sive and up-to-date resource for practising community mental health nurses and community mental health nursing students in the UK, those with responsibilities for teaching community mental health nurses, and pre-qualifying students of mental health nursing for whom learning to work in community settings is a major part of their educational preparation.

The context of community mental health care has provided an unarguable rationale for the choice of contributors to this text. Many chapter authors are mental health nurses with contemporary experience of community care. The book, however, also includes contributions from academics, service users and other professionals involved in mental health care and in this sense recognises the multidisciplinary and service user context of our work. It is not possible, however, to produce a text that remains up-to-the-minute, and this book should be treated as a jumping-off point, a place to start from and then track down further useful material. With this in mind, chapter authors have provided details of key suggested reading in addition to their already highly relevant reference lists. The appendices also contain numerous further resources for readers to locate organisations and academic and professional journals. These lists, of course, will never be complete, but they do provide, again, a point from which to start your journey. Chapters are organised around three linked themes: context, practice, and education and research. Each section is introduced to provide a quick and easy summary of what you should expect to find there.

This book is by no means the last word on community mental health nursing practice. Mental health nursing in the community is too diverse and complex an activity to imagine that we could provide such. Community mental health nursing has defied definition, sought professional status, and now treads a fine line between providing genuinely empowering care and participating in the social control of the mentally ill. It has done these things in a context of indifference and neglect by a wider nursing profession that appears ignorant of the needs of people with mental health difficulties and the specialist contribution that properly prepared mental health nurses can offer. We believe that it is of absolute importance that community mental health nurses articulate the specialist nature of their practice so that the fallacy of 'generalist nursing' is seen for what it is.

Community mental health nursing, as can be seen within these pages, extends beyond the narrow confines of policy, political fashion and topical campaigns. These nurses provide care to people with mental health problems in a multitude of settings and often regardless of whatever or whoever categorises them. This text recognises these tensions, celebrates the diversity and most importantly challenges us to provide community mental health care that is helpful despite the winds of change.

At this point, a note on terminology. Many contributors to this book, including us, have chosen to use the term 'community mental health nurse' in their chapters. This term has become increasingly popular in recent years to describe nurses who work with people with mental health problems living in community, rather than hospital, settings. Other contributors, however, have elected to use the older term 'community psychiatric nurse'. We have deliberately chosen not to 'standardise' the term in this book, and for the purposes of this volume have treated the two options as being interchangeable. However, we also speculate that the ongoing use of these two titles may say something about a continued lack of clarity over the identity, role and expectations of this group of practitioners.

In producing a text of this size we are indebted to our contributors. They have provided without exception compelling, thoughtful, and often provocative chapters. We were frequently excited by reading these as they arrived, and we have felt a frank gratitude and privilege that authors have taken the time to produce such excellent work. They have provided this material to us in a timely fashion and responded to our requests for revisions with professional diligence and good nature. Some have done so despite difficult personal circumstances and we are grateful for their efforts here.

## REFERENCES

Brooker, C. and White, E. (1997) *The fourth quinquennial national community mental health nursing census of England and Wales*, Manchester and Keele: Universities of Manchester and Keele.

Hannigan, B., Burnard, P., Edwards, D. and Turnbull, J. (2001) 'Specialist practice for UK community mental health nurses: the 1998–99 survey of course leaders', *International Journal of Nursing Studies*, 38 (4): 427–435.

# PART 1

## CONTEXT

## INTRODUCTION

It is now almost half a century since mental health nurses first began leaving the psychiatric hospitals to ply their trade in the community. Much has changed in the intervening years, and more change lies ahead. In this opening section, contributions address important historical, social, political and professional issues which have relevance for all community mental health nurses, whatever their particular field of practice.

In his chapter, Peter Nolan provides a lively account of the origins and early development of community mental health nursing. He writes about how, from the 1950s onwards, the work of nurses was increasingly acknowledged as being a therapy in its own right. From this, Peter writes, 'it was only a small step to recognising that they might be equally effective outside the hospital'.

Paul Godin also starts his chapter in the 1950s, and offers a sociological analysis of the development of community mental health nursing. Whilst Paul sees some evidence of professionalisation, he argues that CMHNs continue to be characterised by a willingness to put themselves in the 'frontline' of mental health care.

Chapter 3 is an analysis of the policy and legal context. Here, Ben Hannigan considers the components of mental health care 'modernisation', including work launched in the late 1990s to introduce national standards of care and treatment, and work to review the UK's mental health laws. Ben argues that, taken together, emerging mental health policies reveal both tensions and inconsistencies.

In his chapter, Chris Chaloner urges CMHNs to engage in 'ethical reflection'. Chris makes the point that the everyday practice of community mental health nurses is shot through with ethical dilemmas, and that – for example – even if something *can* be done, it may not be 'right' that it *is* done.

In their chapter, Rachel Perkins and Julie Repper point out the many ways in which people who use mental health services experience social exclusion and discrimination. The aspirations that people with mental health problems have are no different from the aspirations that everyone has, and Rachel and Julie suggest ways in which CMHNs can assist people to achieve these.

It is now a commonplace that community mental health nurses work in teams alongside members of other professional groups. However, as Edward Peck writes in his contribution, the multidisciplinary community mental health team model has never been free from criticism. New solutions to the difficulties of delivering multiprofessional community care include a move away from 'locality' teams in favour of 'functional' teams.

In her chapter, Elizabeth Armstrong begins by highlighting the extent of mental health need encountered in primary care, and makes the point that the majority of people with mental health problems are cared for in this setting. Elizabeth urges community mental health nurses to forge close links with their primary care colleagues, and suggests a number of strategies to accomplish this.

Peter Campbell writes about how, despite changes in policy and practice which have brought mental health users and providers of care together in a spirit of collaboration, there is still much that has to be done. Peter writes that, whilst the status of service users within the mental health care system has improved, the position of people with mental health problems in wider society has diminished.

Men and women experience mental health problems differently, and are treated differently by mental health service providers. In her chapter, Anne Fothergill offers some explanations for this, and makes a case for community mental health care which is more sensitive to the particular needs of women.

In his contribution, Suman Fernando argues that mental health services are failing to meet the needs of black and Asian people. He makes a powerful case that the mental health care system is institutionally racist, and ends his chapter by suggesting ways in which this major problem might be addressed.

Working in community mental health care is stressful, and in her chapter Deborah Edwards reviews the evidence which has demonstrated this. However, as Deborah argues, knowledge about the causes of stress has not been matched by an awareness of how stress can be managed, at both the 'primary' and 'secondary' levels.

This first section of the book ends with a chapter by John Cutcliffe on clinical supervision and reflective practice. John makes the point that the work of CMHNs is inherently isolating, making opportunities for a 'reflective space' vitally important for both personal support and professional development.

# CHAPTER 1

# THE HISTORY OF COMMUNITY MENTAL HEALTH NURSING

*Peter Nolan*

## SUMMARY OF KEY POINTS

This chapter focuses mainly on early developments in community psychiatric nursing. By the end of the chapter, the reader will:

- be aware of the multiple complex factors that led to the emergence of community psychiatric nursing in the late 1950s;

- understand the types of work undertaken by the first community psychiatric nurses;

- appreciate the problems now confronting community mental health nurses.

## INTRODUCTION

The birth of community mental health nursing in the late 1950s took place during a troubled period in mental health care. The asylum system, a highly ambitious attempt to manage mentally ill people, which had been founded almost one hundred years previously, was close to collapse. The therapeutic optimism that had produced it and the ardour which had driven its chief architect, Lord Shaftsbury, had become muted. In the mid-nineteenth century, the magnificence of some of the asylums and their superb facades had been symbols of civic pride and social concern; one historian remarked that in France such buildings were used to house royalty, not pauper lunatics (Porter 1987). However, by the 1950s, the system that had once held out hope to the marginalised and the stigmatised had been undermined by overcrowding, bureaucracy and loss of the original vision of providing compassionate accommodation for the mentally ill away from the prisons, workhouses and private madhouses.

Overcrowding meant that 155,000 patients were being accommodated in buildings designed to cater for less than half that number (Shorter 1997). In 1956, Claybury Hospital near London admitted 1,360 patients (560 males and 800 females) compared with 215 in 1937 (Pryor 1993). Overcrowding stifled efforts to create a therapeutic environment. Griffiths (2001) contends that over-diagnosis of psychiatric conditions, coupled with the belief that compulsory institutionalisation was the only solution to mental illness, contributed largely to this glut of patients. In their role as guardians of social order, psychiatrists operated with relatively inclusive nosologies of psychopathology; yet many of the problems with which clients presented were no more than normal reactions to difficult life events. Also contributing to overcrowding was the fact that psychiatric hospitals tended to admit disruptive patients whom relatives and support agencies were very reluctant to re-assume responsibility for on discharge. The burden shouldered by the mental hospitals was only matched by the burden on primary care professionals, relatives and carers of people with mental health problems, who struggled on, receiving little or no statutory assistance (Freeman 1999).

Morale amongst psychiatric staff was further depressed by criticisms such as those made by Peter Townsend in *The Observer* of 5 April 1964. Townsend described how conditions in the hospitals degraded both staff and patients. He did not blame the staff, but suggested that society should take responsibility for the care provided for its mentally ill. Echoes of Townsend were heard at the 1964 Annual Conference of the Chief Male Nurses Association when attendees were told that the psychiatric nursing profession was 'despondent'. Delegates heard that approximately 70 per cent of student nurses left before completing their training, not because of the nature of the work but because of the way in which they were treated. Split shifts, long days, scant notice of 'off-duty', and 'heavy-handed and insensitive management' contributed to low morale. The conference also heard that training was largely irrelevant to the work nurses were being asked to do on the wards, and yet nurses were being blamed for low standards. One delegate asked:

> What can nurses do about the appalling conditions that still persist in mental hospitals? Nurses are asked to remedy the situation, but how can they when they have no power in the organisation and have no presence on any decision making committee?
>
> (quoted in Nolan 1993, p. 127)

In July 1948, the National Health Service (NHS) came into being. The first Minister of Health was also the Minister of Housing, to emphasise the relationship between living conditions and health (Webster 1998). Psychiatry, which was predominantly based in psychiatric hospitals, came under the aegis of the NHS. The hospitals were encouraged to remain independent of the acute sector and were funded to provide their own pathology laboratories, X-ray departments and other investigative and medical facilities. This expansion of services elevated the standing of psychiatry within the NHS, and yet isolated it from other health services. Policy-makers appeared to believe that relatively minor changes could reform the mental health system (Rogers and Pilgrim 2001), although dissenting voices argued that the infrastructure of care had to be tackled if there were to be real and ongoing improvements in the services provided (Martin 1984).

Within a decade of its inauguration, the Guillebaud Report (1956) confirmed that the NHS was proving far more costly than originally envisaged. The Report also noted, with regret, that the NHS had become a national *hospital* service rather than a national *health* service, with pre-eminence given to the acute sector to the detriment of other areas of health care, including mental health services. By the 1960s, mental health services were in crisis, as the first of eighteen public inquiries revealed. Authors such as Szasz (1960) decried the way in which patients were excessively medicated and confined within soulless institutions. The Manchester Regional Hospital Board (1956) summarised the problems it faced when asked to take over mental health care in their area:

> The Board inherited mental hospitals some of which were in the neighbourhood of 100 years old, and most of them were victims of damage and bombings during the last war. In addition, they were . . . generally ill adapted to the needs of patients under treatment within them. The patient population in the hospitals was predominantly composed of chronic long-stay patients in various stages of deterioration resulting from prolonged hospitalisation.

Szasz suggested that psychiatrists were colluding with the State to control non-conformist, 'awkward' citizens. Shepherd *et al.* (1966) advised that mental health care could be improved by strengthening the role of general practitioners. Treating mental health problems in general practice would reduce stigma for clients and have a significant impact on the number of patients in psychiatric hospitals. Primary care personnel were ideally placed to identify the early signs of mental ill health and to initiate treatment. Over thirty years later, the central role of primary care has been enshrined in the National Service Framework for Mental Health (Department of Health 1999).

## REFORM FROM WITHIN

It would be a mistake to presume that reform of the mental hospitals was dependent on the arrival of the NHS. In 1935, the 'kind and benevolent Welshman', T.P. (Percy) Rees, superintendent at Warlingham Park Hospital, had embarked on a crusade against 'locks and keys'. All the wards were unlocked including, to the horror of staff, the doors confining the suicidal patients (Shorter 1997). Rees strove to reduce the time patients spent in his hospital, recognising that there were only limited benefits to be gained from removing people from their homes and social networks. By the 1950s, attitudes were changing in line with Rees's thinking. New policies and innovative care included: adoption of the open-door policy by some superintendents (Dr MacMillan at Mapperly

Hospital, Nottingham, 1954; Dr Stern at Central Hospital, Warwick, 1957; Dr Mandelbrote at Coney Hill Hospital, Gloucester, 1957); part-time hospitalisation; provision of easily accessible out-patient care; industrial therapy; hostels for people with mental health problems; therapeutic social clubs; locating psychiatric units in general hospitals; and mental health staff carrying out home visits (Shorter 1997). The discovery of powerful new psychotropic medication assisted these changes by controlling the symptoms of major mental illness. For many, the introduction of Largactil (chlorpromazine) refuted the conjecture that schizophrenia was irreversible and deterioration inevitable.

During the 1950s, it began to be recognised that nursing care might in itself be therapeutic and that nurses could be used more effectively than simply to subdue and control patients. Cameron and Laing (1955) reported the transformation that took place at Glasgow Royal Infirmary when nurses and patients started talking to each other more. Patients got to know their nurses, were able to feel relaxed with them, and, as a result of their attention, began to take an interest in themselves and their futures. At De La Pole Hospital near Hull, Dr Bickford (1955) reformed the way in which nurses worked with and related to patients and found that many patients could then be discharged with very little input from doctors (Nolan 1993). Such changes indicated a gradual shift away from the medical model of psychiatry, with its emphasis on biogenic approaches, and towards a social model which gave the conditions in which patients lived equal weighting with what was assumed to be happening to them at a biological level. The rise of community care was part of the search for social explanations of mental illness and a further repudiation of psychiatrists and the value-laden language of degeneration.

The 1959 Act introduced voluntary status admission and placed a strong emphasis on community care. The therapeutic community strategy, originally deployed at Mill Hill during the war under the direction of Maxwell Jones, became one of the foundation stones of social psychiatry and played a significant part in the search for alternatives to hospitalisation. It was revolutionary at a time when treatment for mental illness was firmly rooted in the biological domain. Interestingly, therapeutic communities did not meet with similar success in America, as Ken Kesey's novel, *One flew over the cuckoo's nest* (1962), so graphically illustrates.

## THE FIRST CPNs

If nurses could transform the culture of the hospital ward and exercise a therapeutic effect in their relationship with patients, it was only a small step to recognising that they might be equally effective outside the hospital. Stan Moore, chief male nurse at Warlingham Park Hospital, near Croydon, certainly came to this conclusion. Moore chose to work at Warlingham because of the reputation of its superintendent, Dr Rees. Both men had served in the medical corps during the war and had seen what could be achieved with patients suffering from even the most severe psychiatric conditions. They were convinced that containing patients in overcrowded wards did not enable them to be treated effectively.

Furthermore, they shared a conviction that psychiatric hospitals were over-regulated and that many of the interventions employed there had little to commend them. Moore's post-war vision for mental nurses was that their influence should stretch well beyond the mental hospital. His first step towards realising a community brief for nurses was to second Lena Peat, a senior ward sister, to the social work department at Warlingham Park Hospital. In Peat, Moore recognised someone committed to improving services for patients and who had the courage and vision to challenge the status quo. Initially, Peat worked as an aide to the social workers, but she soon developed a new role as 'out-patient nurse', providing psychological support for patients and relatives, supervising medication and dealing with difficulties before they became entrenched. One of the psychiatrists at Warlingham Park commented:

> Domiciliary mental nursing is playing a useful role in community care within a framework of joint clinical social services. The trained nurse is invaluable in that she is able to make an appraisal of the patient, which is of fundamental value to the psychiatrist. In addition, the nurse can give direct support to patients and relatives, which frequently results in preventing relapse.
>
> (May 1965)

A year later, Moore identified another nurse to join Lena Peat. Working in the community, the nurses were able to appreciate, as they had not done before, the destructive effects of mental illness on the social and family lives of patients (Moore 1964).

John Greene also served during the war and then played a significant part in the development of community mental nursing when he became chief male nurse at Moorhaven Hospital near Plymouth. His considerable abilities coupled with those of the matron, Belle Briton, and the medical superintendent, Francis Pilkington, soon made the hospital a flagship of progressive psychiatric practice in the UK. Pilkington was committed to reforming the mental hospitals, and was prepared to consult widely on how best to do it. Greene was encouraged to use the vast experience he had amassed in the Navy to transform psychiatric nursing, and the collaborative relationship he developed with Pilkington had repercussions throughout mental health services in the UK. Greene visited Moore at Warlingham Park in 1954 and was instantly convinced of the advantages for patients and their families of having nurses working in the community, particularly as psychiatric social workers were beginning to diminish in number. He saw community psychiatric nurses not as social work aides, but rather utilising their skills to support people who had recently left hospital. Nurses, he believed, were far more effective in the local community than they had ever been on the wards (Greene 1989).

During his first year at Moorhaven, Greene demolished the high walls around the male and female airing courts. Patients were encouraged to walk in the grounds, to visit shops in the nearby town, and to go on trips. Theatre groups, lecturers from nearby Dartington Hall, and children from local schools were invited into the hospital. Staff were encouraged to welcome outsiders who could do so much to brighten the lives of the patients. Greene then appointed the first part-time community psychiatric nurse at Moorhaven. Here he records how the nurse helped one client with mental health problems:

> A naval pensioner, living alone in deplorable conditions, gradually began to deteriorate and refused all contact with social services. He agreed initially to talk to the nurse but only through the letter-box. After a few days and many reassurances, he allowed the nurse to enter his home. The nurse bathed him, provided clean clothes, cooked him fresh food and reviewed his medication. He was visited daily for about ten days after which the visits became infrequent. Though he never regained his former state of health, yet he lived an active social life for many years until his death and was never admitted to hospital. The demand for mental nurses increased almost immediately and there was insufficient to meet the needs in the locality.
>
> (Greene 1989)

Despite the demonstrable benefits of community psychiatric nurses, hospital boards were not disposed to make resources available to extend the service. The early service survived on the motivation of the nurses, who were prepared to work long hours, far in excess of their colleagues on the wards. John Greene's records demonstrate how the nurses' commitment to community psychiatric nursing led to a rapid escalation in the number of patients seen during the first ten years at Moorhaven (Table 1.1).

Table 1.1 Development of community psychiatric nursing at Moorhaven Hospital, Devon

| Year | No. of nurses | No. of patients | No. of visits |
| --- | --- | --- | --- |
| 1957 | 2 | 44 | 740 |
| 1960 | 2 | 116 | 1589 |
| 1964 | 5 | 165 | 2878 |
| 1966 | 5 | 182 | 3142 |

Reproduced by kind permission of the Royal College of Nursing.

Greene noted that approximately 50 per cent of clients had a primary diagnosis of schizophrenia, while the other 50 per cent had a history of severe and recurrent depression. Over 50 per cent had been taking medication for many years and were likely to continue in the future.

Greene and Pilkington were frequently challenged about the community psychiatric nursing 'experiment'. Social workers, general practitioners, health visitors and district nurses all expressed concern that the new community psychiatric nurses were trespassing on their territory. Some wanted clarification of the nurses' role and to ensure that they were limited to certain categories of patient. Greene bore the brunt of these criticisms, but was not deflected from his vision of providing better care for psychiatric patients following discharge. He realised that while other professional groups might claim to be providing aftercare, in reality, the majority of these patients received little support. In 1968, in response to the need to define the role of the community psychiatric nurse so that other groups could work effectively with them, Greene formulated a job specification (Box 1.1).

---

**Box 1.1    Greene's formulation of the role of the community psychiatric nurse in 1968**

Community psychiatric nurses should:

- provide psychiatric nursing care of a physical or psychological nature for patients discharged from hospital and in need of continuing care;
- work in close liaison with doctors and social workers as professional members of a therapeutic team;
- extend to the patient and his family such support as may reasonably be regarded as part of a nurse's work;
- play a preventive role in relation to patients whose illness does not require treatment in a clinic or hospital;
- be available in a consultative capacity to non-psychiatric nurses with patients showing symptoms of mental disorder.

---

Others committed to the groundbreaking work of initiating a community psychiatric nursing service at this time were Peter Barry, chief male nurse at St Francis Hospital, Haywards Heath, and a long-time member of the Standing Mental Health Advisory Committee; and Peter Dawson, chief male nurse at St Ebba's Hospital in Epsom, and a founder member and chair of the Society of Mental Nurses. Algie Whitmore, chief male nurse at Horton Hospital in Surrey, was another who championed the cause, and also John Corbett, who became chief nursing officer in York. By 1966, there were approximately 225 community psychiatric nurse whole-time equivalents, employed by 42 psychiatric hospitals. As the service became established, managers developed their understanding of who were the best nurses to work in community settings, recognising that:

- not all qualified nurses could make the transition from hospital to community work;
- CPNs must have the ability to communicate with a wide variety of people;
- they must be able to work and make decisions independently;
- they must respect the skills and understand the role of other health professionals;
- they must avoid being seen as an elitist group, superior to their hospital-based colleagues.

Managers also saw that:

- there was an urgent need for specialist nurse training and ongoing education.

The work of CPNs gradually gained in status and the reduction in numbers of hospital patients was attributed largely to them. Some were given their own offices at their hospitals and had secretarial time allocated to them. In many places, CPNs were no longer seen as an extension of ward-based nursing, but as providing an entirely separate service. Where hospital-based nurses still adhered to the biological model of mental illness, community nurses tended to espouse the newly-emerging psychosocial model. The *Expert Committee on Mental Health* (WHO 1965) made reference to the vital work being carried out by CPNs in keeping patients in touch with their families. Shepherd *et al.* (1966) remarked that, were it not for CPNs, community care would never have got off the ground in the UK, although they had little professional power and limited access to educational resources.

The issue of specialist training for community psychiatric nurses proved difficult to address, principally because the General Nursing Council was, in the 1960s, focused on basic rather than post-basic training. Moorhaven Hospital and Plymouth Polytechnic put forward a pioneering training course for CPNs which built upon the close working relationships that existed between nurses, social workers, psychiatrists, voluntary organisations, the clergy, the police and welfare services. However, nothing came of this initiative. The establishment of the Joint Board of Clinical Nursing Studies (JBCNS) in the early 1970s signalled a new era in post-basic training for nurses, especially those working in child care, care of older adults and mental health. Plymouth Polytechnic's course for CPNs was accredited and others soon came on stream around the country. The term *community psychiatric nurse* (CPN) was now widely recognised in the UK. Although all these courses followed a syllabus drawn up by the JBCNS, there was little uniformity in either form or content and great variation both in the competence of lecturers and in the degree of supervision students received on clinical placements. The course at Plymouth was specifically designed for nurses and drew upon the expertise of mental health professionals already involved in community care, while the course at Chiswick College adapted the Diploma in Nursing and existing courses for health visitors.

By the mid-1970s, CPNs had become part of specialist community teams, working in rehabilitation and with various client groups including older people, children and adolescents, acute psychotic patients, those with behavioural problems and substance abusers. By building up alternatives to in-patient services, CPNs were playing a central role in developing the community services the government wanted, and *Better services for the mentally ill* (Department of Health and Social Security 1975) acknowledged the importance of their work.

From the 1980s onwards, governments increasingly emphasised the importance of community mental health care, and the work of community mental health nurses became a legitimate subject for research. For the first two decades of their existence, CPNs had worked almost exclusively with people with schizophrenia and older people with mental health problems. Their role was essentially to prevent relapse and reduce re-admission rates. The first major study of the work of CPNs was carried out by Paykel *et al.* (1982) who showed that they were as effective as doctors in providing aftercare for patients. Marks (1985) found that nurses who had trained in behavioural therapy had excellent outcomes with clients with phobic and obsessive disorders. Such research convinced GPs that

CPNs had much to offer their non-schizophrenic patients, and they became increasingly keen to see them working in primary care. At the beginning of the 1980s, the establishment of district general hospitals and reorganisation of NHS management structures gave added impetus to the move to primary care (Gournay 2000). Many CPNs were delighted to escape the stigma associated with psychiatric hospitals and the control of psychiatrists. By the 1990s, they were taking as many referrals from GPs as they were from psychiatrists. Twenty-five per cent did not have anyone with schizophrenia on their caseload (White 1990). Instead, they were working with people with adjustment disorders and other neurotic conditions, and using counselling-type approaches.

Recent research found that there were approximately 7,000 CPN whole-time equivalents working in England and Wales in 1996 (Brooker and White 1997). This seems a very small number considering that the majority of people with mental health problems were then being cared for either by community mental health teams or in primary care, and that there were approximately 57,000 mental health nurses registered with the UKCC (United Kingdom Central Council for Nursing, Midwifery and Health Visiting). In fact, the majority of mental health nurses were still employed in in-patient services where 80 per cent of the resources available for mental health care were still directed.

Reorganisation of the mental health services in the 1990s stimulated debate about the role of the CPN. Who were the clients they should be working with? Should they be based in community or primary care? The report *Working in partnership* (Department of Health 1994) advised CPNs to refocus their work on people with serious and enduring mental illness and to relinquish their work with primary care. Gournay and Brooking (1995) found that CPNs' work in primary care was not cost-effective, although they were not in favour of abandoning the link completely. Fewer than half of CPNs had appropriate training for the work they were doing and this aroused concerns that they might be an obstacle to the implementation of new approaches to mental health care. Gournay (2000) was fiercely critical of the training and education of CPNs (see Box 1.2).

Repper (2000) argues that nurses' contribution to mental health care has never been properly evaluated. Because their work underpins all services, it is easy to overlook it when service evaluation is being undertaken by other professionals.

---

**Box 1.2   Criticisms of CPN training in the early 1990s**

- Theory- rather than practice-based
- No emphasis on skills acquisition
- Academic content not supported by apprenticeship component
- Nursing lecturers out of touch with current practice
- Anti-psychiatry bias in most courses; promotion of prejudice regarding 'malevolent medical model'
- Huge variation in form and content of courses nationally
- Absence of any reference to assertive community treatment, medication management or psychological and family interventions.

(Gournay 2000)

There has been a tendency to attribute successful mental health outcomes entirely to interventions; indeed, the design of some studies has been constructed to confirm this. The reality is that the factors which have the greatest impact on the recovery of clients may be their relationships with carers, the manner in which information is imparted to them, and being encouraged to draw on their own resources. Repper also points out that nurses, even though the largest group in mental health care, are far from united in their thinking about what they should be doing and where they should be working. Mental health nursing is divided by passionate ideological debates, she argues, with opposing camps competing for academic supremacy.

## CONCLUSION

Few would deny that community mental health nurses (CMHNs) have played a significant part in the provision of mental health services since the 1960s. Shepherd *et al.* (1966) noted that it was nurses who carried the burden of developing community mental health services in the UK and, in many places, services would have collapsed without them. Nonetheless, they are highly vulnerable to criticism because of lack of quality education and training. While well organised in comparison to other groups of mental health nurses (CMHNs have their own professional journal and hold regular professional seminars and annual conferences), they are perceived to be academically weak by those from the high-status mental health disciplines.

### Problems facing community mental health nursing

• Community mental health nursing came into being to ease a desperate situation in the psychiatric hospitals – it was not a planned strategic response. The General Nursing Council was noticeably lacklustre in supporting both CMHNs and the development of mental health nursing services in general.
• The number of CMHNs has not increased commensurate with the numbers of people with mental health problems being cared for in the community. The reason for this remains unclear. Nor is it clear why untrained practice nurses are assuming more and more responsibility for mental health care in the community.
• Ironically, CMHNs appear to be more highly valued by GPs and primary care personnel than by other mental health professionals.
• The rivalry between groups of mental health nurses from contrasting ideological positions is damaging. It leads to a lack of clarity regarding the models and interventions which they can be expected to implement.

As discussion continues regarding the merits of generic and specialist nurses, it remains to be seen whether CMHNs will eventually merge with other community nurses. This and other current issues for community mental health nurses are considered in the following chapters.

# REFERENCES

Bickford, J. (1955) 'The forgotten patient', *The Lancet*, 1: 543–557.

Brooker, C. and White, E. (1997) *The fourth quinquennial national community mental health nursing census of England and Wales*, Manchester and Keele: Universities of Manchester and Keele.

Cameron, J.L. and Laing, R.D. (1955) 'Effects of environmental change in the care of chronic schizophrenics', *The Lancet*, 106: 1384–1386.

Department of Health (1994) *Working in partnership: a collaborative approach to care. Report of the Mental Health Nursing Review Team*, London: HMSO.

Department of Health (1999) *National service framework for mental health: modern standards and service models*, London: Department of Health.

Department of Health and Social Security (1975) *Better services for the mentally ill*, London: HMSO.

Freeman, H. (1999) 'Community psychiatry', in Freeman, H. (ed.) *A century of psychiatry*, London: Mosby-Wolfe.

Gournay, K. (2000) 'Role of the community psychiatric nurse in the management of schizophrenia', *Advances in Psychiatric Treatment*, 6: 243–251.

Gournay, K. and Brooking, J. (1995) 'Community psychiatric nurses in primary care', *British Journal of Psychiatry*, 165: 231–238.

Greene, J. (1989) *The beginnings of community psychiatric nursing*, London: The History of Nursing Group at the Royal College of Nursing, 2: 14–20.

Griffiths, L. (2001) 'Categorising to exclude: the discursive construction of cases in community mental health teams', *Sociology of Health and Illness*, 5: 678–700.

Guillebaud Report (1956) *Report of the Committee of Enquiry into the Cost of the National Health Service*, London: HMSO.

Kesey, K. (1962) *One flew over the cuckoo's nest*, London: Picador.

Manchester Regional Hospital Board (1956) *The work of the mental nurse*, Manchester: Regional Hospital Board.

Marks, I. (1985) *Nurse therapists in primary care*, London: Royal College of Nursing.

Martin, J.P. (1984) *Hospitals in trouble*, London: Basil Blackwell.

May, A.R. (1965) 'The psychiatric nurse in the community', *Nursing Mirror*, 31 December.

Moore, S. (1964) 'Mental nursing in the community', *Nursing Times*, 10 April.

Nolan, P. (1993) *A history of mental health nursing*, London: Chapman and Hall.

Paykel, E., Mangen, S.P., Griffiths, J.H. and Burns, T.P. (1982) 'Community psychiatric nursing for neurotic patients: a controlled trial', *British Journal of Psychiatry*, 140: 573–581.

Porter, R. (1987) *Mind-forged manacles*, London: Athlone Press.

Pryor, E.H. (1993) *Claybury – a century of caring 1893–1993*, Forest Healthcare Trust: The Mental Health Care Group.

Repper, J. (2000) 'Adjusting the focus of mental health nursing: incorporating service users' experiences of recovery', *Journal of Mental Health*, 9: 575–587.

Rogers, A. and Pilgrim, D. (2001) *Mental health policy in Britain*, 2nd edn, Basingstoke: Palgrave.

Shepherd, M., Cooper, B. and Brown, A.C. (1966) *Psychiatric illness in general practice*, Oxford: Oxford University Press.

Shorter, E. (1997) *A history of psychiatry*, Chichester: Wiley.

Szasz, T. (1960) 'The myth of mental illness', *The American Psychologist*, 15: 1113–1118.

Webster, C. (1998) *The National Health Service – a political history*, Oxford: Oxford University Press.

White, E. (1990) 'The work of the community psychiatric nurses association: a survey of the membership', *Community Psychiatric Nursing Journal*, 10: 30–35.

World Health Organization (1965) *Expert Committee on Mental Health*, Geneva: WHO.

# FURTHER READING

Smith, L.D. (1999) *Cure, comfort and safe custody*, London: Leicester University Press.
This book shows how the tensions between custody and care were expressed in the asylums and contrasts the rationale behind the asylum system with that underpinning community care.

Webster, C. (1998) *The National Health Service – a political history*, Oxford: Oxford University Press.
This invaluable book provides insights into how mental health services were incorporated into the NHS at its inception. Mental health nurses will gain from it an understanding of the origins of many of the problems the service faces today.

Freeman, H. (ed.) (1999) *A century of psychiatry* (2 vols), London: Mosby-Wolfe.
This book offers a detailed account of changes in mental health care over the past century. Of special interest is its description of the different therapeutic approaches that have been adopted at various times and its understanding of mental health care in a world-wide context.

# CHAPTER 2

# THE FRONTLINE WORKFORCE OF COMMUNITY MENTAL HEALTH CARE

*Paul Godin*

---

## SUMMARY OF KEY POINTS

- Though in their history CPNs have engaged in professionalising strategies they have more characteristically demonstrated a willingness to assume a position in the frontline of community mental health care.

- Since the early 1990s a new regime of specialist community mental health care has prioritised the care of long-term service users.

- As care programme approach (CPA) care co-ordinators, CPNs are subject to policy directives that require them to risk-assess and risk-manage their clients in a way that may not be entirely in their clients' best interests.

---

## INTRODUCTION

The numerical growth of CPNs in Britain over the past fifty years has been remarkable. From a mere handful in the 1950s they grew to an estimated 6,739 in England and Wales, when last enumerated in 1996 (Brooker and White 1997). By the 1990s CPNs outnumbered any other occupational group within specialist community mental health services (Onyett *et al.* 1994). As with any new occupational group, it might be asked whether or not the growth of community psychiatric nursing was the result of a process of 'professionalisation'. There is a wealth of sociological theory associated with health care professions, which cannot be adequately explained in this short chapter. Professionalisation is a term widely used by neo-Weberian theorists, such as Freidson (1970). It refers to a process that health care occupational groups engage in to achieve professional status. This typically involves strategies of credentialism (establishing a knowledge base that others will regard as assuring competent practice) and legalism (getting laws passed to ensure that only appropriately educated and accredited persons can practise as a member of the occupational group). If, as in medicine, they are successful, then professional status is achieved as they gain a monopoly within a particular area of health care work, which enables them to act autonomously and dominate others. Professional autonomy is a rather vague term. However, Elston (1991) suggests that it can be used in three senses. First, economic autonomy refers to the ability of a profession to determine its level of remuneration. Second, political autonomy refers to the power a profession has to influence government policy decisions. Third, clinical autonomy refers to the power that professionals have to set their own standards of work and to control their clinical performance. Both Elston (1991) and Freidson (1970) emphasise that professional autonomy is a relative rather than absolute property. Even medicine has limited autonomy in all these three areas.

I contend that, though strategies of professionalisation are discernible within the development of community psychiatric nursing, CPNs have achieved little professional autonomy. Rather their history is characterised by their willingness to do the work that other occupations would not or could not do. This not only enabled CPNs' numerical growth but also ensured that they worked at the 'frontline' of community care, in a position comparable to that of traditional mental hospital nurses. The work of both involves a high level of contact with service users, which is of a less bounded and specified nature than that of other mental health care occupations. CPNs have assumed various tasks of community mental health care (aftercare, injection administration, counselling, case management, care co-ordination, assertive outreach, supervision, court and prison diversion, etc.), which were, for the most part, fundamental to the operation of the specialist community mental health services. Though these tasks generally afforded little or moderate status, they enabled CPNs to grow in number and develop as an essential, core part of community mental health care services. To illustrate my contention I consider further the history of CPNs, described by Nolan in the previous chapter, in four broad phases to the present day.

## MODEST BEGINNINGS

It was in the 1950s that a few of the about 40,000 mental nurses then in Britain began to work in the community. CPN practice began at Warlingham Park Hospital in 1954 and at Moorhaven Hospital in 1957, and by the early 1960s a number of other hospitals were also operating such schemes. This very minimal nature of community psychiatric nursing reflects the minimal nature of community mental health care at this time. Mental health services almost exclusively attended to the needs of patients within large and overcrowded mental hospitals. Extramural services, such as day care and out-patient clinics, only began to increase in number in the 1950s and 1960s.

From accounts of the early ventures of community psychiatric nursing it is clear that CPNs were only attempting to do work that no other profession wished to do, which, however, could be claimed to be necessary. They ran clubs in the day hospital, attended to administration in out-patient clinics, checked up on patients who failed to keep appointments, provided personal physical care to patients in their own home, and gave support to caring relatives. What is also particularly striking about all the early articles discussing community psychiatric nursing is how modestly and deferentially they describe and attempt to justify the aftercare role of the CPN. They explain how it complemented the work of psychiatrists and how it did not intrude upon that of psychiatric social workers. Moore, chief nurse at Warlingham Park, clearly emphasised that community psychiatric nursing should not involve work that might be regarded as social work, as he explained: 'Detailed investigation of the patient's family situation or modification of his environment and of difficult interpersonal relations is not expected' (1964, p. 469). The reasons for such a modest approach are perhaps explained in a retrospective history of community psychiatric nursing by Greene, nursing officer at Moorhaven Hospital, in which he describes the bureaucratic obstacles and professional opposition that confronted the development of community psychiatric nursing:

> I had to justify using a scarce nursing resource for work outside the hospital without an increase in establishment. There was a violent reaction from individual members of the District Nursing and Health Visiting services. Local Authority Social Workers who were mostly unqualified, complained that the nurses were doing social work. The Regional Health Authority disclaimed knowledge of what we were trying to do, would provide no extra funds, and refused to recognise that the nurses working outside the hospital were part of the official establishment. The use of cars and travelling expenses seemed to pose great problems for the finance officers. The right of entry to a patient's home was questioned, and there were problems about insurance. In some situations, District Nurses insisted that only they could administer drugs to patients in their homes, resulting in two nurses visiting the same patient. Some General Practitioners welcomed the assistance of the psychiatric nurses, while others would have nothing to do with them. Even the Consultant Psychiatrists were divided. At case conferences before a patient's discharge, one would ask for a follow-up by a nurse, while another could not see a role for the nurse at all.
>
> (Greene 1989, p. 16)

Greene's comments also illustrate a salient feature about CPNs' development, namely that it was assisted by the divided support of both GPs and psychiatrists. However, the main point I seek to highlight is that pioneers of community psychiatric nursing, such as Greene, did not boldly claim the terrain of the community, pushing aside other occupations, but rather found areas of aftercare for nurses to work in that other occupations could be persuaded to allow and even support.

# INJECTIONS AND PSYCHOSOCIAL NURSING

It was between the 1960s and the mid-1970s that community psychiatric nursing developed from the rare activity of a handful of mental nurses working out of a few mental hospitals into the full-time activity of a discrete sub-discipline of mental nursing. This rise of community psychiatric nursing can be associated with the development of two main approaches towards mental health care, each of which found ways to generalise the work of the hospital-based specialist mental health care services into the community. On the one hand, the biomedical approach promised to eradicate chronic mental illness with its new psychotropic drugs. In 1962 the *Hospital plan* (Ministry of Health 1962) announced that psychiatric units within new district general hospitals could now replace large mental hospitals. This policy was justified as a response to a decline in the number of chronic patients in mental hospital, which was claimed to be the result of the new drugs that now arrested mental illness at its early stages. These new drugs were increasingly prescribed to people beyond the walls of the mental hospital. Neuroleptic depot injections were introduced in the late 1960s as a means of securing compliance to drug treatment amongst patients discharged from hospital. They were first administered by psychiatrists in out-patient clinics, but this task was soon delegated to CPNs, who grew in number to undertake the administration of this form of treatment in the community. In an early study of CPNs in the 1960s, Hunter (1978, p. 90) noted how disappointed a number of patients and their carers were when the new Moditen treatment was introduced, for this was associated with the stopping of conversation with the nurse. As one patient said of her CPN: 'She used to talk with me about the family, household jobs and my marriage. Now she just calls and gives me an injection' (Hunter 1978, p. 71). The clinical task of depot injection administration seemingly redefined CPN aftercare. Previously emotional support was very often all the CPN had to offer. Now the administration of the depot injection defined the main purpose of their visit, as medication was identified as the patient's primary treatment. The administration of depot injections by CPNs soon became a depersonalising and homogeneous task of mass production. As one CPN in an interview study recollects of what his practice was like in the early 1970s:

> all we [CPNs] did was inject people. There were three of us and we had roughly 600 people who were on injections, and had depot clinics nearly every day of the week, plus home visits. On Wednesday we had a clinic from 9 a.m. until 7.30 p.m. and if you were doing the clinic – there was always two people doing the clinic – you could end up doing as many as 80 injections.
>
> (Godin and Scanlon 1997, p. 79)

However, on the other hand, to a lesser extent, CPNs became involved in psychosocial methods of care. Models of 'crisis intervention', and 'preventive psychiatry', which had been developed in the USA as part of its policy of community mental health, began to inform mental health practices in Britain and helped to secure a place for the emerging occupation of community psychiatric nursing. Crisis intervention had been pioneered by Lindemann (1944), and preventive psychiatry originated from the mental hygiene movement. Both were consolidated into a coherent model by Caplan (1964), which in the USA informed the community mental health centre approach. From the late 1960s crisis intervention teams began to operate out of a number of British hospitals, orientated towards social psychiatry, intervening in the social world of patients in the community. At Dingleton Hospital CPNs became members of its crisis teams working in the community (Stobie and Hopkins 1972a, b). Haque (1973), a CPN attached to the Cassel Hospital, coined the term 'psychosocial nursing' to describe the crisis, preventative and family work in which she and other CPNs were engaged. Psychosocial nursing clearly went beyond the limits of the modest aftercare role CPNs had hitherto sought to claim. Though psychosocial nursing amongst CPNs developed mainly within crisis intervention teams, in the 1970s a few CPNs began to employ it in independent ventures into primary health care. Such a project was established in Oxford. Its responsible nursing officer attempted to justify the scheme by explaining how it embodied principles of crisis intervention and preventive psychiatry (Leopoldt 1974).

In conclusion, what can be said about this period is that the administration of depot injections gave a task to CPNs that promoted their growth in number towards their consolidation as a new occupation within community mental health care. However, CPNs also engaged in psychosocial methods of mental health care, which enabled CPNs to resist biomedical domination and to move beyond their traditional aftercare and injection administration role.

## EXPANSION AND PROFESSIONALISATION

Between the mid-1970s and early 1990s community psychiatric nursing not only continued to expand and develop but some CPNs also engaged in what could be regarded as distinctly professionalising activities, though by the end of this period CPNs had achieved little clinical or economic autonomy. However, they became a standard feature within what was called the 'district service' for mental health care by the White Paper *Better services for the mentally ill* (Department of Health and Social Security 1975). This White Paper became the major policy to shape mental health care services of this era. It recognised growing criticisms of mental health care, acknowledging that drugs could not, as was proclaimed in the 1960s, eradicate chronic mental illness and by themselves bring about community care. Instead *Better services* set targets for an increase in mental health care services and staffing. However, no recommendations were made about the size and precise function of district community psychiatric nursing services and no special money was set aside for their development. Yet the number of CPNs increased substantially, from 717 in 1975 (Parnell 1978), to 4,351 in 1990 (White 1991). I suggest that this increase was largely the result of the activities of members of the Community Psychiatric Nursing Association (CPNA). The CPNA was formed in 1976 as a nationwide association for the representation and promotion of CPNs' professional interests. From its early existence members of the CPNA struggled to establish a national standard CPN-to-population ratio. Such a ratio had already been established for health visiting and district nursing. CPNs sought to achieve the same. The CPNA initiated a census of CPNs in 1980, which was repeated in 1985, 1990 and 1996. Not only did these censuses draw attention to the presence and position of CPNs within community mental health care services, but they also helped to expose variations. The information was used to argue for an upward standardisation of CPN service provision, education and practice. Though these demands were never endorsed by the Department of Health and Social Security, the dissemination of the census data permeated and influenced service planning at a more local level towards increasing the number of CPNs (White 1993).

In addition to CPNs' quest for expansion, a professionalising strategy of credentialism and legalism can also be identified in their actions during this era. In 1980, the CPNA established the *Community Psychiatric Nursing Journal*, which was later renamed *Mental Health Nursing*. In the same year a textbook on community psychiatric nursing practice, written by nurse-teachers involved in CPN training at Manchester, was published (Carr *et al.* 1980). The CPNA also attempted to make CPN post-registration training, established in 1970, mandatory for CPN practice (though this was never achieved).

Despite general nursing's history of constraining mental nursing's development (Nolan 1993), Carr *et al.* (1980) seemingly felt a need to stress CPNs' generalist nursing identity. They embraced the new enthusiasm for nursing theory and the nursing process, recently imported from the USA, which general nursing regarded as its route to credible independent professional practice, arguing that it provided a means to bring about more individualised and less medically focused care. Carr *et al.* stressed the value of CPNs being generalists before specialists: 'It is important to achieve the overall aim of community psychiatric nursing service which should be the comprehensive delivery of psychiatric nursing skills to the community, before this specialisation is realised' (1980, p. 25). Seemingly they thought that generic care was the key to nursing and that CPNs' association with nursing was key to their future development. In contrast, Mangen and Griffith (1982) argued that the development of a generalist role would not foster the development of CPNs' professional expertise but rather trap them in a role sphere at a level of performance less than their potential. Though generalism threatened to inhibit CPNs' development of professional expertise it assisted their objective of widespread growth into becoming a ubiquitous occupational group.

Though psychiatrists often supported the development of CPN services, psychiatrists frequently obstructed them. Psychiatrists feared a loss of control and domination over CPNs as they moved into primary care. By taking referrals directly from GPs, CPNs were effectively usurping psychiatrists' monopoly over access to treatment from specialist mental health care services. In White's (1990) retrospective study of the recollections and experiences of nursing officers involved in establishing CPN services in the 1970s and early 1980s, only 13.8 per cent reported positive memories of local psychiatrists' influence on the development of their CPN service. Most (78.2 per cent) reported negative memories, largely related to consultants' objections to CPNs' intentions to take referrals directly from GPs. The Royal College of Psychiatrists (1980) attempted to reassert their monopoly over access to treatment by demanding that CPNs should be regarded as members of the psychiatric team and that any referrals they took from GPs should be viewed as referrals to the psychiatric team. However, the mandate for the development of district mental health care, given by the 1975 White Paper, enabled CPNs to disregard psychiatrists' opposition to the setting up of CPN services and their development of open referral systems. Furthermore, the Short Report (Department of Health and Social Security 1985), which in its introduction proclaimed the CPN to be the most important single profession in bringing about community care, encouraged psychiatrists to approve of CPNs taking referrals directly from GPs. In short CPNs during this period had been able to exert a degree of political influence to secure a considerable growth in their numbers and policy approval of their autonomous involvement in primary health care.

By 1990 CPNs were taking 39.7 per cent of their referrals from GPs and other primary care professionals (White 1993). CPNs could enjoy more respect and clinical freedom in primary care than was available to them within specialist mental health teams. The difference in the way in which GPs, compared to consultant psychiatrists, regarded CPNs is apparent in Morrall's (1998) study of referrals to CPNs. GPs were more inclined to approach CPNs in a consultative capacity, as fellow professionals, than were psychiatrists, who were more inclined to delegate work to CPNs.

However, CPNs' professional autonomy within primary care was very limited. CPNs could only get access to patients in primary health care through GPs or other primary health care professionals who had first assessed the patient and deemed them to be in need of CPN care. Yet CPNs' limited professional autonomy was perhaps more an issue of credibility than of doctors having a monopoly over access. People experiencing disabling mental health problems might well seek non-medical help, which they could access independently of their GP. Apart from the solace of friends, they might seek out a counsellor or psychotherapist. However, it is unlikely that people in mental distress would specifically seek out the services of a nurse, unless they knew the nurse to have expertise in counselling or psychotherapy. Consequently, it was the generalist connotations of nursing, more than anything else, that precluded CPNs from having direct access to this client group and operating any form of economic professional autonomy.

By the end of the 1980s CPNs had become a ubiquitous and generalist workforce in frontline mental health care work, both within specialist mental health care and primary care services, in part at least through exerting political influence. Though they had slightly more clinical autonomy within the latter, they had little professional autonomy in other respects.

## KEYWORKERS/CARE CO-ORDINATORS

In the 1990s British community mental health care policy again followed the example of the USA, which had in the previous decade abandoned its ambitions to provide comprehensive preventive mental health care from community mental health centres in favour of the case management of the most seriously mentally ill. In Britain a new framework for the delivery of community mental health care, based on case management, took shape, as a result of the NHS and Community Care Act, pushing CPNs away from their involvement in primary care and back into the specialist mental health care services. The 'care programme approach'

(CPA) (Department of Health 1990), introduced in 1991 as an NHS-led system of case management, became the cornerstone of this new regime. It required a community 'keyworker' (later renamed care co-ordinator) to be allocated to each mental patient in the community. The keyworker was to ensure that their client received an individually tailored package of care from the specialist mental health services. This role required considerable time, effort and ongoing contact with patients to co-ordinate and deliver care. By default, the role of 'community keyworker' fell to CPNs, partly because they were by now the most numerically dominant occupational group involved in specialist community mental health care, and partly because psychiatrists, social workers and psychologists would or could not take on this role. Thus, the frontline work of CPA case management fell mainly into the laps of CPNs, which promoted their numerical growth yet further.

## CONCLUSION

I conclude this chapter by drawing attention to three main issues that are key to understanding contemporary community mental health care and the role of the CPN. First, specialist mental health services now concentrate on patients with severe and long-term problems. A number of research studies and reports strongly encouraged CPNs in this direction (White 1993, Audit Commission 1994, Department of Health 1994, Gournay and Brooking 1994). The role they played in the care of people with less severe mental illness within primary care was increasingly taken over by practice nurses, who have, since the 1980s, grown in number even more dramatically than CPNs (Kendrick *et al.* 1993, Nolan *et al.* 1999). The renewed interest in and priority given to patients with severe and long-term problems certainly enabled CPNs to value working with such clients. However, the prioritised care of such clients led to a two-tier service. People with less severe mental health care problems were largely denied specialist mental care, though the New Labour government's 'modernisation' of mental health care promises to reverse this situation. Meanwhile, long-term patients under CPA became increasingly subject to methods of control towards minimising the risk they were increasingly seen to pose.

Secondly, as I have just indicated, there has been a growing preoccupation with the perceived risk of mental patients in the community. A number of high-profile cases of homicides by mental patients in the community helped amplify public concerns and made for the introduction of community supervision and proposals for compulsory treatment orders to be applied within the community. In addition to these measures of control over patients in the community, government directives have progressively pushed CPNs and other mental health workers into making risk assessment and risk management an integral and central part of their work. They have had to problematise and treat their clients as objects of risk, which subordinates clinical or more general need assessment. I suggest there is a serious danger of CPNs becoming so preoccupied with minimising the risks their clients pose that they will fail to recognise the risks that their clients face. Securing compliance to drug therapy is commonly seen as a major means of avoiding relapse of illness in mental patients which may lead them to become a danger to themselves or others. However, how much concern is there to protect patients from the iatrogenic effects of such treatment? How much concern is there amongst CPNs and other mental health care workers to protect their clients from the harm that may be inflicted upon them from members of the community? Furthermore, as is suggested by Alaszewski in Chapter 16, to always regard risk as a hazard that should be minimised can have disempowering consequences, for risk-taking offers opportunities to learn and develop. Are CPNs able to support positive risk-taking amongst their clients? CPNs have traditionally been willing to take risks in providing nursing care beyond the restraints and controls of the asylum for the freedom it offered their clients. Let us hope that the present preoccupation with risk minimisation does not lead CPNs to create an asylumised community.

Finally, I contend that the present regime of community mental health care has involved a general decline in mental health care workers' professional power. Though CPNs have been pushed back into specialist mental health care services, the domination they now experience is not so much from psychiatrists as from the policies that direct the practices of all mental health workers. An abundance of government directives instruct them on the practice of CPA and the assessment and management of the risk their clients pose. As Castel (1991) argues, power has passed to a level above clinicians, to those who administer the system. CPNs and other mental health care workers are now merely operatives of the system. However, CPNs have lost least as they only ever minimally achieved professionalisation. Despite the primacy given to psychiatrists as 'responsible medical officers' within the CPA, this does not secure their professional dominance. Their examination and diagnosis of the patient, which once largely directed the patient's treatment and care, is now of secondary importance. The primary focus of the work of mental health care services is now on risk assessment and risk management, which mostly involves organising practical mundane things, such as making sure that patients continue to take medication, maintain links with services and avoid homelessness and illicit drugs. What has developed is what Rose describes as the 'quotidian' clinic, in which CPNs are key frontline operatives (1996, p. 16). CPNs might therefore at least be assured of a very secure position within the mental health care division of labour.

# REFERENCES

Audit Commission (1994) *Finding a place: a review of mental health services for adults*, London: HMSO.

Brooker, C. and White, E. (1997) *The fourth quinquennial national community mental health nursing census of England and Wales*, Manchester and Keele: Universities of Manchester and Keele.

Caplan, G. (1964) *Principles of preventive psychiatry*, New York: Basic Books.

Carr, P., Butterworth, C. and Hodges, B. (1980) *Community psychiatric nursing*, Edinburgh: Churchill Livingstone.

Castel, R. (1991) 'From dangerousness to risk', in Burchell, G., Gordon, C. and Miller, P. (eds) *The Foucault effect: studies in governmentality*, London: Harvester Wheatsheaf.

Department of Health (1990) *The care programme approach for people with a mental illness referred to the specialist psychiatric services*, HC(90)23/LASSL(90)11, London: Department of Health.

Department of Health (1994) *Working in partnership: a collaborative approach to care. Report of the Mental Health Nursing Review Team*, London: HMSO.

Department of Health and Social Security (1975) *Better services for the mentally ill*, London: HMSO.

Department of Health and Social Security (1985) *Community care: with special reference to adult mentally ill and mentally handicapped people*, House of Commons Select Committee Report, House of Commons Paper 13 (1) (The Short Report), London: HMSO.

Elston, M.A. (1991) 'The politics of professional power: medicine in the changing health service', in Gabe, J., Calnan, M. and Bury, M. (eds) *The sociology of the health service*, London: Routledge.

Freidson, E. (1970) *Profession of medicine, a study of the sociology of applied knowledge*, New York: Harper and Row.

Godin, P. and Scanlon, C. (1997) 'Supervision and control: a community psychiatric nursing perspective', *Journal of Mental Health*, 6 (1): 75–84.

Gournay, K. and Brooking, J. (1994) 'Community psychiatric nurses in primary health care', *British Journal of Psychiatry*, 165: 231–238.

Greene, J. (1989) *The beginnings of community psychiatric nursing*, London: The History of Nursing Group at the Royal College of Nursing, 2: 14–20.

Haque, G. (1973) 'Psychosocial nursing in the community', *Nursing Times*, 69 (2): 51–53.

Hunter, P. (1978) *Schizophrenia and community psychiatric nursing*, Surbiton: National Schizophrenia Fellowship.

Kendrick, T., Sibbald, B., Addington-Hall, J., Brenneman, D. and Freeling, P. (1993) 'Distribution of mental health professionals working on-site within English and Welsh general practices', *British Medical Journal*, 307: 544–546.

Leopoldt, H. (1974) 'The role of the psychiatric community nurse in the therapeutic team', *Nursing Mirror and Midwives Journal*, 138 (5): 70–72.

Lindemann, E. (1944) 'Symptomatology and management of acute grief', *American Journal of Psychiatry*, 101: 141–148.

Mangen, S. and Griffith, J. (1982) 'Community psychiatric nursing services in Britain: the need for policy and planning', *International Journal of Nursing Studies*, 19 (3): 157–166.

Ministry of Health (1962) *A hospital plan for England and Wales*, London: HMSO.

Moore, S. (1964) 'Home care from Warlingham Park hospital', *Nursing Times*, 60 (15): 468–470.

Morrall, P. (1998) *Mental health nursing and social control*, London: Whurr.

Nolan, P. (1993) *A history of mental health nursing*, London: Chapman and Hall.

Nolan, P., Murray, E. and Dallender, J. (1999) 'Practice nurses' perceptions of services for clients with psychological problems in primary care', *International Journal of Nursing Studies*, 36 (2): 97–104.

Onyett, S., Heppleston, T. and Bushnell, D. (1994) 'National survey of community mental health teams. Team structure and process', *Journal of Mental Health*, 3 (2): 175–194.

Parnell, J.W. (1978) *Community psychiatric nurses: an abridged version of the report of a descriptive study*, London: The Queens Institute of Nursing.

Rose, N. (1996) 'Psychiatry as a political science: advanced liberalism and the administration of risk', *History of the Human Sciences*, 9 (2): 1–23.

Royal College of Psychiatrists (1980) 'Community psychiatric nursing: a discussion paper of the social and community psychiatry section working group', *Bulletin of the Royal College of Psychiatrists*, 4 (8): 114–118.

Stobie, G. and Hopkins, D. (1972a) 'Crisis intervention 1: a psychiatric community nurse in a rural area', *Nursing Times*, 68 (43) supplement: 165–166.

Stobie, G. and Hopkins, D. (1972b) 'Crisis intervention 2: a psychiatric community nurse in a rural area', *Nursing Times*, 68 (44) supplement: 169–172.

White, E. (1990) 'Psychiatrists' influence on the development of community psychiatric nursing services', in Brooker, C. (ed.) *Community psychiatric nursing: a research perspective*, London: Chapman and Hall.

White, E. (1991) *The third quinquennial community psychiatric nursing survey: research monograph*, London: Department of Health, University of Manchester.

White, E. (1993) 'Community psychiatric nursing 1980 to 1990: a review of organisation, education and practice', in Brooker, C. and White, E. (eds) *Community psychiatric nursing: a research perspective*, vol. 2, London: Chapman and Hall.

## FURTHER READING

A fuller account of sociological theory about health care professions related to CPNs can be found in: Morrall, P. (1998) *Mental health nursing and social control*, London: Whurr. For more detailed discussion about the nature of frontline work in mental health nursing and how CPNs operate power in their relationships with their clients see: Godin, P. (2000) 'A dirty business: caring for people who are a nuisance or a danger', *Journal of Advanced Nursing*, 32 (6): 1396–1402.

# CHAPTER 3

# THE POLICY AND LEGAL CONTEXT

*Ben Hannigan*

---

## SUMMARY OF KEY POINTS

- Health policy shapes the context in which community mental health nurses work.

- Mental health continues to be a priority health policy area in the UK. New initiatives, such as England's National Service Framework for Mental Health, are intended to improve the quality of mental health services and reduce unacceptable variations in standards of care and treatment.

- Elements of the government's new approach to community mental health care, and particularly its concern to construct a more coercive legal framework, have been subject to sustained criticism.

---

## INTRODUCTION

Health care is political. Over the years, governments in the UK have grappled to find answers to questions such as: how should the National Health Service (NHS) be organised and managed? How should resources for health care be allocated? What sort of relationship should the health service have with other organisations, such as local authority social services departments, voluntary agencies and the private health care sector? What should be the roles and responsibilities of the different health professional groups, and how should they be regulated?

Just as health care is political, so too is nursing. However, despite the grow-ing interest in politics and policy analysis in nursing from the 1980s onwards (Robinson 1997), it is likely that many practising mental health nurses still perceive that these are matters far removed from the practical realities of providing everyday nursing care. In reality, however, policy impacts on nursing at a number of levels, from the 'macro' through to the 'micro' (Masterson and Maslin-Prothero 1999).

This chapter begins with a brief review of why policy analysis is important for nurses. The larger part of the chapter is then devoted to a critical account of the mental health policy and legal context as this has emerged since the beginning of the 1990s. Particular attention is paid to the development of themes in mental health policy since the election of the Labour government in 1997. Specific areas addressed include: policy responses to the problems of providing community mental health care; the pursuit of quality and national standards; and the relationships between policy and community mental health nursing practice.

## CRITICAL POLICY ANALYSIS

Critical policy analysis in nursing includes exploration of the relationships between nursing and wider health and welfare policies, the socioeconomic context in which policy-making occurs and in which specific policy emerges, ideology, and power relationships (Robinson 1997). The mental health field is a fascinating one in which to conduct a critical policy analysis of this sort. Mental health remains a highly contested area, in which a range of different – and sometimes competing – ideas and 'stakeholders' exist (Pilgrim and Rogers 1999). Not all ideas or interests are equally represented at policy-making level, however. Through critical analysis, it is possible to identify how different constellations of ideas and different groups of stakeholders exercise greater or lesser influence on the development of mental health policy themes and specific policy initiatives.

## COMMUNITY CARE POLICY FROM 1990

Modern community mental health care emerged in the UK in the 1950s and 1960s. Early landmarks included Health Minister Enoch Powell's 'Water tower speech' of 1961, and the Hospital Plan of the following year. This initiated plans to close the Victorian asylums, and develop in their place a combination of general hospital in-patient psychiatric services, and care in the community (Rogers and Pilgrim 2001). Community mental health nursing owes its early origins to these develop-ments. From the 1950s to the present time the number of CMHNs working in the UK has grown considerably. Throughout this period, mental health policy has continued to shape and re-shape the context in which CMHNs practise, with some of the most significant changes taking place in the last decade and a half.

The NHS and Community Care Act 1990 initiated a new system of organis-ing community care. The Act was passed by a Conservative government committed to the introduction of market principles into the provision of publicly-funded health and welfare services. Under the Act, local authority social services departments were given 'lead responsibility' for community care. Following the full implementation of 'care management' in 1993, social services departments were also required to assume an 'enabling', rather than a solely 'providing', role (Means and Smith 1998). The Act also brought changes to the way in which health services were organised. Health authorities assumed the responsibility for purchasing health care, with NHS trusts taking the responsibility to provide services. General practitioner (GP) fundholders were also able to purchase care for their patients, alongside providing primary health care to individuals and families.

The introduction of the NHS and Community Care Act was significant for CMHNs in a number of ways. As employees of NHS trusts, the services of many CMHNs came to be purchased by two agencies: health authorities and GP fundholders. However, the purchasing priorities of these two groups were often quite different. Health authorities tended to emphasise the importance of specialist mental health workers providing care primarily to people identified as experiencing 'severe' or 'serious' mental health problems. Many GPs, however, also wanted primary-care-based mental health services to be available to people experiencing a wider range of mental health difficulties (Muijen and Ford 1996).

One important driver for the NHS and Community Care Act 1990 was a desire on the part of central government to clarify the roles and responsibilities of the different agencies that contributed to the provision of health and social care. Care management, therefore, became the social services-led vehicle through which community care was to be organised for all groups of service users. However, alongside the introduction of care management, separate guidance issued by the Department of Health in England introduced a new 'care programme approach' (CPA) for the organisation of community care for people accepted by specialist mental health services (Department of Health 1990).

The care programme approach, the implementation of which was to be led by the health service, obliged health and other agencies to: assess the needs of mental health service users; construct care plans to meet these needs; and identify a keyworker to oversee each individual plan of care. Confusingly, both care management and the CPA were introduced as mechanisms through which multidisciplinary and multi-agency community care could be organised and delivered. In many areas, the lack of integration between these two systems of 'case management' (Bergen 1992) resulted in a duplication of effort, excessive bureaucracy and the construction of a barrier to effective joint working (Hancock and Villeneau 1997).

Many CMHNs became keyworkers following the introduction of the CPA, and as a consequence assumed responsibility for overseeing multiprofessional plans of care. Other important policy initiatives in the 1990s also propelled CMHNs towards closer multiprofessional working. Alongside the introduction of new frameworks for organising and delivering care was the widespread appearance of the multidisciplinary and multi-agency community mental health team (CMHT). Guidance such as *Building bridges* (Department of Health 1995) identified CMHTs as the most appropriate means of providing locally-available community mental health services. CMHNs became core, and the most numerous, members of CMHTs throughout the UK (see, for example, Onyett *et al.* 1994).

However, CMHTs have had their critics. Galvin and McCarthy (1994), for example, criticised CMHTs for lacking in focus, for being inefficient and for delivering services that tended to be poor in quality.

## 'NEW LABOUR' AND THE NATIONAL HEALTH SERVICE

After eighteen unbroken years of Conservative party administration, a Labour government was elected to power in Britain in 1997. During its years in opposition and in the run-up to the election, Labour had campaigned for a new approach to publicly-funded health and welfare services. However, this did not mean that Labour planned to completely undo all that the Conservative Party had done in the years to 1997. For example, in relation to the purchaser–provider split in the health service, Labour wrote in its 1997 election manifesto that there would be 'no return to top-down management . . . [with] the planning and provision of care . . . necessary and distinct functions' (The Labour Party 1997, p. 20). In health policy as in other areas of policy, Labour proposed a 'third way': a path between bureaucratic, top-down central planning and the use of market mechanisms (Ham 1999).

NHS 'modernisation' under Labour has included a range of far-reaching general health policy initiatives. In the 'new' NHS, the long-standing tension between central control and local autonomy appears to have shifted in favour of the centre. Many of the Labour government's earliest initiatives were designed to reduce local variation in the quality of health care, and establish instead new, nationally-applicable, standards of care (Baker 2000). White Papers for the reorganisation of the health service published by the government in its first term of office, such as England's *The new NHS: modern, dependable* (Secretary of State for Health 1997), included proposals for a number of new bodies, with novel and wide-ranging responsibilities. For example, the National Institute for Clinical Excellence (NICE) was established in 1999 with a remit to provide health service professionals and users of health services in England and Wales with guidance on 'best practice'. The guidance produced by NICE is widely available, in order to maximise the chances that good practice becomes incorporated into everyday clinical care. Areas that NICE has recently focused on which have direct relevance to mental health care include the management of depression (NICE 2001), and the management of schizophrenia (NICE 2002).

Other important new national bodies introduced by the Labour government include the Commission for Health Improvement (CHI). CHI commenced its programme of work in April 2000, and has the task of monitoring and improving the quality of health care in England and Wales. Each NHS organisation in these two countries can expect a 'clinical governance review' led by CHI every four years. CHI also has the responsibility of investigating health organisations in instances where 'serious service failures' have occurred (CHI 2002). At the request of the Secretary of State for Health, CHI's first task on assuming its new responsibilities in April 2000 was to commence an investigation into standards of care for older people at North Lakeland NHS trust, an organisation which provided mental health and community services (CHI 2000). Further health care reforms announced in spring 2002 will see the work of CHI extended to include, for example, the inspection of private health care organisations. Reflecting its new role, CHI will also change its name to become the Commission for Healthcare Audit and Inspection (CHAI).

A third component of the Labour government's approach to reducing variation in health care has been the introduction of National Service Frameworks (NSFs). NSFs specify national standards of care and models of service delivery for particular care groups, or for service areas (Secretary of State for Health 1997). Significantly for community mental health nurses working in England, one of the first NSFs published by the Department of Health was the NSF for Mental Health (Department of Health 1999a), details of which are discussed both below and in many of the other chapters appearing in this book.

Whilst these new organisations and frameworks have exerted a powerful centralising influence within the health service, the devolution of political power to elected bodies in Scotland, Wales and Northern Ireland has exerted a significant influence in the opposite direction (Baker 2000). Although differences in health policy have always existed within the four countries of the UK, the appearance of the new assemblies has magnified the potential for difference. Evidence already exists of significant post-devolution divergence. For example, the Scottish Parliament's decision to centrally fund both personal and social care for older people marked a clear shift away from English social policy developed in Westminster (Pollock 2001). Important differences in mental health policy and law also exist throughout the countries of the UK. Although space in this chapter does not permit a thorough review of these differences, the reader is nonetheless alerted to the dangers of assuming that just one 'UK' mental health policy framework exists.

## MENTAL HEALTH POLICY FROM 1997

New Labour has made the 'modernisation' of mental health services a priority area. Shortly after the election of 1997, senior members of government made a series of significant, and controversial, statements about the state of mental health care. In a press release issued in July 1998, Frank Dobson, Secretary of State for Health in England, announced that:

> Care in the community has failed. Discharging people from institutions has brought benefits to some. But it has left many vulnerable patients to try to cope on their own. Others have been left to become a danger to themselves and a nuisance to others. Too many confused and sick people have been left wandering the streets and sleeping rough. A small but significant minority have become a danger to the public as well as themselves.
>
> (Dobson 1998)

In this press release, the Health Secretary also announced the specific measures which the government planned to take in order to modernise mental health care.

First, plans were announced for a new overarching mental health strategy, with increased funding, to be issued by the end of 1998. Also announced was the creation of an External Reference Group, chaired by Professor Graham Thornicroft of the Institute of Psychiatry, London. This group had the task of making recommendations to government on the creation of new national standards for mental health care throughout England. Finally, the Health Secretary announced plans for a 'root and branch' review of the Mental Health Act (1983) for England and Wales. The press release included the Health Secretary's promise that this review of legislation would:

> cover such possible measures as compliance orders and community treatment orders to provide a prompt and effective legal basis to ensure that patients get supervised care if they do not take their medication or if their condition deteriorates.
>
> (Dobson 1998)

The first part of the government's new strategy for mental health services in England was launched at the end of 1998. *Modernising mental health services: safe, sound and supportive* (Department of Health 1998) reasserted the claim that 'care in the community' had failed. This document also drew attention to a number of other pressing areas, including: the burden faced by families caring for people with severe mental health problems; the problem of stigma; difficulties in the recruitment and retention of mental health staff; and the unacceptable variation in standards of mental health care found throughout different parts of the country. *Modernising mental health services* argued that the quality of mental health care would improve with the operation of new frameworks such as clinical governance, and through the work of new organisations such as CHI and NICE. However, echoing the Health Secretary's press release of earlier that year, the document also made the case for wide-ranging changes in the policy and legal contexts specifically relating to mental health care. Finally, *Modernising mental health services* also acknowledged the need to increase the resources available for the delivery of mental health care.

Rogers and Pilgrim (2001) have argued that, taken as a whole, *Modernising mental health services* made for very contradictory reading. The document included explicit recognition of the association between mental ill health and experiences such as poverty and physical illness. Tackling social exclusion, tackling the causes of mental ill-health and promoting the integration of people with mental health problems into communities were therefore presented as important aims. In this same document, however, plans for an increasingly coercive legal framework were also set out, with future legislation aiming to 'address the responsibility of individual patients to comply with their programmes of care' (Department of Health 1998, p. 40).

Work by Professor Thornicroft's External Reference Group (ERG), which had the task of making recommendations to government in support of a National Service Framework (NSF) for Mental Health in England, continued alongside the separate task of reviewing the English and Welsh Mental Health Act (1983). This latter work was taken up by a specially-commissioned expert group, chaired by Professor Genevra Richardson of London University. With respect to the former of these two tasks, a considerable period elapsed between the ERG producing its report for government, and the English NSF for Mental Health finally appearing in September 1999. This delay may have reflected the tensions between the interests and aspirations of the ERG, which drew its membership from a wide range of mental health 'stakeholder' groups, and the specific interests of government, with its narrower concern for public safety and rectifying the 'failure' of community care (Peck 1999).

When it appeared, England's National Service Framework for Mental Health (Department of Health 1999a) contained seven national standards for mental health services, backed up by a range of measures to assess performance and progress in the achievement of key 'milestones'. These seven standards were associated with five areas, which were:

- mental health promotion;
- primary care and access to services;
- effective services for people with severe mental illness;
- caring about carers;
- preventing suicide.

Each standard and its associated interventions were underpinned by explicit reference to the evidence base, and examples of good practice. For example, the first standard urged health and social services to 'promote mental health for all' and 'combat discrimination against individuals and groups with mental health problems, and promote their social inclusion'. Underpinning this standard was reference to studies which have investigated the importance of social networks, the importance of 'healthy workplaces' and the impact of unemployment on mental health. Examples of good practice in promoting mental health which were included in this section of the NSF included interventions targeted at schools, and workshops aimed at reducing stress.

The NSF for Mental Health is a highly significant document, which when published set out a long-term strategy for mental health services in England. The strategy did, however, attract criticism. Rogers and Pilgrim (2001) criticised both the process through which the document was produced, and specific areas of content. Rogers and Pilgrim (ibid., p. 215) found examples of 'crude political rhetoric', sitting awkwardly alongside the more measured, 'academic' sections of the document. This, they argued, reflected the tension between the work and aspirations of the External Reference Group and the more overtly 'political' interests of the civil servants and politicians who had the final responsibility for drafting and publishing the document. Other criticisms raised by Rogers and Pilgrim included the selective use of evidence to support the points that were made.

The promised 'root and branch' review of mental health legislation in England and Wales began with the establishment of Professor Richardson's expert committee in 1998. In *Modernising mental health services* (Department of Health 1998), the government had described the Mental Health Act (1983) for England and Wales as being 'outdated', and no longer appropriate for an era of community, rather than hospital-based, care. As with the NSF for Mental Health in England, an analysis of the way in which mental health law in England and Wales has been reviewed reveals significant tensions in the policy-making process.

Professor Richardson and her team presented their report to ministers in July 1999. However, the full 170-page document (Department of Health 1999b) was not published until the end of that year, alongside the government's Green Paper, *Reform of the Mental Health Act 1983: proposals for consultation* (Secretary of State for Health 1999). This simultaneous publication, Rogers and Pilgrim (2001) argued, made it difficult for the expert committee's report to be given proper consideration, without also having to consider the government's response to it. In many places, it was clear that there was concordance between the recommendations set out in the Richardson report and the recommendations made in the Green Paper. For example, the government accepted the expert review team's proposal that any future Mental Health Act should include a statement of the principles that underpinned it. However, there were also areas of significant difference. In the committee's view, the decision to proceed or not to proceed with compulsory treatment should take account of the capacity of the person with mental disorder. In the opinion of the expert committee, a person who possessed capacity but who also had a mental disorder would need to present a greater level of risk before compulsory treatment was ordered than would a person who had a mental disorder but who *lacked* capacity. However, the government questioned this 'capacity-based' model, arguing instead that the level of risk presented by an individual should be the overriding criterion in making decisions regarding the use of compulsory powers.

A further period of consultation in 2000 followed the publication of the government's Green Paper. Throughout this whole period, the government's interest in finding ways of making sure that people with mental health problems complied with their programmes of care and treatment continued to cause considerable alarm to both campaigning mental health organisations and some professional groups. The Mental Health Alliance, which included MIND, the Royal College of Nursing (RCN) and the Community Psychiatric Nurses' Association (CPNA), continued a vigorous campaign against the possible introduction of 'community treatment orders' (for example, see MIND (and others) 1999).

When the White Paper *Reforming the Mental Health Act* was published in December 2000 (Secretary of State for Health and Home Secretary 2000a, b), it was clear that many of the proposals contained in the Green Paper which the Alliance had lobbied against remained in place. Amongst the White Paper's proposals was, again, confirmation of the government's plan to extend the use of compulsory powers to people with mental health problems living in the community. However, in response to concerns expressed by campaigning and professional groups, the White Paper did make clear that medication would only be given to people who were 'actively resisting treatment' in hospital settings. Also contained in Part 1 of the White Paper was the suggestion that, in the future, the task of applying for the use of compulsory orders might not fall just to approved social workers (ASWs), but to 'a social worker or another mental health professional with specific training in the application of the new legislation' (Secretary of State for Health and Home Secretary 2000a, p. 25). For the first time, this seemed to suggest, some community mental health nurses might have a role in making decisions over the initial use of compulsory powers.

After the initial flurry of government-inspired activity, extending from the autumn of 1998 (the setting up of the Richardson committee) to the end of 2000 (the release of the two-part White Paper), all suddenly became very quiet. To the surprise of many, the government did not announce plans to make further progress towards an Act of Parliament at any point in 2001. Instead, a draft mental health bill eventually appeared in June 2002, alongside a call for a further period of public consultation (Department of Health 2002). The publication of the document was greeted by considerable media interest. National newspapers, television and radio stations carried the news, and gave space to the debate over the bill's content. However, for those who had hoped that the lobbying of recent years might have modified the government's concern to extend compulsory treatment into the community, the draft bill proved to be a bitter disappointment. As the White Paper had earlier proposed, the bill suggested that, once the criteria for the use of compulsory powers were satisfied, compulsory orders could be equally applied to people detained in hospital and to those who were to be treated in the community. Mental health nurses, too, were explicitly mentioned for the first time as having a possible part to play in the operation of any new Act. The consultation document accompanying the draft bill (Department of Health 2002, p. 22) suggested that the role of the approved social worker disappear in favour of the new role of 'approved mental health professional' (AMHP). This person – who could be a social worker, a nurse, a psychologist, an occupational therapist, or some other qualified mental health practitioner – would be required to co-ordinate the 'preliminary examination' of a person liable to be treated under a compulsory order, and to provide a non-medical assessment alongside the assessment of two medical practitioners.

## CONCLUSION

At the start of this chapter the suggestion was made that, despite sometimes appearing far-removed from everyday practice, policy and legal frameworks exert a powerful influence on nursing from the 'macro' through to the 'micro' level. Through a critical analysis of UK mental health policy, I hope to have illustrated the ways in which the policy-making process is subject to competing ideas and interests. In discussing specific policy initiatives, this chapter has shown how emerging mental health policy and law continue to set the context and parameters for mental health nursing practice.

Health and social policy is a fast-moving area. Since 1997, the pace of change has, if anything, increased. Simultaneously, mental health care appears to have become an increasingly politicised area. Inevitably, aspects of this chapter will soon appear outdated, as the cumulative impact of new policy frameworks is felt and as new initiatives are introduced. A challenge for community mental health nurses is to remain engaged with debates over policy development and implementation, at both national and local levels, in order that the 'voice' of nurses is heard alongside those of other, often more powerful, groups.

# REFERENCES

Baker, M. (2000) *Making sense of the NHS White Papers*, 2nd edn, Oxford: Radcliffe.

Bergen, A. (1992) 'Case management in community care: concepts, practices and implications for nursing', *Journal of Advanced Nursing*, 17: 1106–1113.

Commission for Health Improvement (CHI) (2000) *Investigation into the North Lakeland NHS Trust: report to the Secretary of State for Health*, London: CHI.

Commission for Health Improvement (CHI) (2002) About CHI. Online. http://www.chi.nhs.uk/eng/about/index.shtml

Department of Health (1990) *The care programme approach for people with a mental illness referred to the specialist psychiatric services*. HC(90)23/LASSL(90)11, London: Department of Health.

Department of Health (1995) *Building bridges: a guide to arrangements for interagency working for the care and protection of severely mentally ill people*, London: Department of Health.

Department of Health (1998) *Modernising mental health services: safe, sound and supportive*, London: Department of Health.

Department of Health (1999a) *National service framework for mental health: modern standards and service models*, London: Department of Health.

Department of Health (1999b) *Review of the Mental Health Act 1983: report of the expert committee*, London: Department of Health.

Department of Health (2002) *Mental health bill: consultation document*, London: The Stationery Office.

Dobson, F. (1998) *Frank Dobson outlines third way for mental health*, Press release 98/311, London: Department of Health.

Galvin, S.W. and McCarthy, S. (1994) 'Multidisciplinary community teams: clinging to the wreckage', *Journal of Mental Health*, 3: 167–174.

Ham, C. (1999) 'The third way in health care reform: does the emperor have any new clothes?' *Journal of Health Services Research and Policy*, 4 (3): 168–173.

Hancock, M. and Villeneau, L. (1997) *Effective partnerships: developing key indicators for joint working in mental health*, London: The Sainsbury Centre for Mental Health.

House of Commons (1990) *National Health Service and Community Care Act*, London: HMSO.

The Labour Party (1997) *Election manifesto: new Labour – because Britain deserves better*, London: The Labour Party.

Masterson, A. and Maslin-Prothero, S. (1999) 'Preface', in Masterson, A. and Maslin-Prothero, S. (eds) *Nursing and politics: power through practice*, London: Churchill Livingstone.

Means, R. and Smith, R. (1998) *Community care: policy and practice*, 2nd edn, Basingstoke: Macmillan.

MIND (and others) (1999) *10 Questions about compulsory treatment in the community*, London: MIND.

Muijen, M. and Ford, R. (1996) 'The market and mental health: intentional and unintentional incentives', *Journal of Interprofessional Care*, 10 (1): 13–22.

National Collaborating Centre for Mental Health (commissioned by the National Institute for Clinical Excellence) (2002) *Schizophrenia: core interventions in the treatment and management of schizophrenia in primary and secondary care, National Clinical Practice Guideline Number 1*, National Collaborating Centre for Mental Health.

National Institute for Clinical Excellence (NICE) (2001) *Clinical guidelines in progress: depression*. Online. http://www.nice.org.uk/cat.asp?c=20093

National Institute for Clinical Excellence (NICE) (2002) *Schizophrenia: core interventions in the treatment and management of schizophrenia in primary and secondary care,*

*National Clinical Practice Guideline Number 1, Second consultation*, London: NICE/National Collaborating Centre for Mental Health.

Onyett, S., Heppleston, T. and Bushnell, D. (1994) *The organisation and operation of community mental health teams in England*, London: The Sainsbury Centre for Mental Health.

Peck, E. (1999) 'Tensions in mental health policy?', *Journal of Mental Health*, 8 (3): 213–214.

Pilgrim, D. and Rogers, A. (1999) *A sociology of mental health and illness*, 2nd edn, Buckingham: Open University Press.

Pollock, A.M. (2001) 'Social policy and devolution', *British Medical Journal*, 322: 311–312.

Robinson, J. (1997) 'Power, politics and policy analysis in nursing', in Parry, A. (ed.) *Nursing: a knowledge base for practice*, 2nd edn, London: Arnold.

Rogers, A. and Pilgrim, D. (2001) *Mental health policy in Britain*, 2nd edn, Basingstoke: Palgrave.

Secretary of State for Health (1997) *The new NHS: modern, dependable*, London: The Stationery Office.

Secretary of State for Health (1999) *Reform of the Mental Health Act 1983: proposals for consultation*, London: The Stationery Office.

Secretary of State for Health and Home Secretary (2000a) *Reforming the Mental Health Act. Part 1: the new legal framework*, London: The Stationery Office.

Secretary of State for Health and Home Secretary (2000b) *Reforming the Mental Health Act. Part 2: high risk patients*, London: The Stationery Office.

## FURTHER READING

There are many books and journals which deal with general health policy in the UK. However, books which deal specifically with UK mental health policy are few and far between. An exception is:

Rogers, A. and Pilgrim, D. (2001) *Mental health policy in Britain*, 2nd edn, Basingstoke: Palgrave.

This excellent book provides a critical account of the process of mental health policy-making in the UK, and an analysis of substantive mental health policy up to and including the early years of the new Labour government.

# CHAPTER 4

# ETHICAL ISSUES

*Chris Chaloner*

## SUMMARY OF KEY POINTS

- Community mental health nurses are faced with many and varied ethical issues in their day-to-day practice.
- The process of considered ethical reflection is vital in responding to ethical questions and situations encountered within practice.
- Ethical issues such as relationship formation, confidentiality, consent and autonomy lie at the heart of community mental health nursing.

## INTRODUCTION

Community mental health nursing gives rise to complex ethical questions and decisions. Central to the ethics of a community mental health nurse's (CMHN's) practice may be issues relating to consent and treatment acceptance (or 'compliance' – an ethically questionable term in itself), professional autonomy and the use of power and control.

Indeed, the function of the CMHN – together with that of many other mental health professionals – may be considered an ethical endeavour in that its primary aims are basically either to do 'good' or to avoid 'harm'; of course, defining 'good' and 'harm' is an ethical issue in itself.

The potential influence that a CMHN can have on their patients' lives is wide-ranging and the access such nurses have to the 'real lives' of their patients can be considerable. It is essential therefore that any exploration of the CMHN's role considers its ethical character.

For example, what is the ethical nature of the CMHN–patient relationship? To what extent is practice affected by issues such as consent and confidentiality? Should patients be coerced into receiving treatment that the nurse believes will be of benefit to them? How can a CMHN assist their patients to exercise individual autonomy? Underpinning such questions is the ability (or willingness) of the CMHN to participate in the often demanding process of ethical reflection.

Although trying to do 'good' and avoid 'harm' provides a simple definition of the ethical nature of a CMHN's practice, identifying 'good' and 'harm' may not always be a simple task – e.g. a patient wants to terminate her relationship with mental health services (in order to obtain the 'good' of independence) but her clinical team want to maintain contact (in order to obtain the 'good' of treatment). Alternatively, there may be no 'goods' in the choices CMHNs face, only lesser harms – e.g. a CMHN wishes to discourage his patient's reliance on medication (to minimise the 'harm' of dependence) but the patient is requesting an increase in medication (to avoid the 'harm' of distressing thoughts). It is possible that 'good' can only be achieved by inflicting 'harm' – e.g. a CMHN feels that enforced treatment ('harm') may be the only means of achieving a positive clinical outcome ('good').

Ethical decisions are further complicated by the legal permissibility of interventions that may be claimed, in some instances, to be 'unethical', i.e. just because CMHNs are legally empowered to do something – e.g. under the powers of 'supervised discharge' – does that mean that, ethically, they *should*?

## ETHICS

In order to enable ethical practice it is essential that an understanding of ethics is acquired.

Ethics is basically concerned with considerations of 'right' and 'wrong' or 'good' and 'bad' in relation to the decisions and actions taken by people. Ethical questions usually contain a morally evaluative component, e.g. 'Is "A" a *good* person?' They frequently incorporate '*should*', a word that is commonly used and has significant ethical implications, e.g. '*Should* we tell "B" the full facts regarding her prognosis?'

In our daily lives we face many 'should' questions. For example, '*Should* I go to work today?', '*Should* I phone my mother?' Such questions rarely demand a great deal of consideration – it would make life extremely difficult if we indulged in lengthy contemplation of *every* ethical issue. For a CMHN, however, a practice-based question such as 'I am aware that my patient may have committed a criminal offence – should I disclose confidential information?' demands more measured ethical reflection.

In response to such an 'ethical dilemma' it is usual either to consider the potential *consequences* of doing or not doing something ('What will happen if I breach confidentiality?', 'What will happen if I don't?'), or to base one's decision on a perception of ethical *duty* ('I have a duty to avoid harm – I must therefore disclose confidential information as it is the right thing to do – regardless of the consequences – not to do so would simply be wrong'). These responses reflect two broad ethical approaches that, among several competing ethical theories, are the most commonly applied (Box 4.1). Ethical responses may also be informed by a consideration of how specific ethical principles apply to a situation, e.g. a principle that states we should try to avoid harm whenever possible (Box 4.2).

Both theories and principles *assist* in the assessment of an ethical dilemma. They do not, however, provide a substitute for considered ethical reflection (Box 4.3). This requires the ability to identify morally relevant aspects of a situation (in the example above, breakdown of trust, avoidance of harm, etc. may be thought relevant) and to carefully consider what ethical concepts are involved (moral obligations towards this patient and society as a whole, the patient's right to privacy, etc.).

Ethics and ethical practice are closely associated with:

- the use of the terms 'right' and 'wrong'/'good' and 'bad' (when applied in a morally evaluative sense, i.e. 'he/she is a *good* person, not in a morally neutral sense, i.e. 'it is a *good* car');
- attitudes and values held by individuals and groups (personal, cultural, societal);
- considerations of how people *ought* to act in a particular situation;
- the ability to think, make decisions and act independently (autonomy);
- the concept of 'rights' – one's own and others';
- moral duties owed to others and duties owed to ourselves;
- attempting to bring about the 'best outcome';
- avoiding 'harm';
- trying to do what is 'right'.

---

### Box 4.1   Two ethical theories

**1 *Utilitarianism*** (outcome-based approach) – a consequentialist theory concerned with the effects of actions, i.e. for the utilitarian the ethically correct act is the one that aims to achieve the best overall outcome (in simple terms it is concerned with producing the most 'good' or the most 'benefit' at the cost of least suffering) (Gillon 1985, ch. 4).

A utilitarian will claim that what matters morally is ends and that 'the ends justify the means'. For example, a utilitarian view may support the withdrawal of expensive treatment from an individual with serious mental illness who shows little sign of improvement if resources can then be distributed more widely, thereby increasing overall benefit. The individual patient may be 'harmed' as a result of this action but overall benefit will be maximised if others, with a greater chance of improvement, can be treated. Utilitarianism states that 'good' actions maximise overall happiness, or minimise overall pain, and 'bad' actions are those that do the opposite.

**2 *Deontology*** (duty-based approach) – concerned with adhering to moral *rules* or moral *duty**, i.e. the deontologist views the ethically correct act as

*continued*

the one that is 'right in itself' – regardless of the consequences (Fletcher *et al.* 1995). According to a deontological view the moral agent must act out of a *duty* to do right (and avoid wrong) and not because of any inclination, emotion, etc. Such an approach may offer ethical justification for telling the truth, even if harm is caused by so doing. In such an instance, truth telling is regarded as being right in itself – regardless of its potential consequences.

To demonstrate how these theories are applied in our day-to-day lives, consider why you would (or would not) offer your seat on a bus to a frail elderly lady. Would you do so because of the potential *consequences* of your action (the lady will be safer/more comfortable/grateful, etc., other people on the bus will think I am a good person etc.), or would the offer be made out of a sense of *duty*, i.e. because it is the 'right thing to do'?

---

\* It is generally accepted that most moral rules cannot be *absolute* – they are prima facie rules that can be broken in certain circumstances, e.g. self-defence, when killing may be permitted (the threat must equal the action and vice versa). A rule of thumb is that not doing harm takes priority over doing harm.

---

## Box 4.2    Ethical principles

Ethical principles can provide a framework for ethical thinking and decision-making (Beauchamp and Childress 2001). They help to identify the ethical aspects of a situation or decision. None of the following principles should be regarded as unconditional but they can usefully inform ethical thinking and ethical practice:

- *Beneficence*: requires that we actively contribute to the welfare of others, i.e. we should 'do good'. Defining 'good' may be problematic and a requirement to do 'good' is very demanding.

- *Non-maleficence*: requires that we do not inflict harm intentionally. Possibly an easier principle to adhere to than the principle of beneficence – it is generally the case that we are not intentionally harming another person.

- *Respect for autonomy*: we are obliged to respect others' ability to self-determination. This principle holds that individuals should be able to exercise their autonomy freely, the only limit being the extent to which their autonomy infringes upon the autonomy of others.

- *Justice*: requires that we treat all others fairly and equally. Problems arise when trying to determine 'fairness', particularly with regard to the allocation of limited resources (see below).

**Box 4.3   Ethical reflection**

Robert is an experienced CMHN whose patient 'Francis', a 35-year-old man with long-standing mental health problems, has recently told him that he has been stealing from his part-time employer. Robert is unsure what is the 'right thing to do' in this situation. He is aware that Francis has only recently acquired his job after many frustrating attempts to gain employment.

Robert must consider the morally relevant aspects of the situation. For example:

- Theft – although legally 'wrong', can it ever be ethically justified?
- What has been stolen and for what purpose?
- His relationship with his patient – what is the purpose of this relationship? How is the relationship affected by what he has been told?
- How may the theft be affecting Francis's employer?

He must also consider what ethical concepts are relevant to the situation. For example:

- His ethical (and professional) duty – does he have a duty to inform someone about the theft? That is, none of the above aspects should inform his decision-making – he should simply report the theft.
- Respect for autonomy – could Robert justify overriding Francis's autonomy by informing others of the possible theft?
- The best interests of Francis (and the best interests of Robert).
- Rights – does Francis have the right to confidentiality? Do others (e.g. Francis's employer) have a right to be told this information?
- Avoidance of harm – if Robert seeks to avoid or at least minimise harm, what is the most appropriate action for him to take? How can he define 'harm' in this instance?

By carefully considering the morally relevant aspects and key ethical concepts it may be possible for Robert to reach an ethical conclusion. This does not have to be one that is agreed by others but it must be one that Robert himself can ethically justify.

# EXAMPLES OF THE ETHICAL ASPECTS OF A CMHN's PRACTICE

## The relationship between the nurse and patient

Relationship formation and development lie at the heart of ethical practice, and the ability of CMHNs to gain their patient's trust is a crucial factor in the therapeutic process. Although the identification of mutually agreed goals is frequently promoted as being desirable, it may not always be achievable in practice where the expectations of nurses and their patients may differ. It may be necessary to consider the application of ethical theories and/or principles in justifying an action that is apparently at odds with what may be considered an ethical ideal.

Boundaries between nurses and their patients are established via their roles within the therapeutic process. If, however, these boundaries become blurred or are transgressed, it may be necessary to carefully explore the 'rights' and 'wrongs' via the process of ethical reflection (see above).

Trust formation is generally accepted as an ongoing process, dependent upon the length of contact and specific circumstances of the relationship. Dibben *et al.* (2000) examined the process of trust formation within the professional–patient relationship. They described how 'dispositional trust' (a psychological trait to be trusting) is dominant in the early stages of a relationship, but that ultimate co-operation is dependent on the development of a 'secure situational trust' which emerges and is carried forward and modified as the relationship develops.

## Confidentiality and privacy

Confidentiality is generally perceived to be implicit within professional–patient relationships. A professional duty of confidentiality is based upon an obligation to respect autonomy and an acknowledgement of patients' rights to privacy. Although such a duty is strict, any guarantee of confidentiality is inevitably constrained by the CMHN's need to share information with their colleagues. Complete confidentiality may not serve the interests of the nurse or their patient – it could even lead to serious harm occurring if, for example, a nurse became aware of a threat that they were unable to act upon as a result of a strict confidentiality rule (see comments regarding respecting autonomy below).

The sharing of confidential information is a feature of a CMHN's practice, and a patient's consent to such disclosure is usually implicit (although the majority of patients may be unaware of the number of people who may ultimately gain access to their confidential records). Disclosure for non-clinical purposes without the patient's consent is generally considered 'unethical' unless serious harm is threatened.

Tensions may arise between a professional's duty to maintain confidentiality and their obligations to society as a whole. It may be claimed that where serious harm is threatened society has a vested interest in the disclosure of what may otherwise be regarded as 'confidential' information. The 'public interest' or a 'duty to warn' provides the greatest justification for non-consensual disclosure (Griffith *et al.* 1999). For example:

- Doctors have a statutory requirement to give notification of an infectious disease (Public Health (Control of Disease) Act (1984)).
- Threatened or actual criminal activity – the interests of justice may be claimed to outweigh those of the individual, depending on the seriousness of the crime.
- When some aspect of an individual's health implies a threat of harm to others – for example, a patient who has poor eyesight but is determined

to go on driving (this raises questions regarding the extent of a professional's duty of care, i.e. is it solely to the patient or does it extend to others?).

Gaining access to patients' homes is a feature of a CMHN's role. Such a potentially intrusive measure must be supported by considered ethical reflection. It is perhaps a commonly accepted aspect of community practice that receives insufficient ethical examination. Magnusson and Lützén (1999) studied the process of ethical decision-making in patients' homes. One of the questions they asked community mental health professionals to consider was 'Am I an intruder in the patient's home, or am I a professional?' Although, arguably, these terms are not mutually exclusive, the authors found that nurses expressed concerns about the nature of their role in this environment. For example, participants in the study described the unique dynamics of their relationships within the patient's home where: 'In situations where nurses experienced that they did not have the "upper hand", the "power" relationship [between nurse and patient] would be reversed' (p. 403).

## Autonomy – of both nurse and patient

Autonomy ('self-rule' or 'self-determination') lies at the heart of many ethical questions, decisions and actions. It is particularly relevant to practice-based issues such as:

- encouraging patients to make informed choices, e.g. with regard to their participation in therapy;
- demonstrating respect (in order to acknowledge the patient as a self-determining individual);
- maintaining confidentiality (in order to protect a patient's privacy);
- acknowledging one's own and others' rights (protecting justified claims, e.g. to respect).

Being autonomous requires having the ability to:

- think for oneself, believe things, have preferences (autonomy of *thought*);
- make decisions and plans, freely and independently based on autonomous thought (autonomy of *will*);
- act freely and independently in response to one's thoughts and decisions (autonomy of *action*).

(Gillon 1985, ch.10)

The ethical principle of respect for autonomy demands that autonomous individuals should be allowed to make decisions about what they do and what is done to them. However, an additional requirement for autonomy is the ability to recognise other autonomous individuals. Therefore, although being autonomous implies freedom from personal limitations, it does not mean doing whatever you please, as the autonomy of others must also be considered.

If any one of the above criteria is absent or impaired, then autonomy is diminished. Consider, for example, a man suffering from a physical disability

– how might his autonomy of action be affected? Alternatively, consider the woman who gives her verbal consent to therapy but does not fully understand what is going to happen to her – is she able to make an autonomous decision if she is not fully informed? In other words, is she able to make a free and independent choice?

A community patient's autonomy may appear to be enhanced by virtue of the fact that they reside in their own home (rather than in a hospital) and therefore take responsibility for many of their day-to-day activities. However, it has been suggested that, rather than strengthening individual autonomy, the pressures of community-based living serve to repress autonomous actions: 'there may be reason to believe that, for mentally ill persons, self-determination weakens when attempts at social integration and rehabilitation are made' (Magnusson and Lützén 1999, p. 400). Autonomy can be enhanced and/or diminished by a number of factors (Box 4.4).

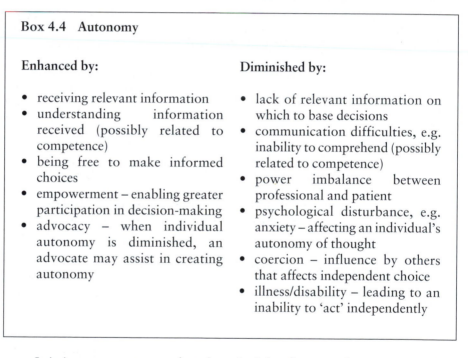

**Box 4.4   Autonomy**

**Enhanced by:**

- receiving relevant information
- understanding information received (possibly related to competence)
- being free to make informed choices
- empowerment – enabling greater participation in decision-making
- advocacy – when individual autonomy is diminished, an advocate may assist in creating autonomy

**Diminished by:**

- lack of relevant information on which to base decisions
- communication difficulties, e.g. inability to comprehend (possibly related to competence)
- power imbalance between professional and patient
- psychological disturbance, e.g. anxiety – affecting an individual's autonomy of thought
- coercion – influence by others that affects independent choice
- illness/disability – leading to an inability to 'act' independently

It is important to note that the principle of respect for autonomy does not only apply to patients; it applies to all autonomous individuals – including the CMHN. Therefore, if an autonomous individual claims a moral right to receive a certain form of service, this does not imply that a nurse has an automatic duty to provide it. The professional's autonomy must also be respected and they must be permitted to make autonomous decisions about the service they supply. The professional autonomy of CMHNs was explored by Morrall (1995) who examined the degree of autonomy that nurses experienced working within multiprofessional community mental health teams.

Many areas of community mental health practice reflect an increasingly autonomous (and accountable) role. With increasing autonomy comes greater accountability; the more independence a professional enjoys, the more answerable they become. Autonomy and accountability are closely aligned in relation to issues such as consent and confidentiality, where the nature of *what* a nurse did and *how* they acted may be subject to ethical scrutiny.

Being 'autonomous' is not a static state; levels of autonomy vary in accordance with circumstances and environment. In addition to respecting autonomy, it has been suggested that health professionals should also seek to *create* autonomy in those whose autonomy may be impaired. The justification for this is made clear if you consider *why* it is important to gain a patient's informed consent prior to initiating some course of action – isn't the main reason to allow them the opportunity to exercise their individual autonomy? Seedhouse (1998) describes an 'autonomy spectrum' ranging from point 'A' – no autonomy – to point 'B' – complete autonomy. Professional practice, he suggests, should be aimed at assisting individuals to move along this spectrum in the direction of point 'B'. The creation of autonomy, i.e. assisting individuals to play a greater part in decision-making and to have control over their own lives, can be viewed as an essential aspect of community mental health nursing.

Problems may arise when the CMHN's strongly-held desire to respect their patient's autonomy clashes with an equally stringent requirement – for example, when respecting the autonomy of one individual may threaten harm to another. Consider the nurse who is informed by her HIV-positive patient that he (the patient) intends to continue having unprotected sex with his partner who is unaware of his diagnosis. The nurse wishes to respect the autonomy of her patient but is aware that this may lead to harm occurring to the patient's partner. It may be claimed that the patient's autonomous decision should be overridden and that rights to personal safety are more basic than an obligation to respect autonomy.

## Consent, refusal and compliance

Consent is the means by which patients authorise health professionals to intervene in their care. For consent to be meaningful (i.e. both ethically and legally valid) it must be informed. Beauchamp and Childress (2001, p. 78) define informed consent as 'an individual's autonomous authorisation of a medical intervention', and the process of seeking and gaining a patient's informed consent to participation in a treatment programme is closely linked to the ethical requirement to respect individual autonomy (see above).

Valid consent amounts to more than a verbal agreement or the signing of a piece of paper. The consenting individual must be competent and receive sufficient information relevant to their specific circumstances. They should understand what they have been told, i.e. the features, consequences and alternatives associated with the proposed intervention, and their decision must be made independently, i.e. free from interference or coercion by others. Any person giving consent on a patient's behalf, e.g. an adult for a child, must be in a legal position to do so.

The principal benefits of informed consent are that it enables patients to act autonomously and obliges CMHNs to make appropriate disclosure of relevant information. When consent is given, if possible, it should be the culmination of a *process* of information giving, understanding and decision-making rather than a one-off event.

Acceptance of treatment does not necessarily indicate that a patient has freely given their consent. Other factors may influence treatment acceptance, not least of which is the CMHN's desire to act in the best interests of the patient, which may possibly encourage some degree of 'beneficent coercion' into their practice. Although patients' participation may be reliant on some degree of coercion (Chaloner 1998), it should, of course, be closely constrained by the need to act at all times in the patient's best interests.

'Compliance' is a frequently used term to describe a patient's participation in treatment. This term, however, has undoubted ethical undertones and possibly indicates a one-sided approach to care delivery.

> One cannot ignore the moral and ethical problems of the use of the term compliance. . . . It indicates a dictatorial and subordinate relationship between the professional and the service user. At its worst is an ideology based on the person (patient) being passive and to blame. The issues of power and status are central.
>
> (Gardner *et al*. 1999, p. 20)

Compliance may even be used as a 'bargaining tool' for CMHNs to use when seeking a patient's 'co-operation' in treatment. If the patient can see some sort of 'reward' for their co-operation, e.g. maintenance of disability benefit, they may be encouraged to participate in treatment (whilst also reinforcing their perception of themselves within a 'sick' role) in order to achieve a desired end (Godin 2000, p. 1401).

Assessing competence to make informed decisions can be a contentious issue within mental health practice. Although the Nursing and Midwifery Council (2002, Clause 3.4) states that 'You should presume that every patient and client is legally competent unless otherwise assessed by a suitably qualified practitioner', ongoing assessments of competence may be required within mental health settings. A further issue relating to competence is the potential for subjective discrimination (by the health professional), i.e. is the patient deemed 'competent' if they agree with a proposed form of treatment and 'non-competent' if they do not?

In summary, valid informed consent requires:

- *Competence* – is the patient *able* to make an autonomous decision? Has their competence been assessed?
- *Information* relevant to the individual – how much information does he/she require? What non-clinical issues, e.g. personal circumstances, might influence their decision-making?
- *Understanding* – does the patient understand what they have been told, i.e. the nature, consequences and alternatives associated with the proposed intervention?
- *Independence* – has the patient made an autonomous decision, free from interference/coercion by others?

## Paternalism

Increasing attention is paid to involving patients in decision-making and ensuring that informed consent is sought. However, in promoting the human good (beneficence), traditional health care practice has emphasised the treatment process over respect for autonomy. Therefore, the two principles (beneficence and autonomy) may clash when what the CMHN – applying their skills, knowledge and experience – believes is 'good' for their patient conflicts with what the patient themselves wants or is prepared to accept. In overriding a patient's wishes, supposedly in their best interests, the CMHN may be accused of paternalism:

> intentional overriding of one person's known preferences or actions by another person, where the person who overrides justifies the action by the goal of benefiting or avoiding harm to the person whose preferences or actions are overridden.
>
> (Beauchamp and Childress 2001, p. 178)

Although paternalism may be claimed to be incompatible with modern-day practice, it could be justified as a means of *enabling* the patient to exercise autonomy at a later date, i.e. the CMHN's paternalistic intervention could be viewed as a means of *creating* autonomy prior to *respecting* it.

## Allocating limited resources

The distribution of limited health resources (i.e. personnel, treatments, equipment, buildings, etc.) is a source of contentious debate. The ethical principle of justice demands *fair* distribution, but how can this be achieved? Does it mean giving everyone an exact share? Does it mean giving in accordance with need? Does it mean that we should give in accordance with merit, i.e. the one who deserves the most gets the most?

Which, if any, of the following indicates an ethical means of resource allocation?

- Allocate according to age – prioritise treatment for the young rather than the old.
- Allocate resources according to clinical need, i.e. give most resources to the most 'ill'.
- Allocate more to those who have a greater potential for recovery.
- Ensure that the most vulnerable in society are cared for, i.e. those least able to look after themselves.
- Meet the needs of the greatest number (can the competing needs of individuals/groups be compared?).
- Prioritise preventative over curative care strategies as this make the most sense in the long term.

Individual nurses may feel they are unable to contribute to resource allocation decisions. However, if the most fundamental resource, i.e. the individual nurse's time and attention, is considered, it becomes apparent that nurses are in fact at the forefront of resource distribution and make 'resource allocation' decisions on a daily basis. From such a subjective perspective it is possible that additional criteria may be applied to the allocation process, e.g. allocate to the patient who is most demanding, or to the patient who the CMHN enjoys spending time with/ gains most professional satisfaction from.

## CONCLUSION

CMHNs are faced with a variety of potentially complex ethical issues. Their ability to provide an effective response to these issues relies on their being able to participate in the process of ethical reflection. Some of the ethical aspects of a CMHN's practice have been explored within this chapter, which I hope will assist practitioners and others in clarifying both the meaning of ethics and the nature of ethical practice.

Although, having considered the ethics of community mental health nursing practice, it would appear essential that CMHNs are encouraged to develop the skills of ethical reflection and the ability to identify and respond to the ethical aspects of their practice, there is little evidence that ethics is regarded as a significant factor within educational activities (Simpson 1999a, b).

Ultimately, for many CMHNs (if not all), identifying what is 'right' and 'wrong' within their practice and 'doing the right thing' will remain a difficult task. Ethical reflection is not easy and no one has the 'right' answers. Indeed, it has not been the aim of this chapter to provide answers, only to indicate that ethics is a vitally important area for consideration within community mental health nursing.

## REFERENCES

Beauchamp, T.L. and Childress, J.F. (2001) *Principles of biomedical ethics*, 5th edn, Oxford: Oxford University Press.

Chaloner, C. (1998) 'Working in secure environments: ethical issues', *Mental Health Practice*, 2 (2): 28–35.

Dibben, M.R., Morris, S.E. and Lean, M.E. (2000) 'Situational trust and co-operative partnerships between physicians and their patients: a theoretical explanation transferable from business practice', *QJM: Monthly Journal of the Association of Physicians*, 93 (1): 55–61.

Fletcher, N., Holt, J., Brazier, M. and Harris, J. (1995) *Ethics, law and nursing*, Manchester: Manchester University Press.

Gardner, B., Owen, L. and Thompson, S. (1999) 'Compliance: the need for a fresh approach', *Mental Health Nursing*, 19 (5): 18–22.

Gillon, R. (1985) *Philosophical medical ethics*, Chichester: Wiley.

Godin, P. (2000) 'A dirty business: caring for people who are a nuisance or a danger', *Journal of Advanced Nursing*, 32 (6): 1396–1402.

Griffith, R., Tengnah, C. and Grey, R. (1999) 'Keeping secrets: CPNs and the duty of confidence', *Mental Health Nursing*, 19 (4): 9–12.

Magnusson, A. and Lützén, K. (1999) 'Intrusion into patient privacy: a moral concern in the home of persons with chronic mental illness', *Nursing Ethics*, 6 (5): 399–410.

Morrall, P. (1995) 'Clinical autonomy and the community psychiatric nurse', *Mental Health Nursing*, 15 (2): 16–19.

Nursing and Midwifery Council (2002) *Code of professional conduct*, London: NMC.

Seedhouse, D. (1998) *Ethics: the heart of health care*, Chichester: Wiley.

Simpson, A. (1999a) 'Focus on training', *Nursing Times*, 95 (47): 66–68.

Simpson, A. (1999b) 'Creating alliances: the views of users and carers on the education and training needs of community mental health nurses', *Journal of Psychiatric and Mental Health Nursing*, 6: 347–356.

# FURTHER READING

Dickenson, D. and Parker, M. (2001) *The Cambridge medical ethics workbook*, Cambridge: Cambridge University Press.

Although a medically orientated text, this book provides an extremely useful and practical exploration of many of the ethical issues and dilemmas that may be encountered within all areas of health care practice.

Fletcher, N., Holt, J., Brazier, M. and Harris, J. (1995) *Ethics, law and nursing*, Manchester: Manchester University Press.

A straightforward and easily accessible book which provides a general overview of ethics and law within nursing.

Bloch, S., Chodoff, P. and Green, S.A. (eds) (1999) *Psychiatric ethics*, 3rd edn, Oxford: Oxford University Press.

A comprehensive exploration of the ethical aspects of mental health practice.

# CHAPTER 5

# SOCIAL EXCLUSION, DISCRIMINATION AND SOCIAL ISOLATION

*Rachel Perkins and Julie Repper*

## SUMMARY OF KEY POINTS

- People with mental health problems experience discrimination and exclusion in all areas of daily life, work, education and access to services.

- Discrimination and exclusion are probably the greatest barriers to recovery from mental health problems.

- Community mental health nurses can help to decrease exclusion, and thereby facilitate recovery, by: focusing on people's strengths and possibilities rather than their deficits and dysfunctions; fostering hope; and facilitating access to valued opportunities.

## INTRODUCTION

The isolation and exclusion of people with mental health problems is not new. Community care initiatives may have ended most exclusion in large remote asylums, but the discrimination and rejection experienced by people with mental health problems continue. People may live within communities, but this physical presence does not mean that they are included as a part of those communities. Indeed, people who experience more serious or long-standing mental health problems are amongst the most excluded in British society (Sayce 2000, 2001a).

Traditionally, treatment and cure have been the focus of mental health services, but recovery involves a great deal more than this. It is about people doing the things they want to and growing within and beyond the limits of ongoing problems (Deegan 1988, 1993, Anthony 1996). But people can only rebuild meaningful and satisfying lives if they have access to opportunities – roles, relationships, activities and facilities – that they value. And it is increasingly recognised that discrimination and social exclusion severely limit such opportunities, and are at least as disabling as the problems that led to the diagnosis in the first place (Sayce and Measey 1999, Sayce 2000, 2001b, Bates 2002, Perkins and Repper 2003).

The social inclusion of marginalised groups has been a key tenet of UK government policy since 1997, a focus reflected in the Mental Health National Service Framework (Department of Health 1999). Standard 1 requires that we 'combat discrimination against individuals and groups with mental health problems and promote their social inclusion'. Standard 5 requires that all enhanced care plans for people with more serious mental health problems include action necessary to ensure that people have access to adequate housing, employment, training or other occupation, and social relationships and activities. In this chapter we will explore the reality, nature and origins of discrimination and social exclusion and the ways in which practitioners might facilitate the inclusion and community participation of people with mental health problems.

## THE REALITIES OF SOCIAL EXCLUSION

> There is mounting evidence of the discrimination experienced by people with mental health problems in Britain. This discrimination results in their systematic exclusion from society. Social exclusion operates in all areas of life – daily living, work, training and access to services.
>
> (Dunn 1999)

Read and Baker's (1996) survey of 778 people gives an insight into the extent of such exclusion:

- 34 per cent had been dismissed or forced to resign from jobs.
- 69 per cent had been put off applying for jobs for fear of unfair treatment.
- 47 per cent had been abused or harassed in public (11 per cent had been physically attacked) and 26 per cent had been forced to move home because of harassment.
- 50 per cent felt they had been unfairly treated by physical health services.
- 33 per cent complained that their GP had treated them unfairly.
- 25 per cent had been turned down by insurance or finance companies.

Feeling different and being ostracised and rejected are too often a daily reality for people who have experienced mental health problems. Sometimes this can be quite subtle:

> I talk to the people at the bus stop but they ignore me, they talk to each other but they reject me.
>
> (cited in Rose 1996)

> Friends, family, people you meet everyday – people treat you differ-
> ently. Like they are treading on eggshells . . . they think that if they say
> the wrong thing you're going to flare up or whatever.
>
> (cited in Repper *et al.* 1998)

But it may also take on a more sinister form. Read and Baker (1996) found people
who had been teased, taunted and even physically attacked simply because they
were known to have mental health problems.

Such rejection readily leads to a diminution of social networks. Former
friends and social contacts drift away, too often leaving the person alone and
isolated:

> Friends avoided me and would not let their children play with my
> children any more.
>
> (cited in Read and Baker 1996)

> I feel alone on the estate – they know about me and they shut me out.
>
> (cited in Rose 1996)

One survey of people with ongoing mental health problems showed that 40 per
cent of those living in the community had no social contacts outside mental health
services (Ford *et al.* 1993).

Lack of social contact and support are disabling in and of themselves, but
they also exacerbate mental health problems. Social support can prevent mental
health problems by buffering the effects of stressful events (Gourash 1978).
Friends can raise a person's self-esteem and overcome a sense of helplessness
(Schradle and Dougher 1985). Social isolation has been associated with the development of depression (Brown and Harris 1978), a deterioration in social skills
(Birchwood 1992), and more extreme reactions to life events and stress (Cohen
and Willis 1985). Social isolation is also exacerbated by unemployment.

Work is central to social inclusion. The work we do is an important way in
which we define ourselves. Work links us with, and enables us to contribute to,
the community in which we live. Not all work is paid work: our economy relies
on numerous forms of unpaid work, such as bringing up children, as well as
various sorts of political, religious and other volunteering activities. As well as an
income, work provides: social contact and support; social status and identity; a
means of structuring and occupying time; activity and involvement; and a sense
of personal achievement (Shepherd 1989, Nehring *et al.* 1993, Pozner *et al.* 1996).

People who are already excluded because of their mental health problems
are particularly sensitive to the loss of structure, purpose and identity and the
social isolation that unemployment brings:

> It boosts self-esteem and provides a sense of purpose and accomplish-
> ment. Work enables people to enter, or re-enter, the mainstream after
> psychiatric hospitalisation.
>
> (Rogers 1995)

Most people with mental health problems attach a high priority to work (Secker
*et al.* 2001) but discrimination and lack of support combine to ensure that it is a

luxury enjoyed by very few: only 18 per cent of those with mental health problems lasting more than one year are in employment (Office for National Statistics 2000).

> I had a cleaning job for three years, but when I mentioned an appointment with a psychiatrist I received a letter the next week to say my services were no longer required.

> I was employed as a social worker, but after six months I went into hospital with depression . . . my contract of employment was terminated despite reports provided by my GP and psychiatrist which stated that my illness didn't affect my work and they were prepared to sign me fit to return to work.
>
> (cited in Read and Baker 1996)

The experiences of service users are reflected in surveys of employers which reveal a reluctance to consider employing people with a history of mental health problems (see Manning and White 1995, Department of Work and Pensions 2001).

The consequences of unemployment – poverty, limited social networks, poor physical and mental health (Warner 1994, Steward 1996, Warr 1987) – are all factors implicated in social exclusion (Social Exclusion Unit 1999). Thus unemployment is excluding in and of itself, but also leads to a range of other problems that aggravate this exclusion. In particular, unemployment is linked to poverty and the low incomes forthcoming from welfare benefits. Almost all social activities – going out with friends, using the local sports centre, going to the pictures – require money.

Discrimination also impacts upon family life. Many people gain a great deal of support from relatives, but family relationships can also be damaged and distorted.

> My in-laws wouldn't have me in the house for 10 years after my mental illness. My wife and daughter visited them, but I was not permitted.
>
> (cited in Sayce 2000)

> My father won't give me a key to my own front door.

> They want me to stay away.
>
> (cited in Rose 1996)

However, the greatest area of discrimination in terms of family life occurs in relation to parenting (Sayce 1997, 2000). Read and Baker (1996) found that 48 per cent of women and 26 per cent of men with mental health problems felt their parenting abilities had been unfairly questioned and/or had had children taken into care. And this can have a devastating impact on the parents involved (Perkins 1992).

> My ex-husband's got them and won't let me see them. The courts gave him custody because I've been in hospital. I want to see them so much.
>
> (cited in Rose 1996)

Typically such actions are deemed to be in the interests of the children, but Hardman (1997), herself the daughter of a mother with severe and enduring mental health problems, has described the negative impact of enforced separation and the absence of contact with her mother.

The literature is also replete with examples of people with mental health problems being debarred from a range of services and activities, including the police, housing and benefits agencies, community organisations, churches, clubs and physical health:

> This man was sexually harassing me and I went to the police station for help. I said I wanted to take out an injunction. They said I couldn't because I was a mental patient. I don't think it's right.

> I've changed my church because at the last one they were terrible about mentally ill people.

> I moved house when I was eight months pregnant, and my midwife wrote 'hypomanic' in large red letters across my notes. No GP in my new area would take me on.

> Every genuine illness I have had over the last twenty years has been dismissed as anxiety, depression or stress.
>
> (all cited in Read and Baker 1996)

In the face of the discrimination and exclusion that exist, it is not surprising that many people choose to keep very quiet about their mental health problems:

> I always lied, no-one ever knew. On the health forms I always ticked 'No' in the box that says 'Have you ever had mental health problems?'
>
> (cited in Perkins *et al*. 2000)

> I was working in a solicitor's as a trainee receptionist. I couldn't tell my boss I had to see a psychiatrist every week, so I told him I was on a training scheme one day a week.
>
> (cited in Dunn 1999)

However, maintaining silence can have negative effects. There is the constant fear of being found out; and people are likely to be dismissed, rejected or excluded should their difficulties come to light. Yet to tell the truth is all too often likely to have the same result . . . the devil or the deep blue sea.

Exclusion from opportunities within their communities understandably leads some people to exclude themselves: to give up trying to engage in order to avoid further rejection. And this is a course of action too often encouraged by mental health practitioners.

> In 1971, I was 19 and had the same abilities and ambitions as any other 19-year-old. I hoped to make a place in the world for myself. But instead I was a patient in a state hospital. . . . One day I was summoned

to the office of the vocational rehabilitation counsellor . . . he looked up and said 'Well, there's nothing much I have to offer you; I can see from your chart that you'll never be capable of holding a job. . . . At the age of 19, when most people are eagerly anticipating and planning for the future, I had been told that I had nothing to look forward to but a 'career' as a ward of the state.

(Rogers 1995)

In fact, this man has enjoyed a successful career and now occupies a very senior position. A survey almost thirty years later echoes this experience. Rinaldi (2000) found that of those people with mental health problems who had successfully gained and sustained employment, 44 per cent had been told by a mental health worker that they would never be able to work. Similarly, the highly successful researcher and professor of psychiatry Kay Jamison, who also has a diagnosis of manic depression, remembers:

In an icy and imperious voice that – I can hear to this day he [the doctor] stated – as though it were God's truth, which no doubt he felt it was – 'You shouldn't have children. You have manic depressive illness'. I felt sick, unbelievably and utterly sick, and deeply humiliated. . . . I asked him if his concerns about my having children stemmed from the fact that, because of my illness, he thought I would be an inadequate mother or simply that he thought it best to avoid bringing another manic-depressive into the world. Ignoring or missing my sarcasm, he replied 'both'.

(Jamison 1995)

Often mental health workers justify pessimism about service users' ability to work on the grounds of 'being realistic'. However, as well as engendering a despair that exacerbates exclusion, such 'realism' is not always grounded in evidence. With appropriate support, at least 50 per cent of people with serious ongoing mental health problems can gain and sustain employment (Bond *et al.* 1997, 2001, Crowther *et al.* 2001).

## THE NATURE AND ORIGINS OF EXCLUSION

In relation to people with mental health problems, Sayce (2001a) has described social exclusion as:

the inter-locking and mutually compounding problems of impairment, discrimination, diminished social role, lack of economic and social participation and disability. Among the factors at play are lack of status, joblessness, lack of opportunities to establish a family, small or non-existent social networks, compounding race and other discriminations, repeated rejection and consequent restriction of hope and expectation.

The relationship between mental health problems and social exclusion is complex. Many elements associated with social exclusion, like low income, unemployment, poor housing, high crime environments, family breakdown (Social Exclusion Unit 1999), can be both a cause and a consequence of mental health difficulties. The MIND Enquiry into social exclusion (Dunn 1999) describes a number of factors that interact with mental health problems to promote and maintain social exclusion:

- Media stereotyping
- Discrimination at work
- Lack of access to educational and training opportunities
- Unemployment
- Poor income
- Homelessness and poor housing
- Lack of informal job contacts
- Contact with the criminal justice system
- Ostracisation by the wider community
- Disrupted family and social networks
- Adverse effects of prescribed drug treatments
- Drug misuse
- Physical health problems
- Stigmatising health and social services.

In considering the nature of stigma, Link and Phelan (2001) offer an analysis of the processes which result in discrimination and exclusion. The process begins with the distinguishing and labelling of human differences. But labelling of difference alone does not result in the exclusion: some differences (like hair colour) are salient only in a few situations, while others (like IQ, skin colour and mental health status) are highly salient. The next step therefore involves stereotyping – linking labelled people with undesirable characteristics – like dangerousness, unpredictability and incompetence. Next comes the separation of 'them' from 'us'. Those to whom negatively loaded labels are attached are seen as a distinct class of person different from the rest of society, and 'they' become the thing that they are labelled: not 'people with schizophrenia', but 'schizophrenics' and 'manic depressives' (Estroff 1989). This then results in a loss of status and discrimination, which lead to exclusion.

## PROMOTING ACCESS AND INCLUSION

If we are to promote inclusion, we must first foster hope and self-belief in those with whom we work. In the face of the discrimination and exclusion that many people with mental health problems have experienced it is very easy to lose hope. And if a person can see no possibility of a positive future, then it is all too easy for them to give up trying to do anything at all (Lovejoy 1982, Deegan 1988, 1993, 1996). Russinova (1999) has described a number of 'relationship skills' that are important in developing effective hope-inspiring relationships that can enable people to gain the confidence and self-belief that are critical if they are to rebuild their life and access the opportunities that they value. These include:

- believing in the person's potential and strength;
- valuing them as a unique human being;
- listening non-judgementally to their experiences and trusting their authenticity;
- tolerating the uncertainty about the future developments in the person's life;
- accepting setbacks and failures as part of the recovery process;
- expressing a genuine concern for the person's well-being;
- using humour appropriately.

These skills are central to the development of strong trusting relationships that inspire hope and promote confidence. Building on the foundation of such relationships, Bates (2002) and Perkins and Repper (2003) have outlined a number of strategies that can be adopted to facilitate inclusion and access opportunities that are valued. At a general level, these include:

- *Collecting information* about the facilities, opportunities and services available in the local area.
- *Creating links* with local facilities to facilitate access. This involves getting to know key people at the local college, leisure centre, church or job centre; and understanding the demands and expectations of these facilities and the sort of people who use them.
- *Capacity building*: increasing the ability of community organisations and facilities to accommodate people who have experienced mental health problems. Breaking down prejudice and suspicion about mental health problems and providing the support that they feel is necessary.

At an individual level there are a number of different strategies that practitioners might use to assist a person to access the opportunities and activities that they seek. These include:

- *Providing information* about facilities, opportunities and services in the area.
- *Finding out what people really do* when using the facility – this is far more helpful and realistic than what the formal descriptions and rules say they should do!
- *Planning and target setting*: helping people to think about their goals and ambitions. Break these down into manageable steps and plan the necessary interim goals and targets on the way.
- *Practice*: helping the person to rehearse what they are going to do until they feel comfortable doing it.
- *Skills development*: using a variety of techniques – instruction, prompting, modelling, guided practice, feedback – to help a person to develop the skills they need to do the thing they want to do.
- *Graded exposure* to help people overcome specific anxieties that stop them doing what they want to do.

- *Graded return* to roles, activities and facilities following a period of absence.
- *Visiting* a place or activity beforehand to find out how to get there and what to expect.
- *Time-limited experience* (such as work experience or sitting in on a college class): enabling someone to try something out before deciding whether it is what they want to do.
- *Providing transport* to help the person to get to the activity.
- *Doing with*: helping someone to do something by doing it alongside them. This may involve friends, relatives, volunteers, someone already engaged in the activity or others who experience mental health difficulties.
- *Subsidy*: helping to meet the costs of the activity and/or exploring sources of subsidy.
- *Creating special groups within ordinary settings*, e.g. special groups or classes to introduce people with mental health problems to the local sports centre, library or college.
- *Deliberately integrating groups*: creating specific settings where people with mental health problems and those who do not experience such difficulties can do things together.
- *Staff from different facilities coming into mental health facilities* to familiarise people with the activities involved before going to the community facility.
- *Mentoring*: support and help from someone already involved in the setting to provide information about what will be expected before they enter the setting and advice and encouragement when they are there.
- *Helping people to make new friends* by enabling them to access activities where they are likely to meet people who share their interests; accessing internet chat-lines and e-groups (some of which are designed specifically for people with mental health problems, like the Yahoo 'uksurvivors' e-group); befriending; or facilitating contact between service users who share interests/aspirations.
- *Self-help and support groups* where people with mental health problems can get together and gain encouragement and support from each other.
- *Negotiating adaptations and adjustments on the part of the provider*: changing the physical or social environment, and/or the expectations of the person, so that they are able to engage in the activity. The UK 1995 Disability Discrimination Act requires that employers and providers of education, goods and services make 'reasonable adjustments' to ensure that people with such difficulties can access the opportunities they offer.
- *Helping people to obtain their rights under the law*. The 1995 Disability Discrimination Act has been used by people with mental health difficulties to good effect (see Sayce 2001a). Sayce (2001a, 2002) has suggested that mental health practitioners can usefully:

  ➥ be aware of the rights and protection that the Disability Discrimination Act provides for people with mental health problems;*

* Disability Rights Commission Help Line: 08457 622633, text phone: 08457 622644. Disability Rights Commission website: www.drc-gb.org

- ➔ provide information about the assistance available from the DRC Help Line;*
- ➔ help employers, colleges and the providers of services to decide what 'reasonable adjustments' people with mental health problems might need to facilitate access;
- ➔ provide advocacy initiatives in relation to employment, education, leisure and other services.

This list is not exhaustive: facilitating access and promoting inclusion depend upon the creativity and ingenuity of the practitioner and service users involved. Any assistance must be tailored around the individual's needs/preferences and the possibilities and constraints of the opportunity they wish to access. Most of all, practitioners should aim to enable people to access those opportunities which they value rather than those that are deemed by others to be good for them. This is critical if attempts to facilitate inclusion are to be successful (Bond *et al.* 1997, 2001): people are more likely to stick with things they want to do.

## CONCLUSION

Repeatedly, research has shown that people with mental health problems are concerned about having somewhere decent to live, an adequate income, a satisfying sex life, meaningful work, a satisfying social life, intimacy and privacy (Estroff 1993, Sainsbury Centre for Mental Health 1997, Dunn 1999). These aspirations are no different from those of most citizens, yet they are things from which people with mental health problems are often excluded. People with mental health problems want the opportunity to participate as equal citizens and enjoy the opportunities available to non-disabled citizens. With the right sort of assistance and support these do not have to be impossible dreams.

## REFERENCES

Anthony, W.A. (1996) 'Recovery from mental illness: the guiding vision of the mental health system in the 1990s', *Innovations and Research*, 2 (3): 17–24.

Bates, P. (ed.) (2002) *Working for inclusion. Making social inclusion a reality for people with severe mental health problems*, London: Sainsbury Centre for Mental Health.

Birchwood, M. (1992) 'Early intervention in schizophrenia: theoretical background and clinical strategies', *British Journal of Clinical Psychology*, 31: 257–258.

Bond, G.R., Drake, R.E., Meuser, K.T. and Becker, D.R. (1997) 'An update on supported employment for people with severe mental illness', *Psychiatric Services*, 48: 335–346.

Bond, G.R., Becker, D.R., Drake, R.E., Rapp, C.A., Meisler, N., Lehman, A.F., Bell, M.D. and Blyler, C.R. (2001) 'Implementing supported employment as an evidence based practice', *Psychiatric Services*, 52 (3): 313–322.

Brown, G.W. and Harris, T. (1978) *Social origins of depression: a study of psychiatric disorder in women*, London: Tavistock.

Cohen, C. and Willis, T.A. (1985) 'Stress, social support and the buffering hypothesis', *Psychological Bulletin*, 98: 310–357.

Crowther, R.E., Marshall, M., Bond, G.R. and Huxley, P. (2001) 'Helping people with severe mental illness to obtain work: systematic review', *British Medical Journal*, 322: 204–208.

Deegan, P. (1988) 'Recovery: the lived experience of rehabilitation', *Psychosocial Rehabilitation Journal*, 11 (4): 11–19.

Deegan, P. (1993) 'Recovering our sense of value after being labeled', *Journal of Psychosocial Nursing*, 31 (4): 7–11.

Deegan, P. (1996) 'Recovery as a journey of the heart', *Psychosocial Rehabilitation Journal*, 19 (3): 91–97.

Department of Health (1999) *National service framework for mental health: modern standards and service models*, London: Department of Health.

Department of Work and Pensions (2001) *Recruiting benefit claimants: qualitative research with employers in one pilot area*, Research Papers Series No. 150, prepared by Bunt, K., Shury, J. and Vivian, D., London: Department of Work and Pensions.

Dunn, S. (1999) *Creating accepting communities. Report of the MIND inquiry into social exclusion and mental health problems*, London: MIND Publications.

Estroff, S.E. (1989) 'Self, identity, and subjective experiences of schizophrenia: in search of the subject', *Schizophrenia Bulletin*, 15 (2): 189–196.

Estroff, S.E. (1993) 'Community mental health services: extinct, endangered or evolving?', paper presented at the *Mental health practices in the nineties: changes and challenges* conference, Silver Springs, MD.

Ford, R., Beadsmore, A., Norton, P., Cooke, A. and Repper, J. (1993) 'Developing case management for the long term mentally ill', *Psychiatric Bulletin of the Royal College of Psychiatry*, 17 (7): 409–411.

Gourash, N. (1978) 'Help-seeking: a review of the literature', *American Journal of Community Psychology*, 6: 499–502.

Hardman, K. (1997) 'My busy mother', *Women and Mental Health Forum*, 2: 8–9.

Jamison, K.R. (1995) *An unquiet mind: a memoir of moods and madness*, New York: Alfred A. Knopf.

Link, B.G. and Phelan, J.C. (2001) 'Conceptualising stigma', *Annual Review of Sociology*, 27: 363–385.

Lovejoy, M. (1982) 'Expectations and the recovery process', *Schizophrenia Bulletin*, 8 (4): 605–609.

Manning, C. and White, P.D. (1995) 'Attitudes of employers to the mentally ill', *Psychiatric Bulletin*, 19: 541–543.

Nehring, J., Hill, R. and Poole, L. (1993) *Work, empowerment and community*, London: Research and Development in Psychiatry (now the Sainsbury Centre for Mental Health).

Office for National Statistics (2000) *Labour force survey 1999/2000*, London: Office for National Statistics.

Perkins, R.E. (1992) 'Catherine is having a baby . . .', *Feminism and Psychology*, 2: 56–57.

Perkins, R.E. and Repper, J.M. (2003) *Recovery and social inclusion: a model for mental health practice*, London: Baillière Tindall.

Perkins, R.E., Evenson, E. and Davidson, B. (2000) *The Pathfinder User Employment Programme*, London: South West London and St. George's Mental Health NHS Trust.

Pozner, A., Ng, M.L., Hammond, J. and Shepherd, G. (1996) *Working it out*, London: Sainsbury Centre for Mental Health.

Read, J. and Baker, S. (1996) *Not just sticks and stones. A survey of the stigma, taboos and discrimination experienced by people with mental health problems*, London: MIND Publications.

Repper, J.M., Perkins, R.E. and Owens, S. (1998) '"I wanted to be a nurse . . . but I didn't get that far": women with serious ongoing mental health problems speak about their lives', *Journal of Psychiatric and Mental Health Nursing*, 5: 505–513.

Rinaldi, M. (2000) Personal communication concerning a survey conducted by Merton Mind, London.

Rogers, J. (1995) 'Work is key to recovery', *Psychosocial Rehabilitation Journal*, 18: 5–10.

Rose, D. (1996) *Living in the community*, London: Sainsbury Centre for Mental Health.

Russinova, Z. (1999) 'Providers' hope-inspiring competence as a factor optimizing psychiatric rehabilitation outcomes', *Journal of Rehabilitation*, 16 (4): 50–57.

Sainsbury Centre for Mental Health (1997) *Pulling together: the future roles and training of mental health staff*, London: Sainsbury Centre for Mental Health.

Sayce, L. (1997) 'Motherhood: the final taboo in community care', *Women and Mental Health Forum*, 2: 4–7.

Sayce, L. (2000) *From psychiatric patient to citizen. Overcoming discrimination and social exclusion*, Basingstoke: Macmillan.

Sayce, L. (2001a) 'Social inclusion and mental health', *Psychiatric Bulletin*, 25: 121–123.

Sayce, L. (2001b) 'Not just users of services, but contributors to society: the opportunities of the Disability Rights Agenda', *Mental Health Review*, 6 (3): 25–28.

Sayce, L. (2002) 'Psychiatric disability and the disability rights agenda', *HAS Rehab Good Practice Network Newsletter*, 5: 3–5, London: Health Advisory Service.

Sayce, L. and Measey, L. (1999) 'Strategies to reduce social exclusion for people with mental health problems', *Psychiatric Bulletin*, 23: 65–67.

Schradle, S.B. and Dougher, M.J. (1985) 'Social support as a mediator of stress: theoretical empirical issues', *Clinical Psychology Review*, 5: 641–646.

Secker, J., Grove, B. and Seebohm, P. (2001) *Challenging barriers to employment, training and education for mental health service users. The service users' perspective*, Institute for Applied Health and Social Policy, King's College, London.

Shepherd, G. (1989) 'The value of work in the 1980s', *Psychiatric Bulletin*, 13: 231–233.

Social Exclusion Unit (1999) *What's it all about?* Online. http://www.cabinet-office.gov.uk/seu/index/faqs.html

Steward (1996) 'Unemployment and health 1: the impact on clients in rehabilitation and therapy', *British Journal of Therapy and Rehabilitation*, 3: 360.

Warner, R. (1994) *Recovery from schizophrenia. Psychiatry and political economy*, 2nd edn, London: Routledge.

Warr, P. (1987) *Work, unemployment and mental health*, Oxford: Oxford University Press.

# FURTHER READING

Sayce, L. (2000) *From psychiatric patient to citizen. Overcoming discrimination and social exclusion*, Basingstoke: Macmillan.

This book offers a comprehensive analysis of legal and positive promotion strategies to reduce discrimination and promote the inclusion, rights and citizenship of people diagnosed as mentally ill.

Bates, P. (ed.) (2002) *Working for inclusion. Making social inclusion a reality for people with severe mental health problems*, London: Sainsbury Centre for Mental Health.

This edited collection focuses on ways in which services can support people with mental health problems to engage in a full life in the community.

Perkins, R.E. and Repper, J. (2003) *Recovery and social inclusion: a model for mental health practice*, London: Baillière Tindall.

This book offers an analysis of the challenge of recovery facing people with mental health problems and describes practical ways in which practitioners can facilitate social inclusion and recovery.

# CHAPTER 6

# WORKING IN MULTIDISCIPLINARY COMMUNITY TEAMS

*Edward Peck*

---

## SUMMARY OF KEY POINTS

- Nurses have played a major role in the development of multidisciplinary team working over the past twenty years, although this contribution has served to highlight that nurses have the least defined set of roles of any of the mental health professions.

- Research has consistently suggested that multidisciplinary teams struggle to gain commitment from some potential members, struggle to create consensual aims, and struggle to establish coherent leadership.

- As a consequence, policy-makers have lost confidence in locality-based teams and are requiring the setting up of functional teams serving specific user groups, which may offer nurses the chance to be more selective in the therapeutic role that they adopt, although it is unlikely that these teams will necessarily avoid the problems pinpointed in the research.

---

## INTRODUCTION

Mental health nurses have always plied their trade alongside other professions, and often under their direction. However, it is only since the early 1980s that mental health services – and in particular community mental health services – have been viewed as a team endeavour. For instance, the key mental health policy document of the 1970s (*Better services for the mentally ill*, Department of Health and Social Security 1975) devoted only two out of ninety-one pages to the specialist therapeutic team. Nonetheless, despite the brevity of the discussion, the document was clear about which profession should lead the team: the consultant psychiatrist. Further, it raised the option of 'each consultant led team [having] ultimate responsibility for a particular geographical sector' (or sectorisation as it became known).

So how was it that, by the late 1990s, the multidisciplinary community team – usually known as the community mental health team (CMHT) – had become the cornerstone of the policy for and the practice of mental health services? What was the impact of these teams on the relationship between nurses and other professionals? And what are the prospects for nurses as these teams move from a focus on locality to a focus on function? These are the questions this chapter addresses. In doing so, it draws on a combination of key texts and the author's own experience of management, consultancy and research around CMHTs over the past twenty years. The chapter will focus on teams providing services to adults in England, although most of the themes apply to all varieties of multidisciplinary teams wherever they practice in the UK.

## A SHORT HISTORY OF MULTIDISCIPLINARY WORKING

The introduction of sectorisation discussed in *Better services for the mentally ill* was fundamental to the development of CMHTs. It offered, for the first time, the prospect of the co-ordination of the health and social care resources for the population of a locality. By the late 1970s, CMHTs in the United Kingdom were being initiated – and led – by consultant psychiatrists, their development influenced by enthusiasm for the American experience (see Mosher and Burti 1989). By 1985 there were reported to be 22 CMHTs (Sayce 1989) and by 1990, 122 were in place or planned (Sayce *et al.* 1991). The policy aspiration for these teams was that they would 'provide a service in which the boundaries between primary health care, secondary health care and social care do not form barriers seen from the perspective of the service user' (Department of Health 1990). Five years later the Department of Health decreed CMHTs to be one of the foundations of local, comprehensive mental health services (Department of Health 1995).

However, this pattern of local innovation brought about a lack of consistency between CMHTs in terms of the needs that were met, the services that were offered and the procedures that were followed (see Sayce 1989). At the same time the enthusiasm for creating CMHTs passed from consultants to managers in health and social services, and there emerged the trend of appointing one member – frequently a community psychiatric nurse (CPN) – as team co-ordinator, although the role was often ill-defined.

During this period, primary care teams were rarely consulted prior to the development of CMHTs, although in most cases they provided over 90 per cent of the referrals. Some CMHTs introduced self-referral policies through which users could bypass primary care and directly access secondary health care. Although GPs frequently welcomed this new source of support, in particular the contribution of CPNs, they were often hostile to CMHTs for a number of reasons: CMHTs were organised around social services boundaries which meant that most practices had to deal with more than one; CMHTs, unlike primary care teams, were increasingly not led by doctors; and frequently CMHTs did not observe the formalities of the relationship between primary and secondary care. Further, many CPNs preferred the relative autonomy of working with primary care colleagues. The consequences of this history were to emerge later with the advent of GP fundholding.

Throughout their development, the professional mainstays of CMHTs were CPNs and social workers, and to a much lesser extent occupational therapists. However, CMHTs did not command the support of all members of all professions; for example, the most trenchant critics of CMHTs were psychologists (e.g. Galvin and McCarthy 1994). Even amongst nurses, loyalty to profession remained more powerful than loyalty to team. This was reflected in the majority of CMHTs still containing combined professional and hierarchical leadership. This could result in a CMHT possessing numerous managers of individual professions (including a CPN manager), as well as a co-ordinator and consultant psychiatrists, all potentially attempting to exercise leadership. The effective management of CMHTs was to remain a problem well into the 1990s (Onyett et al. 1997).

An influential study of ten CMHTs in the late 1980s showed a trend away from users with serious and enduring problems towards a client group which had traditionally been served by primary care (Patmore and Weaver 1991). In retrospect, this trend can be largely attributed to the locality focus of CMHTs – the provision of services to a geographical population – rather than a functional focus – the provision of services to a specified client group. This study served to help convince policy-makers that CMHTs should focus on users with serious and enduring problems, and that CMHTs should be the vehicle for the local integration of local authority care management and the care programme approach (CPA), both devices aimed at directing resources to users assessed as being in the most need.

However, in many localities, this policy aspiration was undermined by the introduction of GP fundholding (Department of Health 1989), through which GPs were enabled to purchase community mental health services. As discussed above, some GP fundholders did not hold positive views about CMHTs. Furthermore, many GPs considered themselves entitled to more mental health resources to support their mental health work. As a result, some fundholders used their new financial leverage to achieve their priorities, identified in one survey (Marum 1995) as: protecting or increasing CPN time in the surgery; increasing the availability of practice-based counsellors; and challenging sectorisation. In the light of these priorities, many mental health professionals viewed GP fundholding as the major obstacle to creating comprehensive services (e.g. Lelliot and Audini 1995). Towards the end of the 1990s a more mature relationship was emerging based on an understanding of the aspirations of both primary care and secondary care (Goldberg and Gournay 1997, Greatley and Peck 1999).

What, then, are the key lessons from this short history? First, multi-disciplinary working evolved in a piecemeal fashion in the UK, with many professionals unconvinced about its benefits. Second, much of the research evidence on CMHTs has been at best ambivalent, and often critical. Third, increasing endorsement of teams from policy-makers has been accompanied by frustration at their apparent inability to deliver on policy (e.g. the integration of CPA and care management). Fourth, multidisciplinary team working as envisaged by policy-makers is always vulnerable to being influenced by initiatives that originate outside of the mental health world, and in particular those that empower primary care.

Nonetheless, the balance sheet for community mental health nursing, from being in the vanguard of multidisciplinary working, has been positive overall. The drive to create CMHTs was a major factor in the increase in numbers of CPNs. It offered an opportunity for these CPNs to forge new relationships with colleagues in other professions, beyond the traditional association with doctors which itself started to be transformed. Enhanced links with social workers enabled CPNs to develop the social aspects of their practice, whilst more involvement with psychologists supported CPNs in acquiring new therapeutic interventions (e.g. cognitive therapy). Many created close links with primary health care teams, often achieving considerable professional autonomy. Finally, for numerous CPNs the role of CMHT co-ordinator was the first step on a managerial career; by the late 1990s most of the general managers in mental health services in NHS trusts in London, for instance, were nurses (Peck *et al.* 1999).

## TEAMS AND GROUPS, BOUNDARIES AND BARRIERS

It is important to place CMHTs in the context of what we know about all teams. The grouping of different professionals into one physical space – and the adoption of a collective title for their work – does not constitute the creation of a team. The distinction between groups and teams is a commonplace of management text-books (e.g. Brooks 1999). Teams have characteristics that groups do not have, and there have been attempts to set out the prerequisites of a CMHT as a team: 'clear aims need to be embodied in an operational policy that is informed by strategic planning and implemented as the responsibility of operational managers and professional practitioners' (Onyett and Ford 1995, p. 51). On this argument, without clear aims being established, CMHT members will typically be left feeling inadequate and perhaps vulnerable. However, Onyett and Ford also state that CMHTs are often riven by 'conflicting ideologies, incompatible ways of working and enduring power struggles' (p. 51), apparently suggesting – perhaps realistically – that these obstacles to identifying clear aims can never be entirely overcome.

More specifically, Willshire (1999) suggests that no consensual aims exist for mental services, especially within multidisciplinary teams. This stems from the fact that people who work within mental health services are working with a phenomenon – madness – that defies clear definition. In the literature on CMHTs, the majority of their problems reportedly stem from a lack of consensus between the professions (e.g. Onyett and Smith 1998) and the apparent managerial expectation that when professionals from diverse disciplines are brought together they will immediately coalesce around common, often externally defined, goals (King 2001).

Of course, an alternative account of multidisciplinary teams would suggest that it was the differences between the professions that made them worthwhile. If such difference – the creative tension between perspectives – is not the grit in the oyster that makes the pearl, then why create teams at all? If that is not the aspiration, then surely it would be easier to let distinct professions practise in their own, internally consensual, way (basically the argument put forward by Galvin and McCarthy (1994), although crucially they believe that the pearl will not materialise under any circumstances). In the longer term, some argue, the answer may be to create a generic mental health worker so that such differences and boundaries could not arise (as has been suggested by Holmes (2001) and Basset and Corrigan (2002), among others). Cochrane *et al.* (1999), in the second report of the *Future healthcare workforce* project, put forward scenarios in which a so-called 'healthcare practitioner' would become responsible for the majority of patient care in any care sector. Those based in CMHTs would take on all the aspects of the role of mental health nurses as well as some of the work currently undertaken by doctors, psychologists and occupational therapists. In so doing, Cochrane *et al.* (1999) estimated that these healthcare practitioners would take on around 80 per cent of the workload of the CMHT.

Nonetheless, the prevailing view – endorsed by the report of the Workforce Action Team (WAT) (Department of Health 2001) – is that the current professions will continue to be the bedrock of community mental health services and that more effective collaboration – 'to re-shape professional boundaries' – remains a central goal. Perhaps this is partly a recognition that each of the professions that have arisen over the last two centuries seeks to address an important and distinct aspect of the human condition, although this is arguably less true of nursing than the others (this is a theme to which I shall return later). Partly, it is a pragmatic response to the fact that for the foreseeable future we have the workforce that we have. However, the influence of the generic mental health worker lobby can be seen in the focus in the WAT report on the so-called *capable practitioner* initiative which will provide 'a single agreed set of the knowledge, skills and attitudes required by the mental health practitioner workforce' (Sainsbury Centre for Mental Health 2001).

At a local level, the recent moves towards integrated management of health and social services personnel in the community have only served to highlight that many managers are unsure what they want from professionals in multidisciplinary teams. A study in London revealed that:

> executive managers delivered a slightly contradictory message regarding expectations of their staff. There was a tendency for these managers to state that within the integrated service staff would be more flexible, that is more generic, whilst also stating that they wished to see staff valuing their own discipline within a multidisciplinary setting.
>
> (Field *et al.* 2001, p. 2)

In my study of integration in Somerset, of which more below, I found:

> an apparent ambiguity in Somerset in the outcome being sought in relation to cultural change. Is the desired result one entirely new

culture, albeit comprised of elements taken from all the current professional cultures – the melting pot approach to culture? Or is the desired result the enhancement of the current professional cultures by the addition of mutual understanding and respect – the orange juice with added vitamin 'c' approach to culture?

(Peck *et al*. 2001, p. 325)

For policy-makers the professional boundaries that prevent consensus are often seen as barriers. This view has been revealed in documents, from the Department of Health (1990) document quoted above to *The NHS Plan* (Department of Health 2000). These boundaries come into being through differences in organisational structures and values (Stantham 2000). They are inculcated into individuals through training regimes and sustained by patterns of socialisation (Peck and Norman 1999), and often underpinned by being enacted in discrete physical spaces. Furthermore, they can be conceptualised as crucial to making individuals feel secure in their work. Willshire (1999) describes boundaries as containers for anxiety for mental health staff in their daily interactions with people who have 'severe disturbance of emotional and cognitive function'. She argues that maintaining boundaries poses a particular challenge for mental health organisations due to unclear task definitions. On this view, clear boundaries between professionals are not merely inevitable, they are essential. The challenge for teams is to improve the professional interaction across these boundaries, through the modification of roles and relationships within teams and by the response of these teams to demands from outside (from service users, general practitioners, national policies, etc.).

# THE EXPERIENCE OF CREATING MULTIDISCIPLINARY TEAMS

Given these complexities, what does research tell us about the creation of multidisciplinary teams? The most recent study derives from the work of my colleagues and myself in Somerset (see also Gulliver *et al*. 2000, Peck *et al*. 2002). Here, CMHTs were created as part of a broader integration which involved large numbers of social care staff transferring their employment to an NHS trust.

In the first two years, the balance sheet for staff and their immediate managers was not entirely favourable. There were some reported improvements in the environment for team working as co-location was implemented, and some staff gained from the opportunity to learn new knowledge and skills from team colleagues. On the other hand, workload was perceived to have increased since the integration (for example, from bringing together care management and CPA); the organisation was seen to be more bureaucratic; team managers were seen to be under increased pressure for which they had not been fully prepared; and there were tensions between locality management and the trust leadership.

Perhaps unsurprisingly, therefore, the thrice-repeated staff surveys found a worsening of all quantitative indices measuring job satisfaction, role clarity and morale immediately after the integration in 1999, although by 2001 these findings had stabilised or, in some cases, were showing minor improvements. These changes were associated with the efforts involved in building new relationships with professional colleagues and new ways of working in a period when there was some dissatisfaction with management and difficulty in establishing a clear identity for the new trust as a whole. A finer-grain examination of these issues, utilising a framework developed by Yan and Louis (1999), revealed three activities within the teams: protecting professional difference; making connections with fellow team members; and trying to create commitment to the new teams.

For instance, the case study showed that CMHT managers and members found it difficult to create commitment to these new teams. Team managers argued that commitment might be increased by identifying a shared sense of purpose for the teams, in line with the recommendations of Onyett and Ford (1995). However, they also felt that this should be achieved by the trust laying down clear aims for CMHTs. In so doing, they seemed to be acknowledging that there was too much diversity in the teams for such aims to be generated locally. In this respect, the managers in Somerset were exemplifying the pressures described by Wells (1997): 'managers are required to meet insufficiently delineated central prescriptions while simultaneously retain clinical good will' (p. 336). Perhaps the team managers had an insight that it might not be possible to gain agreement to such core aims, in line with the argument of Willshire (1999), and wished to pass responsibility for any perception of failure elsewhere.

The one exception to these findings in Somerset involved the Psychological Therapies Team (PTT). With a clear focus around which members quickly coalesced, it was apparently adept at creating commitment. On the face of it, this success augurs well for mental health policy in England (Department of Health 1999) with its requirement to create function-focused teams with clear objectives for specific service users (Department of Health 1999), and the apparent demotion of the importance of CMHTs. However, the research in Somerset also contained a warning in the problems that other teams had in making connections with the PTT. A mental health service entirely composed of such focused teams may well develop the same problems of team boundaries that have been alleged for professional boundaries.

# THE EXPERIENCE OF BEING A NURSE IN A MULTIDISCIPLINARY TEAM

So what, then, is it like to be a nurse in a multidisciplinary team? In 1998, Ian Norman and I established an inter-professional dialogue between community mental health care professions in order to identify key problems of inter-professional working in adult community mental health services. This aim was pursued through a programme of facilitated unidisciplinary groups. These groups comprised practitioners from three localities within London recruited from across the range of mental health disciplines. They addressed a series of questions: What are the unique skills of the profession? What is the nature of the collaboration between the profession and other professions? What is the relationship to leadership in the profession? What is the relationship between theory and practice in the profession? The responses were written up as 'stories' and agreed by the groups. Box 6.1 presents the CPNs' story, edited from the version included in Peck and Norman (1999), which includes more details of the methodology and the stories of other professions.

---

### Box 6.1   The CPNs' story

Whatever else happens to patients they will be nursed. Nurses are close to patients; they stand on the boundary of 'wellness–illness' in an ordinary way, taking the emotional labour associated with the management and befriending of people's vulnerability. Nurses are 'travelling companions' with patients, not 'travel agents'.

It is easy to overlook the skills and values in these human contacts and to devalue nursing as if 'anyone could do it'. It is difficult to find clever words and theories to describe it. Of course, nurses have developed sub-specialities, e.g. cognitive behavioural skills; however, it is thought important to maintain the overarching concept of 'nurse' and 'nursing'.

What elements in nursing need to be restated? There is a loss of clarity associated with more diffuse community roles and there were features of institutional care which were important to nursing (without suggesting that the asylum was a good place to be). These elements include: frequent contacts with patients; a domain of psychological containment and practice; development of relationships and community; a critical mass of nurses working together.

There may be lessons for nursing roles in the community in consideration of these elements when addressing key issues for nursing such as: personal and professional qualities and attributes; interpersonal skills; practical applications; and some overarching aspects of the requirements for the role.

Crucial to nursing are personal qualities which might describe any committed and effective mental health professional. Nurses know when they see these qualities, and also notice when they are absent in nurses. Interpersonal skills include listening and talking; instilling confidence and being reassuring; having enabling and facilitative abilities. Practical applications of these qualities and skills manifest themselves in: sustaining relationships over time; relating to different kinds of people at various levels; respecting people's individuality; advocating patients' rights; being practical; making assessments and planning courses of action with patients, families or carer(s); working towards goals; managing complexity; deploying a sound basic knowledge of mental health and illness and associated treatments.

Nurses consider that they need to have a positive outlook, and energy and enthusiasm for life; they must be able to bring hope. They have to see positive strengths in patients and be able to see and be accepting of good and bad in people. They have to be able to maintain boundaries, to be containing and to have the ability to say 'no'. They need to be able to cope with feelings of anger and frustration in others.

> Sometimes nurses feel depleted, vulnerable and exhausted. They report anxiety about being blamed if things go wrong; they also report a sense of loss of clarity in their role, whilst recognising that this must be faced when looking forward to new approaches. The concept of 'nursing' is highly valued by nurses themselves, and by the public, and should be revalued in the mental health context.

I am not suggesting that this story represents the views of all CPNs, either then or now. It is a snapshot of the views of eleven clinicians at one point in time. However, it does raise some interesting questions for mental health nursing in the community. For example, if one of the defining characteristics of nursing is being alongside service users for prolonged periods of time, what replaces this when contact becomes more episodic? If being ordinary is important, what distinguishes the contribution of nurses from the contribution of support workers, which is set to receive a boost from the implementation of the WAT report (where they are called 'Support, Time and Recovery' workers)? If therapeutic interventions are important to the future of community nursing, why are the old ones (e.g. dispensing medication) omitted and new ones scarcely mentioned? Overall, it is difficult to be clear from this account which aspect of the human condition the CPN uniquely addresses (in contrast, for instance, to psychologists). Perhaps it is this very lack of distinct territory, their flexibility, to put it positively, that has made CPNs so central to the multidisciplinary enterprise.

# TEAMS IN THE FUTURE: FROM LOCALITY TO FUNCTION

The PTT in Somerset points the way to the immediate future. The National Service Framework for Mental Health (Department of Health 1999) envisages functional teams with clear aims meeting the needs of specific service users: assertive outreach teams; crisis intervention teams; primary care liaison teams. What will the creation of these teams mean for nurses?

Most importantly, these teams will continue to be multidisciplinary. Although the Somerset PTT was quick to coalesce around its aims, perhaps partly because it was a local initiative comprised of volunteers, the challenges that have faced multidisciplinary working will not disappear overnight. Loyalty to profession will continue, as will professional boundaries, and in my view both are essential components of an effective service. However, the range of teams being created may help professionals – including nurses – select the environment which best suits their orientation. CPNs with a commitment to the social aspect of mental health may gravitate towards assertive outreach teams, whilst those more interested in the psychological dimensions may opt to work in primary care liaison teams (and these teams, of course, inherit the geographical focus of the CMHTs). As a result, inter-professional dialogue may result in more creative tension and less destructive conflict, but only if the professionals involved are nurtured from being groups into becoming teams. The barriers that policy-makers perceive currently between professionals may be seen as having moved to being between teams. Finally, a return to the history serves to underline the fact that policy will continue to evolve.

# REFERENCES

Basset, T. and Corrigan, K. (2002) 'The professions – do we need them?' *Open Mind*, 113: 22–23.

Brooks, I. (1999) *Organisational behaviour: individuals, groups and the organisation*, London: Financial Times/Pitman.

Cochrane, D., Conroy, M., Crilly, T. and Rogers, T. (1999) *The future healthcare workforce: the second report*, Bournemouth: University of Bournemouth.

Department of Health (1989) *Working for patients*, London: HMSO.

Department of Health (1990) *Community care in the next decade and beyond*, London: HMSO.

Department of Health (1995) *Building bridges: a guide to arrangements for interagency working for the care and protection of severely mentally ill people*, London: Department of Health.

Department of Health (1999) *National service framework for mental health: modern standards and service models*, London: Department of Health.

Department of Health (2000) *The NHS Plan: a plan for investment, a plan for reform*, London: The Stationery Office.

Department of Health (2001) *Mental health national service framework (and The NHS Plan) workforce planning, education and training underpinning programme: adult mental health services: final report by the Workforce Action Team*, London: Department of Health.

Department of Health and Social Security (1975) *Better services for the mentally ill*, London: HMSO.

Field, J., Crawford, A., Poxton, R., Hutchison, M. and Mica, M. (2001) *An evaluation of the integrated mental health service in Brent*, London: Institute for Applied Health and Social Policy.

Galvin, S. and McCarthy, S. (1994) 'Multidisciplinary community teams: clinging to the wreckage', *Journal of Mental Health*, 3 (2): 157–166.

Goldberg, D. and Gournay, K. (1997) *The general practitioner, the psychiatrist and the burden of mental health care*, Maudsley Discussion Paper No. 1, London: Institute of Psychiatry.

Greatley, A. and Peck, E. (1999) *Mental health priorities for primary care*, London: King's Fund.

Gulliver, P., Peck, E. and Towell, D. (2000) 'Evaluation of the implementation of the mental health review in Somerset: methodology', *Managing Community Care*, 8 (3): 13–19.

Holmes, C. (2001) 'Editorial', *Journal of Psychiatric and Mental Health Nursing*, 8: 379–381.

King, C. (2001) 'Severe mental illness: managing the boundary of a CMHT', *Journal of Mental Health*, 10 (1): 75–86.

Lelliot, P. and Audini, B. (1995) 'Fundholding and the care of the mentally ill', *Psychiatric Bulletin*, 20 (11): 641–642.

Marum, M. (1995) 'The National Association of Fundholding Practices "straw poll"', *The Fundholding Summary*, February.

Mosher, L. and Burti, L. (1989) *Community mental health: a practical guide*, London: W.W. Norton.

Onyett, S. and Ford, R. (1995) 'Multidisciplinary community mental health teams: where is the wreckage?', *Journal of Mental Health*, 5 (1): 47–55.

Onyett, S. and Smith, H. (1998) 'The structure and organisation of community mental health teams', in Brooker, C. and Repper, J. (eds) *Serious mental health problems in the community: policy, practice and research*, London: Baillière Tindall.

Onyett, S., Standen, R. and Peck, E. (1997) 'The challenge of managing community mental health teams', *Health and Social Care in the Community*, 5 (1): 40–47.

Patmore, C. and Weaver, T. (1991) *Community mental health teams: lessons for planners and managers*, London: Good Practices in Mental Health.

Peck, E. and Norman, I. (1999) 'Working together in adult community mental health services: exploring interprofessional role relations', *Journal of Mental Health*, 8 (3): 231–244.

Peck, E., Hills, B. and Secker, J. (1999) 'Managing mental health services in London', *Journal of Mental Health*, 8 (6): 621–628.

Peck, E., Towell, D. and Gulliver, P. (2001) 'The meanings of culture in health and social care: a study of the combined trust in Somerset', *Journal of Interprofessional Care*, 15 (4): 319–327.

Peck, E., Gulliver, P. and Towell, D. (2002) *Modernising partnerships: an evaluation of Somerset's innovations in the commissioning and organisation of mental health services (final report)*, London: Institute for Applied Health and Social Policy.

Sainsbury Centre for Mental Health (2001) *The capable practitioner*, London: Sainsbury Centre for Mental Health.

Sayce, L. (1989) 'Community mental health centres – rhetoric and reality', in Brackx, A. and Grimshaw, C. (eds) *Mental health care in crisis*, London: Pluto.

Sayce, L., Craig, T. and Boardman, A. (1991) 'The development of community mental health centres in the UK', *Social Psychiatry and Psychiatric Epidemiology*, 26 (1): 14–22.

Stantham, D. (2000) 'Guest editorial: partnership between health and social care', *Health and Social Care in the Community*, 8 (2): 87–89.

Wells, J. (1997) 'Priorities, "street level bureaucracy" and the community mental health team', *Health and Social Care in the Community*, 5 (5): 333–342.

Willshire, L. (1999) 'Psychiatric services: organising impossibility', *Human Relations*, 52 (6): 775–804.

Yan, A. and Louis, M.R. (1999) 'The migration of organisational functions to the work unit level: buffering, spanning and bringing up boundaries', *Human Relations*, 52 (1): 25–47.

# FURTHER READING

There are two readily available journals which regularly carry accessible and informative papers on the topics covered in this chapter. The first is the *Journal of Interprofessional Care* and the second is the *Journal of Mental Health*. The reports of both the Future Workforce Project and the Workforce Action Team are also relevant, and watch out on the Department of Health website for outputs from the Mental Health Care Group Workforce Development Team.

# CHAPTER 7

# MEETING MENTAL HEALTH NEEDS IN PRIMARY CARE

*Elizabeth Armstrong*

---

## SUMMARY OF KEY POINTS

- The majority of people with mental health problems are cared for within the primary care system.

- Mental health care is an integral part of health care, not an optional extra.

- There are new, challenging and interesting roles for community mental health nurses in primary care.

---

## INTRODUCTION

The National Service Framework for Mental Health (Department of Health 1999) was not the first publication to make the point that most people with mental health problems are treated in primary care. This fact has been known for many years. However, whilst it may have been known, it is only relatively recently that the implications have received serious attention.

Primary care is the main 'first contact' service of the NHS. It is normally to their GP that people go when they first feel they need help for some aspect of their health. They may see a GP, a practice nurse, a nurse practitioner or a health visitor. But what all of these professionals have in common is that they are generalists. Their first task is to understand the overall health needs of their patient or client and to help the patient or client gain access to appropriate help.

Sorting out, or assessing, these needs may be no simple task. The patient may have a physical illness, a mental health problem, social difficulties, emotional or relationship problems, or indeed a mixture of all of these. The nature of primary care means that generalists see the full range of illness, from people with a few symptoms to people with serious, life-threatening conditions.

Moreover, the primary care clientele is the whole population. People with mental health problems are not a crazy or mad sub-species. They also have heart disease, diabetes, asthma and cancer. They attend their GP for their cervical smears, for travel health advice or to take their children for immunisation. In other words, mental health care is an integral part of health care in general, not an optional extra. Further, GPs, unlike hospital specialists, do not discharge patients at the end of an episode of care. Anyone can consult their GP at any time and for any reason.

All nurses, primary care nurses as well as mental health nurses, need to be aware of mental health needs as well as physical health needs. In primary care, this is increasingly being recognised. More and more practice nurses, nurse practitioners and health visitors are becoming involved in providing care and support for people who would once have been seen as the province of the mental health nurse.

What, then, are the implications of this for mental health nurses in general, and for those mental health nurses who choose to work in primary care settings? How do mental health nurses and general nurses work together to meet the health care needs of people in primary care?

This chapter will take a fairly detailed look at mental health care at primary care level, discuss the National Service Framework for Mental Health from a primary care perspective and look at collaborative approaches to providing care. However, there is a need for a good deal more nursing research in this field before it is possible to say with any certainty what works and what doesn't.

# MENTAL HEALTH IN PRIMARY CARE

The most common mental health problems seen in primary care are depression, anxiety and eating disorders. For individual GPs, psychotic illness is much less common; the numbers of people with schizophrenia per GP list of about 2,000 patients may vary from about 4 to 12, with about 3 per list with bipolar disorder (Strathdee and Jenkins 1996). The variation depends on a number of factors, but is most marked between rural areas and inner cities.

People suffering from depression and anxiety disorders in primary care are often viewed as the 'worried well'. This label is inaccurate. Studies comparing the symptom levels of depression and anxiety in hospital patients with those attending their GP surgery showed that there was very little difference between the two groups. GP patients may be just as ill as those who are referred to specialists (Mann 1992).

Much of the existing research at primary care level has looked at patients attending their GP surgery, but primary care and general medical practice are not the same thing. A wide range of professionals and others are involved with patients and clients with mental health problems in a variety of settings, not simply health centres and GP surgeries.

Health visitors, for example, may or may not be GP-attached. Many provide services for homeless people, refugees and asylum seekers and travellers. For some of these groups, the health visitor may represent their way in to the health service – for a few, their only source of health care. Most health visitors are involved in screening for postnatal depression, and many also provide treatment for this in the form of a structured programme of listening visits using a counselling-style intervention (Holden 1994). Some also run groups for mothers with postnatal depression, sometimes in collaboration with local community mental health nurses (Foyster 1995). Since they frequently work with disadvantaged groups, health visitors come into contact with many people with mental health problems, not just mothers. Depression, in common with many other health problems, is strongly linked to poverty and deprivation.

District (community) nurses also often have patients with mental health problems. Their clientele is often elderly, suffering from disabling, painful and life-threatening physical illness and therefore at risk of becoming depressed. Community mental health nurses may provide support and care for people with dementia in their own homes. Their role, especially in the support of carers, has been well described by Challenger and Hardy (1998). However, it is often overlooked that much care for people with dementia is actually provided by district nurses, sometimes in collaboration with community mental health nurses but by no means always.

A great deal of care, especially for people with depression and anxiety, is also provided by the voluntary sector, by self-help groups and help lines. A worrying finding of the Clinical Standards Advisory Group study (CSAG 1999) into services for depression throughout the UK was that many people with moderate symptoms attended self-help groups because there was nowhere else for them to go. They were really too ill for groups to be of much help, but, ironically, not ill enough to be referred to overstretched community mental health teams.

School nurses and occupational health nurses can also be seen as part of the primary care system. Both these groups often encounter people with depression or anxiety. Eating disorders will also feature in the school nurse's workload. Other 'first contact' services include accident and emergency departments and NHS Direct.

Within health centres there is also a wide variety of people involved in providing mental health care. In recent years a number of practice nurses have begun to develop collaborative methods of caring for patients with depression, with their GP colleagues. Many practices employ counsellors or psychologists, or both, on a sessional basis. More 'primary care mental health workers' are envisaged under the NHS Plan (Department of Health 2000) but it is not yet clear exactly how this initiative will work.

Freeling and Kendrick (1996) placed the tasks of primary care within a preventive framework. They applied this framework to mental health care, but it is equally applicable to all kinds of health care. It seems to be a useful way of thinking about primary care, where the aim should be to deal with problems as quickly and promptly as possible in order to avoid the consequences of more serious illness and disability. Prevention is normally classified as primary, secondary and tertiary.

Primary prevention includes offering support to people at risk of developing mental illness – for example, unemployed people, bereaved people, new mothers, single parents, isolated elderly people and people who are disabled, including their carers.

Secondary prevention includes early identification of and effective treatment for mental illness. The general practice setting can offer a non-stigmatising environment in which treatment may be given, but it is also essential that there is rapid and easy access to specialist help when required.

Tertiary prevention seeks to provide ongoing care and support ('community care') for those with chronic illness and persistent disability. This usually means that there needs to be effective joint working between the primary care team, specialist services, local authority services and, often, the voluntary sector. It also means that rapid access to help is essential for those whose conditions are liable to relapse or recur.

For the most part, primary prevention may be seen as the province of the primary care team, and often of the nurses on the team. Secondary prevention will involve both the primary care team and the specialist services working in close collaboration. Tertiary prevention may be seen as largely the role of the specialists, but people with severe and enduring mental illness also have physical health needs. It is a very important part of the primary care team's role to ensure that these needs are met.

Goldberg and Gournay (1997) divided mental illness into four diagnostic groups and proposed a model of organising care using these groups.

The model fits in quite well with Freeling and Kendrick's ideas and is not incompatible with the National Service Framework for Mental Health. However, the diagnostic groups used by these authors are not necessarily mutually exclusive and it is well worth remembering that some people with, for example, very severe depression may be more disabled by their condition than some people with schizophrenia.

*Table 7.1* Diagnostic groups and ways of organising care

| Diagnostic group | Recommended care |
| --- | --- |
| **Group 1**<br>Serious mental illness, e.g. schizophrenia, dementia, bipolar disorder, severe eating disorders | Shared care: CMHT with primary care team |
| **Group 2**<br>Mental disorders treatable by drug or non-drug treatments, e.g. depression, panic disorders, anxiety, obsessive compulsive disorder | Care within primary care, not necessarily by GP. CMHT only if no response to treatment |
| **Group 3**<br>Mental disorders responding mainly to non-drug treatments, e.g. phobias, mild eating disorders, post-traumatic stress disorder | Care within primary care, usually by primary care nurses or counsellors |
| **Group 4**<br>Disorders needing time to resolve, e.g. bereavement, adjustment disorders | Supportive care by primary care nurses, voluntary agencies, counsellors, self-help |

Source: adapted from Goldberg and Gournay (1997)

# THE NATIONAL SERVICE FRAMEWORK FOR MENTAL HEALTH

The National Service Framework for Mental Health (NSF) was published by the government in 1999. It focuses on the mental health needs of adults of working age. It is intended to:

- drive up the quality of care;
- remove wide and unacceptable variations in care;
- set national standards and define service models;
- put in place programmes to support local delivery;
- establish milestones and high-level performance indicators against which progress is to be measured.

There is a strong primary care theme running through the whole document, though there was no primary care nursing representation on the external reference group which directed the writing. Therefore, although the document mentions health visitors and practice nurses, it isn't particularly knowledgeable or imaginative in describing their role potential.

The NSF sets seven standards, of which Standards 1, 2 and 3 are particularly important for primary care:

- Standard 1: Mental health promotion – to ensure that health and social services promote mental health and reduce the discrimination and social exclusion associated with mental health problems.
- Standards 2 and 3: Primary care and access to services – to deliver better primary mental health care and to ensure consistent advice and help for people with mental health needs, including primary care services for individuals with severe mental illness.

Primary care organisations are designated leads for Standards 2 and 3, though many may not be ready or have the necessary expertise to fulfil their role. At the time of writing, many primary care trusts are only just coming properly into being, having completed the appointment of their chairs and boards. Since the publication of the NSF the pace of change in primary care organisations (PCOs) has been considerable and seems to have adversely affected the ability to proceed with implementation. For example, most PCOs have probably completed their guidelines and protocols, but how far these have actually been put into practice is highly debatable.

Standard 2 states that any service user who contacts their primary health care team with a common mental health problem should:

- have their mental health needs identified and assessed;
- be offered effective treatments, including referral to specialist services for further assessment, treatment and care if they require it.

The use of the term 'service user' in the primary care context is unfortunate and has led to some misunderstandings. Primary care staff do not refer to their patients as 'service users' – this term being normally reserved for those using secondary mental health care services. GPs and practice nurses refer to everyone on their list as 'patients' even though only a proportion of these people will actually be seeing them at any one time. For health visitors and counsellors, those who use their services are referred to as 'clients'. In the context of Standard 2 of the NSF, it is important to remember that 'service user' means any person using primary care services, not simply someone who is already known to have a mental health problem.

Armstrong and Paton (2001) suggested an eight-point action plan for each primary care team to ensure that the requirements of Standard 2 were met:

- compile, in collaboration with the local community mental health team (CMHT), a register of all patients on their list with severe and enduring mental illness;
- implement protocols for depression, including suicide risk assessment, anxiety disorders, eating disorders and schizophrenia;
- implement practice policies for the prescribing of antidepressants and benzodiazepines, consistent with accepted guidelines;
- provide access to structured psychological therapies;
- provide a range of patient and carer information on common mental health problems;
- ensure appropriate training for all staff;
- provide easily accessible information about local services, including carer support;
- set up and maintain effective liaison with local accident and emergency departments, CMHTs and crisis services especially for people who self-harm.

These authors also suggested that if primary care teams completed this action plan, they would have not only implemented Standard 2, but would also meet most of their obligations under the other standards.

All of these points are designed to help practices develop a planned approach to delivering care. Traditionally, GPs used to work in a reactive way, responding to requests for help rather than anticipating health needs. This has changed dramatically over the last twenty years, in terms of physical health care particularly, following a report on the prevention of cardiovascular disease in general practice published in 1981 (Royal College of General Practitioners (RCGP) 1981a). This report advocated a proactive approach and it is now accepted practice that risk factors are identified and dealt with as early as possible. For example, people are asked about their smoking habits and encouraged to give up. People who have had heart attacks are given advice, help and support in preventing further problems. Planned, structured care for people with cardiovascular disease has been the norm in many practices for more than a decade.

It is interesting that, in the same year, the same organisation also published a report on the prevention of psychiatric disorders in general practice (RCGP 1981b). This latter report disappeared without a trace! Yet, as Gask and colleagues (2000) have emphasised, a planned, systematic style of care, especially for people with severe mental illness, is likely to result in fewer patients falling through the net.

But this is by no means an easy task. GP practices are autonomous businesses with GPs as independent contractors to the NHS. This was the case even before the NHS began, and for the most part remains the case. It implies that individual practices may vary considerably in the scope of services they are able and willing to offer and in the level of support they will require from specialists. It also means that those wishing to change any particular aspect of primary care need to work with a variety of different stakeholders, many of whom will have different ways of understanding the issues.

## NEW APPROACHES TO PROVIDING CARE

Depression is a chronic, relapsing illness. Andrews (2001) pointed out that it is an illness which reduces hope, motivation and treatment adherence and predisposes to suicide. He considered that the traditional reactive model of patient contact was inappropriate for such a condition and suggested that a chronic disease management model, such as is often used for caring for people with asthma or diabetes, might be more effective.

In fact, methods of caring for people with depression based on chronic disease management had been pioneered by nurses and others for several years before Andrews's recent article. In Ipswich, Gardner (1999) devised and evaluated a collaborative model, working alongside the practice GPs, using the skills she had already gained in caring for people with asthma. She points out that chronic disease management skills, such as providing accurate, understandable information, encouraging concordance with medication and monitoring progress, are transferable skills. Her evaluation suggests that attendance at her clinic significantly improved patient outcome.

A group of health visitors based in an area of high social deprivation in Milton Keynes formed a depression support team, with the help of a local community mental health nurse (Scanlan 2002). This area had previously had very high referral rates to the local community mental health team. The patients referred had poor concordance with medication, little information about either their illness or the medication they were taking, and had received little support during their illness. The health visitors provided information, including literature, monitored symptoms and medication, and offered support. Referrals were made to other agencies where appropriate. Patients were seen by a health visitor for a forty-five-minute assessment either at home or at the health centre within two weeks of being prescribed antidepressants by a GP. A further face-to-face appointment was offered at three months, with optional contact in the intervening period, usually by telephone. At three months, 71 per cent were still taking their medication and satisfaction ratings were high. The community mental health nurse offered ongoing training, supervision and support to the health visitors. There is other evidence that telephone support by nurses, of patients with depression, is effective (Simon *et al.* 2000).

A practice team in Northamptonshire has looked in detail at the roles of all the professional members in working with people with depression, as part of an attempt to develop an integrated approach to mental health care. This model acknowledges that any member of the team can meet a depressed patient as part of their day-to-day work. It attempts to provide a framework within which all have a constructive part to play according to their individual skills and training. Table 7.2 is a modified version of the team's approach. They have acknowledged that achieving this level of integration is not painless. They have had to confront the tribalisms which exist in health care. They suggest that one of the benefits is that patients receive a more consistent approach to their care.

This model also reveals that there are opportunities for referral within the practice team, as well as the traditional referral to outside agencies. In this particular practice, the community mental health nurse and the social worker, as well as the counsellor, were seen as members of the team. Both accepted referrals from, and referred back to, other members of the team. This helps to break down the traditional barriers between primary and secondary care services, and can thus benefit not only patients with depression. People with psychotic illness are also likely to benefit from improved collaboration, not least in their physical health care which is often poor.

These developments have largely been driven from within primary care, but there are also initiatives being led by community mental health nurses working with primary care teams. In *Building bridges*, the then government acknowledged the important role of primary care teams in providing care for people with severe and enduring mental illness (Department of Health 1995). This document suggested that specialist services had an important training role with primary care professionals. Goldberg and Gournay (1997) also considered this an important part of the role of community mental health teams. Developments along these lines have been patchy to date, sometimes because of lack of training skills in CMHTs and poor understanding of the training needs of primary care, and also because of lack of management support for the training role even where the skills exist. Nevertheless, there are some interesting initiatives around the country: for example, in Bradford, where the Health Action Zone has funded the employment of primary care liaison nurses, based in CMHTs, one to each of the local primary care trusts (Raistrick and Armstrong 2001). The role of these nurses includes:

- delivering educational packages at practice and primary care trust level;
- assisting individuals to develop skills in cognitive behavioural therapy and solution-focused therapy;
- guideline development and implementation;
- improving communication between primary care teams and CMHTs;
- development of primary care registers for people with severe and enduring mental illness.

An important aspect of this service, and others, is a recognition that whilst those people with severe mental illness have to be a priority for secondary care services, people with less severe problems also need help, and that the latter form the bulk of the primary care clientele. Primary care teams may require help and support to manage the care of the majority of their patients, but this support must not compromise the care of people with severe illness.

Table 7.2 An integrated approach to mental health care

| | Practice nurse | Health visitor | CMHN | Social worker | Counsellor | District nurse | GP |
|---|---|---|---|---|---|---|---|
| Client group | Everyone | Everyone, especially young mothers, families, carers, elderly people | Adults (if over 65 to elderly team; if under 16 to child and adolescent team) | Adults 18–65 – severe and enduring mental illness | Adults 16–65 without psychotic symptoms | Elderly people, people discharged from hospital, carers | Everyone |
| Assessment | Recognition, listening, facilitating, dealing with feelings, using scales | Use of EPDS (Edinburgh Postnatal Depression Scale), GDS (Geriatric Depression Scale) As practice nurse | Scales, coping mechanisms, patient's views, trigger issues, support available | Risk assessment Assessment of needs: social, finance, housing, job, carers | Causes Options for intervention Hypothesis + coping mechanism + suicidality | Use of GDS As practice nurse | Suicidality, severity (scales), patients' views, support, social context, medication |
| Severity | Mild | Mild–moderate | Moderate–severe | Moderate–severe | Moderate–severe | Mild | All |
| When to refer/ liaise | Suicidality Complex issues Failure to improve | Suicidality Complex issues Failure to improve | Neglect Safety issues Failure to improve | Patient wishes Complex social needs Family issues | Suicidality Complex issues Failure to improve | Suicidality Complex issues Failure to improve | Safety issues Failure to improve Patient wishes Family pressures |
| When to receive referrals | For advice and talking through leaflets – an educational role | Mothers of young children Help with postnatal depression, carers and isolated elderly | Moderate to severe risk, especially of self-harm Concurrent psychotic illness | Advice on childcare, benefits, housing Moderate to severe risk, especially of self-harm Concurrent psychotic illness | Problems with personality development, especially people with relationship problems, stress, anxiety | People with other nursing needs impinging on their mood, e.g. physical disabilities, illness | Confirm diagnosis if unclear Multiaxial assessment Concern for other members of team Medication |

Source: Armstrong 2001 (adapted from Clark and Smart 1999); reproduced by kind permission of Radcliffe Medical Press

# CONCLUSION

Notwithstanding the many positive developments in primary care mental health, some of which have been described above, there are many gaps in the mental health knowledge and skills of primary care nurses. Gray and colleagues (1999), in a national survey of practice nurses, found that whilst more than half were administering antipsychotic medication on a regular basis, knowledge of side effects was poor. They also found poor understanding of treatment issues in depression. This is unacceptable, but training opportunities will not improve unless nurses themselves demand that they do. Too often, experience suggests that when cash is short, educational initiatives are the first to suffer, and, in practice, mental health comes a long way down the list of priorities.

There is as yet insufficient nursing research into mental health issues at primary care level, despite much good work going on. It is vital that projects are properly evaluated and, where possible, published. Many nurses are involved in research, especially in evaluating new treatment methods, but this research often fails to focus on nursing itself. Where research evidence does exist, it often takes many years to put effective interventions into practice. There is a great deal of inertia in health care. It may not always be appreciated that even small changes in clinical practice may have profound effects on the system within which the change occurs. Conversely, changes in the system may enable changes in clinical practice which have the potential to improve patient outcome.

Guidelines and protocols, and education and training, whilst necessary, are not enough on their own to do this (Lin and Katon 1998). But there is evidence that where guidelines and protocols and education and training are linked to changes in the way the service is delivered, patient outcome can improve (e.g. Simon *et al.* 2000).

The National Service Framework for Mental Health provides opportunities and challenges to all nurses. It is clear from the document that nurses are key to its implementation, along with colleagues from social services, but unless nurses work to improve understanding and collaboration between the various branches of the profession, little will actually change and care will continue to be patchy and fragmented.

# REFERENCES

Andrews, G. (2001) 'Should depression be managed as a chronic disease?' *British Medical Journal*, 322: 419–421.

Armstrong, E. (2001) 'Developing a team strategy', in Armstrong, E. (ed.) *The guide to mental health for nurses in primary care*, Abingdon: Radcliffe Medical Press.

Armstrong, E. and Paton, J. (2001) *An implementation toolkit for primary care: the National Service Framework for Mental Health*, London: PriMHE.

Challenger, J. and Hardy, B. (1998) 'Dementia: the difficulties experienced by carers', *British Journal of Community Nursing*, 3 (4): 166–171.

Clark, S. and Smart, D. (1999) 'The integrated nursing team and primary care', *Journal of Primary Care Mental Health*, 3: 6–9.

Clinical Standards Advisory Group (CSAG) (1999) *Services for patients with depression*, London: Department of Health.

Department of Health (1995) *Building bridges: a guide to arrangements for interagency working for the care and protection of severely mentally ill people*, London: Department of Health.

Department of Health (1999) *National service framework for mental health: modern standards and service models*, London: Department of Health.

Department of Health (2000) *The NHS Plan: a plan for investment, a plan for reform*, London: The Stationery Office.

Foyster, L. (1995) 'Supporting mothers: an interdisciplinary approach', *Health Visitor*, 68 (4): 151–152.

Freeling, P. and Kendrick, T. (1996) 'Introduction', in Kendrick, T., Tylee, A. and Freeling, P. (eds) *The prevention of mental illness in primary care*, Cambridge: Cambridge University Press.

Gardner, S. (1999) 'Practice nurses in mental health: a changing role?', *Journal of Primary Care Mental Health*, 2: 11–12.

Gask, L., Rogers, A., Roland, M. and Morris, D. (2000) *Improving quality in primary care: a practical guide to the National Service Framework for Mental Health*, Manchester: University of Manchester.

Goldberg, D. and Gournay, K. (1997) *The general practitioner, the psychiatrist and the burden of mental health care*, Maudsley Discussion Paper No. 1, London: Institute of Psychiatry.

Gray, R., Parr, A.-M., Plummer, S., Sandford, T., Ritter, S., Mundt-Leach, R., Goldberg, K. and Gournay, K. (1999) 'A national survey of practice nurse involvement in mental health interventions', *Journal of Advanced Nursing*, 30 (4): 901–906.

Holden, J. (1994) 'Can non-psychotic depression be prevented?' in Cox, J. and Holden, J. (eds) *Perinatal psychiatry: use and misuse of the Edinburgh postnatal depression scale*, London: Gaskell.

Lin, E.H.B. and Katon, W. (1998) 'Beyond the diagnosis of depression', *General Hospital Psychiatry*, 20: 207–208.

Mann, A. (1992) 'Depression and anxiety in primary care: the epidemiological evidence', in Jenkins, R., Newton, J. and Young, R. (eds) *The prevention of depression and anxiety. The role of the primary care team*, London: HMSO.

Raistrick, H. and Armstrong, E. (2001) 'Serious mental illness in primary care', in Armstrong, E. (ed.) *The guide to mental health for nurses in primary care*, Abingdon: Radcliffe Medical Press.

Royal College of General Practitioners (RCGP) (1981a) *Prevention of arterial disease in general practice*, London: RCGP.

Royal College of General Practitioners (RCGP) (1981b) *Prevention of psychiatric disorders in general practice*, London: RCGP.

Scanlan, M. (2002) 'How health visitors can turn a phone line into a lifeline', *Primary Care Report*, 4 (9): 38–39.

Simon, G.E., VonKorff, M., Rutter, C. and Wagner, E. (2000) 'Randomised trial of monitoring, feedback and management of care by telephone to improve the treatment of depression in primary care', *British Medical Journal*, 320: 550–554.

Strathdee, G. and Jenkins, R. (1996) 'Purchasing mental health care for primary care', in Thornicroft, G. and Strathdee, G. (eds) *Commissioning mental health services*, London: HMSO.

# FURTHER READING

World Health Organization (2000) *WHO Guide to Mental Health in Primary Care*,
    London: Royal Society of Medicine. (Available at: www.whoguidemhpcuk.org)
This is the UK version of chapter 5 of the International Classification of Diseases, 10th
edition (ICD-10 PHC). It adapts the primary care version of the classification of mental
disorders for UK use. Many PCOs have used this guide as the basis of their guidelines and
protocols.

Armstrong, E. (ed.) (2001) *The guide to mental health for nurses in primary care*, Abingdon:
    Radcliffe Medical Press.
Though intended mainly for generalist primary care nurses, health visitors and midwives,
this text may help community mental health nurses who want to work in primary care
develop a better understanding of the context. It may also help those CMHNs involved in
training in primary care to identify training needs better.

Blount, A. (ed.) (1998) *Integrated primary care*, London: W.W. Norton.
This is an American text which looks in detail at ways of integrating primary health care
and mental health care. It contains much that is relevant to the UK situation and is highly
recommended for anyone involved in change management in this field.

# CHAPTER 8

# COLLABORATING WITH USERS OF SERVICES

*Peter Campbell*

---

## SUMMARY OF KEY POINTS

- Progress has been made in improving collaboration between mental health workers and service users in the development of services.

- However, there are limits to the degree to which service users are involved in their own care and treatment.

- A conflict exists between ideas of empowerment and partnership, and the urge towards compliance.

---

## INTRODUCTION

We are living and working in an era in which service users are supposed to be at the centre of mental health services. In the 1980s, the market philosophies of Thatcherite governments led to initiatives to create service user- or consumer-led services. Today, the rhetoric may have moved on and become less insistent. Nevertheless, the aspiration emerging from central government and reflected at local level still demands that the wants and needs of service users – expressed both by individuals in relation to their own care and treatment and by collectivities shaping the development, management and monitoring of services – remain fundamental. At the same time, most mental health workers, including mental health nurses, now acknowledge that the relationships between themselves and those receiving their services are among the most important factors in deciding the success of care and treatment. Indeed, in the absence of a constructive relationship, many service users may nowadays refuse to accept the care and treatment being offered, or only co-operate intermittently. In this sense, if in no other, good relationships are a priority. It is not insignificant that the Mental Health Nursing Review of 1994 is entitled *Working in partnership*, or that its executive summary declares: 'The work of mental health nurses rests upon the relationship they have with people who use services. Our recommendations for future action start and finish with this relationship' (Department of Health 1994, p. 5).

Although mental health literature is now full of references to partnership, common agendas, common concerns and collaboration, this is a relatively recent phenomenon and should not prevent us recognising that for the greater part of the history of mental health services the working relationship between care-giver and recipient has been of a slightly different character. For much of the last two centuries, it has been assumed that people with mental illness/madness problems are, by their very nature, not capable of knowing what their best interests are and therefore in fundamental ways are excluded from any real involvement in their own care and treatment. As a result of such attitudes, consent to treatment took a very long time to become an issue of major concern to service providers or society, only starting to gain the attention we now give it during the 1960s. Autonomy is still a problematic concept in mental health care. Available information suggests that from the establishment of the asylum system in the middle of the nineteenth century until the 1940s, service users were usually passive recipients rather than active agents. John Perceval, whose *Perceval's narrative* provides an important insight into asylum conditions in the 1830s, claimed that he was barred from discussion of his treatment and placed into solitary confinement, a strait-jacket or a cold bath when he challenged the care he received (in Hervey 1986, p. 251). Conditions may have improved a little by the time of Montagu Lomax's exposure of asylum care in north-west England in his *The experiences of an asylum doctor* in 1922. But it is clear that at that time attendants controlled their charges through paternalism and fear rather than enlightened care. In his *History of mental health nursing*, Peter Nolan interviewed a number of nurses who were at work in the 1920s and found that they were generally not close to patients: 'Some of the female nurses apparently enjoyed making "homes" on the wards, but the men were for the most part not greatly interested in patient care' (Nolan 1993, p. 94). Diana Gittins, describing the female side in her history of Severalls Hospital, near Colchester, suggests that 'Befriending patients was not considered essential , or even desirable, until well after the Second World War' (Gittins 1998, p. 140).

Such evidence underlines the fact that while mental health nurses have always worked with, and often lived alongside, service users, it is comparatively novel for work to have taken place in close and creative relationships. Moreover, it reminds us that the possibility that service users – the mad, the mentally ill – could make a positive contribution to running mental health services (or even elsewhere) is little short of revolutionary when seen in historical context. Finally, and most importantly, it should suggest to us that such innovatory ideas at this relatively early stage of their development are likely only to have been realised in an incomplete and unsatisfactory fashion. The challenge for mental health nurses and mental health services is not to polish up perfected models and practices but to advance into an area of uncertainty and experiment.

# INCREASING THE INFLUENCE OF INDIVIDUAL SERVICE USERS OVER THEIR OWN CARE AND TREATMENT

Any examination of collaboration with service users must begin by acknowledging the limitation of the term 'service user' in describing people with a mental illness diagnosis. In the past, service use may have occupied the predominant part of their lives. At present, even long-term service users will actually spend a lot less time receiving mental health services and a lot more time doing other things with their lives. They may still be service users but they are also participants in local communities, candidates in the job market, citizens. Any attempt to work with service users that minimises this wider dimension or ignores the complexity of their aspirations risks undermining creative relationships. It is important that mental health nurses work from a starting position that recognises the role (potential and actual) of service users in services and society and understands that, in the eyes of people with a mental illness diagnosis, a major objective of collaboration may be to escape the identity of service user and move on to more fulfilling roles. Few people would choose to be, or be seen as, service users if more positive alternatives were available. Having said that, it remains true that attempts to improve the position of service users in relation to their own care and treatment have been an important aspect of collaboration in the last twenty years. Increasing individual influence in this regard continues to be a priority for service user activists and is often seen as a key test of the success of their actions and a prerequisite for their wider ambitions. If collaboration cannot improve the position of individuals within mental health services, the whole enterprise is fatally compromised. Looking back to the 1980s, there can be little doubt that individuals are now in a more powerful position in relation to the delivery of care and treatment. While claims that service users are centre-stage or are in control of their own care are arguable, they are certainly more likely to be able to influence delivery and thus receive the care and treatment that they want as well as that they are thought to need. The amount of information available to service users has increased, enabling them to be in a better position to make choices. Acute wards will often have displays of relevant information from statutory and voluntary organisations, in a range of languages and formats. Community psychiatric nurses may give service users material photocopied from drug manuals when changes in medication are under discussion. Service users sometimes receive specially-tailored discharge packs to support their return to the community. Overall, the quality and quantity of information have improved greatly. At the same time, service users in most parts of the United Kingdom will have access to independent advocacy, a resource that was barely in evidence in the early 1980s. Collaboration with individuals will now frequently include co-operation with an advocate, a situation which, while presenting new challenges to mental health nurses, gives service users a more effective say in the decision-making process.

Although mental health workers remain the more powerful partner, advocacy can moderate the power differentials. Perhaps the most important single change in the working relationship between providers and recipients has been the introduction of the care programme approach (CPA) in 1991. Although this initiative was largely to do with the targeting and rationing of resources, it also provided service users with a written care plan, subject to regular review, and a keyworker to supervise the implementation of the plan. Most significantly of all, for the development of collaboration, the CPA created definite opportunities when service users would meet with relevant service providers to discuss and agree their care plan. While it would be inaccurate to suggest that service users were excluded from discussions about their care and treatment before 1991, the CPA did give such consultations a status they had not previously acquired. The care programme approach has also proved important by promoting the idea of advance planning, a strategy that has received widespread support from service users and mental health workers. It is now accepted that collaborative written plans about future care are a basic requirement, and the Department of Health has advised that future care plans should cover crisis response and employment planning. In these ways the position of the individual as an agent in their own life is slowly advanced.

## LIMITS TO CHANGE

The above developments have gone some way to altering the basis upon which mental health nurses work with individual service users. However, it is important not to exaggerate what has been achieved, for in each area there is evidence that progress has had clear limits. There have been very real improvements in the quantity and quality of information generally available. Nevertheless, in at least one key area deficiencies are notable. User Focused Monitoring interviewed 500 service users and found that 'access to information about one's mental health problem and medication and its side effects hovered around the 50% mark' (Rose 2001, p. 42). About 500 service users were interviewed for the publication *Experiencing psychiatry* which found that 'of those receiving major tranquillisers, 60% were not informed of their purpose and 70% of this group were unhappy about the amount of information that they had received about their medication' (Rogers *et al*. 1993, p. 165). MIND's Yellow Card survey of 622 service users who had experienced problems with side effects found only 11 per cent who felt they had been given enough information at time of prescription (Campbell *et al*. 1998, p. 12). Clearly, percentages like these must cast doubt not only on whether individuals are meaningfully involved in treatment decisions, but also on their ability to give informed consent. There may be less reason to doubt the positive impact of advocacy. But even here caution is necessary. While we do not yet have enough clear evidence about the effectiveness of advocacy schemes, it seems possible that advocacy may do more to improve the process of decision-making for the service user than to alter the decisions that are finally made. Improving the quality of collaboration may be a worthwhile objective. Yet, in the end, changing outcomes is the primary objective for service users. Limits to change can also be observed in the functioning of the care programme approach, which, even more than ten years after its introduction, has not been effectively implemented in all areas of the country. User Focused Monitoring, operating in five different sites, found that a majority of service users did not know what the purpose of the CPA was. With the exception of one site, the majority of service users did not know who their keyworker was. Service users also tended not to know whether they had a care plan or not (Rose 2001).

Such findings inevitably arouse misgivings about the impact of the whole enterprise and are accompanied by concern that when service users are involved in CPA, their input is much less likely to end up in the completed care plan than the input of mental health professionals. It is also not clear what priority certain professionals attach to the CPA process. Some may even refuse to attend CPA meetings. While the process has the potential to give service users more influence over the care and treatment they receive, numerous professionals view it as a time-wasting nuisance. In some quarters, CPA has been dubbed 'Continuous Paper Accumulation'.

In all areas of involving individuals in their own care and treatment, the last twenty years have seen important progress. Nevertheless, it is important not to exaggerate the speed of progress or overlook the fact that the path has not always been smooth. While practitioners may talk about the empowerment of service users, the truth is that this group remains comparatively powerless and the imbalance of power between individuals and service providers is still quite marked. Moreover, it may not be universally accepted that empowering service users is something that mental health nurses and other professionals can or should do. The tools to increase the influence of individual service users – information, advocacy, care planning – are available. The willingness to exploit them fully may still be lacking.

## THE INFLUENCE OF SERVICE USERS ON THE DEVELOPMENT OF MENTAL HEALTH SERVICES

An examination of the contribution of service users to mental health services must begin with an acknowledgement that there is still a widespread popular belief that people with a mental illness cannot make a positive contribution to anything. If you were to interview passers-by in most streets in the United Kingdom, you would be likely to discover that this group's social contribution is seen to be negative rather than positive. In short, people with a mental illness diagnosis are a burden on society. One of the early advertising slogans of the national mental health charity Sane sums it up quite neatly: 'You don't have to be mentally ill to suffer from mental illness.' In the light of such attitudes and the persistent marginalisation of service users in the day-to-day activities of community life, it is quite remarkable that, over the last twenty years, service users have come to play such an important role in the development of mental health services. In the 1970s and early 1980s, service users were barely involved in deliberations about the shaping of services. They were not stakeholders in the debate. Even within voluntary organisations, where it might be imagined they would have a greater say, their voice was weak, their involvement tokenistic. Agencies spoke on behalf of service users (at that time more likely to be described as 'the mentally ill' or 'mental patients') and acted in their best interests. Service users rarely spoke or acted for themselves. Their absence from the decision-making arena was notable and complete.

The situation has certainly changed. In 2003, it would be almost (but not completely) inconceivable that any important development at national, regional or local level could proceed without consultation with service users. Whereas the voice of service users was scarcely heard during the discussions leading up to the 1983 Mental Health Act, the current debate about a new Mental Health Act significantly includes, and sets out to include, the contribution of service users and service user organisations. It may not be too much of an exaggeration to claim that we are in a completely new era of mental health debate, with service users sharing the platform rather than languishing as a passive audience. Although service user involvement in service development may not be universally desired or welcomed, it has clearly become universally necessary. But, as in the case of individuals' involvement in their care and treatment, caution is needed when assessing what has been achieved. Once again, although real and significant progress has been made, there are also clear limits to progress. Service user involvement has spread through most areas of mental health services but has met with different responses and achieved different degrees of success in different fields of activity. The strength of involvement varies from one part of the country to another. Achievement varies. Complaints about tokenism survive even into the second decade of concerted action by service users.

Consultation is the bread and butter of service user action. Most local action groups will be involved in consultation processes whatever else they may do. Of all the action that service users may be taking, consultation remains the activity that government is most ready to support. Collaboration with service users in the planning and monitoring of services is now essential. Although government initiatives since the early 1990s have ensured that consultation has become regular and widespread, the process is not without problems from the service user point of view. In the first place, consultation mechanisms may not be very friendly to service user or other non-expert participants. Committee procedures, jargon, paperwork, the outnumbering of service user representatives, can all combine to make collaboration an arduous task. While activists in the 1980s called for a change in the way consultation was carried out, the reality is that the process continues to use traditional structures that are not friendly to service users and may help to marginalise their contribution. The resignation of a number of service users from the Reference Groups that informed the National Service Framework is symptomatic of the problems inherent in consultation. But those resignations were also caused by concerns about tokenism – the belief that, although service users are involved, their contributions are not taken seriously or are even ignored. Such concerns have been an aspect of service user action since the upsurge of activity in the mid-1980s and have not disappeared even now. The suspicion remains that decisions are taken elsewhere and that consultation is often window-dressing after the important issues have already been resolved. It may be better to be collaborating with service providers in the development of services than to be left out in the cold. Even so, it is difficult to avoid the impression that service user inputs only have an influence on the margins. But there can be little doubt that service user involvement in the consultative process is secure. Few mental health professionals would now openly deny the value of service user knowledge – essentially the knowledge of using/consuming mental health services – to the development of new and better services. The government is committed to consultation. Although their contributions may not always be put to good use, the right of service users to present consumer evidence is everywhere acknowledged.

The same may not be true when we move from a consideration of service users as providers of consumer evidence to look at service users as providers of new understandings about mental illness. This activity, in which a growing number of service users are involving themselves, presents a more radical challenge to the psychiatric enterprise and as a result may be viewed with less approval or even outright hostility. It is one thing to complain about the lack of nurses in the dayroom or suggest changes to the multidisciplinary ward round, it is quite another to claim that mental health professionals have completely misunderstood the problems they are attempting to deal with. The National Self-Harm Network (NSHN) and the Hearing Voices Network (HVN) are both service user-led organisations that have done pioneering work in promoting new understandings and responses. NSHN has taken a leading role in challenging the traditional approaches to self-harm, arguing that it must be seen as a valid coping mechanism:

> The Network promotes the concept of harm-minimisation; accepting the need to self-harm as a valid method of survival, until survival is possible by other means. This does not condone or encourage self-injury, it's facing the reality of maximising safety in the event of self-harm.
>
> (National Self-Harm Network, no date, p. 6)

HVN have made similar challenges to the understanding and treatment of hearing voices, usually seen as a classic symptom of schizophrenia. They emphasise the need to consider the content of the experience of hearing voices, and promote a much wider range of responses than the usual approach relying on psychotropic medication. At the same time, other service users are presenting their own interpretations of psychotic experiences and opening them out to scrutiny. In these ways some of the major assumptions of psychiatry are put up for debate.

The above developments are some of the more controversial aspects of much wider service user involvement in education and training in recent years. Again there is government support for such activity – the Workforce Action Team's (WAT) final report in August 2001 stated that one of the guiding principles that had informed its work was that service users and carers should be engaged throughout the whole education and training process, and one of the key issues raised was the effective participation of service users and carers in the design, delivery and evaluation of education and training (Department of Health 2001).

Unfortunately, it is at present very difficult to know how far we have travelled in the pursuit of these laudable goals. Little research has been published about the extent or quality of service user involvement in training, so, although we know that service user trainers are working in most areas of the country, the effectiveness of such activity is difficult to gauge. Again, there may be a gap between rhetoric and reality – a gap which, in the absence of more evaluation, it may prove difficult to bridge. Action by service users has spread to most areas of mental health services. Local drop-ins and day services may be run by service user organisations. Advocacy schemes are often provided by service user-led organisations and staffed predominantly or completely by people with direct experience of using services. At the same time, the last few years have seen service users claiming a role in the research field, not just as the subjects of research but as researchers themselves. User Focused Monitoring, developed by the Sainsbury Centre for Mental Health, is one example of a service user-led approach. Another is the *Strategies for living* initiative being carried out by the Mental Health Foundation. In the latter:

> The advertisements for all of the research and interviewer posts made it clear that the posts were for people with direct experience of mental distress and/or mental health services. . . . We aimed to adopt an openly committed 'user perspective' throughout the research and to take what is often termed an 'emancipatory research' approach. This approach is gaining support within mental health research and is reflected in the work of a number of other researchers and research organisations.
>
> (Mental Health Foundation 2000, p. 9)

## DILEMMAS

The mechanisms to allow meaningful collaboration by individual service users in their own care and treatment are largely in place. But mechanisms are not enough in themselves. A crucial consideration is the overall attitudes that inform the use of the available mechanisms. And here there may be cause for concern, because at the same time as there has been an increased emphasis on collaboration there has also been an increased impetus to ensure compliance. At the MIND Annual Conference in 1998, the then minister with responsibility for mental health, John Hutton, declared that the government would not 'tolerate a culture of non-compliance' (Mental Health Foundation 2001, p. 6), and this has set the context for subsequent developments. While there is evidence that non-compliance with medication regimes leads to re-admissions (Perkins and Repper 1998), there must ultimately be a major conflict between the urge towards collaboration and the urge towards compliance. If service users are to be compelled to adhere to their care programme, collaboration can only be a mask for powerlessness. Collaboration between service users and mental health workers can only be effective if the relationship is transparent and recognises the inherent imbalances in power. In this respect, the employment of popular concepts like empowerment and partnership may be a hindrance as much as a help. Although both sound attractive, they can conceal different realities. Empowerment is frequently taken to refer to service use and ignores the wider political and social predicament of service users. It can often mean that service users feel in greater control of their destinies without addressing structural inequalities. Meanwhile, the rhetoric of partnership, while suggesting equality, often conceals the true dynamics of the relationships. How often is there real give and take, how frequently are service users the inviters rather than the invited? It is possible that uncritical use of the concepts of empowerment and partnership actually prevents thorough scrutiny of the service user and service provider relationship.

The dilemma for mental health nurses is how to make collaboration meaningful in a system which is backed up by compulsion and where individuals are seen as not only being ill but also wrong and in the wrong. When it comes to working with service users in the development of services, they must adapt to the need to see service users as providers of expertise and knowledge that may challenge their own certainties.

## CONCLUSION

Misunderstanding is at the centre of the predicament of those diagnosed as mentally ill – misunderstanding about who they are and what their interior experiences signify, misunderstanding about who they might become. It is essential that collaboration – with individuals, with collectivities – penetrates these misunderstandings and enables this social group to be seen in a truer light. People with a mental illness may be service users, but first and foremost they are citizens with rights – the right to be involved in their own care and treatment, the right to participate in society. It is rights of this kind that mental health workers should be promoting. The great irony of the last twenty years is that during a period when the status of service users within services has improved, their position in society has deteriorated. The challenge for all mental health nurses, but particularly those working in the community, is threefold: to recognise and support the expertise, potential and actual, of service users in changing their own lives; to explore, through collaboration in education and research, the reality and diversity of the experience of the diagnosed mentally ill; and to promote and facilitate their contribution to society. After two decades of change, it is no longer enough to concentrate on developing good mental health services. Good mental health services are not sufficient to meet the dreams of service users. Their aspirations now have a wider dimension. Mental health nurses need to recognise the changing identity of people with a mental illness diagnosis and, through collaboration, champion their proper inclusion into society.

## REFERENCES

Campbell, P., Cobb, A. and Darton, K. (1998) *Psychiatric drugs*, London: MIND.
Department of Health (1994) *Working in partnership: a collaborative approach to care. Report of the Mental Health Nursing Review Team*, London: HMSO.
Department of Health (2001) *Mental health national service framework (and The NHS Plan) workforce planning, education and training underpinning programme: adult mental health services: final report by the Workforce Action Team*, London: Department of Health.
Gittins, D. (1998) *Madness in its place*, London: Routledge.
Hervey, N. (1986) 'Advocacy or folly: the alleged lunatics' friend society, 1845–63', *Medical History*, 30: 245–275.
Lomax, M. (1922) *The experiences of an asylum doctor*, London: Allen and Unwin.
Mental Health Foundation (2000) *Strategies for living*, London: Mental Health Foundation.

Mental Health Foundation (2001) *Something inside so strong*, London: Mental Health Foundation.

National Self-Harm Network (no date) *Cutting the risk*, London: National Self-Harm Network.

Nolan, P. (1993) *A history of mental health nursing*, Cheltenham: Stanley Thornes.

Perkins, R. and Repper, J. (1998) *Dilemmas in mental health practice*, Abingdon: Radcliffe Medical Press.

Rogers, A., Pilgrim, D. and Lacey, R. (1993) *Experiencing psychiatry*, Basingstoke: Macmillan/MIND.

Rose, D. (2001) *Users' voices*, London: Sainsbury Centre for Mental Health.

## FURTHER READING

Barnes, M. and Bowl, R. (2001) *Taking over the asylum*, Basingstoke: Palgrave/Mental Health Foundation.
This book is useful in pointing out the achievements and failures of the service user/survivor movement, looking in particular at issues of action and empowerment.

Mental Health Foundation (2001) *Something inside so strong*, London: Mental Health Foundation.
An excellent and very positive publication which includes personal accounts of alternative strategies that service users have adopted to help them cope with their difficulties. A good introduction to the positive skills and energy of people with a mental illness diagnosis.

Rose, D. (2001) *Users' voices*, London: Sainsbury Centre for Mental Health.
User Focused Monitoring of Services (a programme of research devised and carried out by service users) provides interesting angles on how service users really see services, including results that traditional research might overlook.

# CHAPTER 9

# GENDER ISSUES

*Anne Fothergill*

---

## SUMMARY OF KEY POINTS

- Women's mental health needs differ from those of men. The aetiology, manifestation and presentation of mental illness in women are different from those in men.

- Some mental illnesses are viewed as 'gender-specific', in particular, depression, anxiety disorders and eating disorders.

- Gender-sensitive services, especially in the community, need to be provided to ensure that women with mental illness receive care that meets their specific needs.

---

## INTRODUCTION

Community mental health nurses (CMHNs) face increasing challenges in their role, in a dynamic profession. One of these challenges is to meet the mental health needs of disadvantaged groups within society. Women as a social group are not homogeneous in terms of their needs – to suggest so would constitute a form of discrimination – but as a group they face many disadvantages, which impact on their mental health.

This chapter is about gender issues, focusing primarily on women, community services delivery and mental health services delivered within 'the community'. Gender refers to both male and female, but when gender issues are written about and debated in the literature it is usually women rather than men who are the focus. Data on men are used as a comparison to women's experiences. Men and women have different mental health needs; some psychiatric disorders have been noted to be 'gender-specific'. The greatest differential between men and women is seen in the prevalence of depression, anxiety disorders and eating disorders. Sociologists/feminists over the last few decades have attempted to explain the reasons for the differentials in women's and men's mental health, which have included biological differences, gender roles and women's position in society, and differences in help-seeking behaviour. Women are more likely to disclose their emotional distress and seek help for it. They are twice as likely to refer themselves for psychiatric treatment, take on the sick role and define their problems in mental health terms. Men are less likely than women to view their problems in psychiatric terms (Pilgrim and Rogers 1999). An understanding of these theories enables mental health nurses to understand that treatment outcomes and service delivery must reflect the fundamental differences in the aetiology, manifestation and presentation of women's mental health problems. Gender is often ignored in treatment considerations and research (Mowbray *et al.* 1998, ch. 9). Discriminatory practices within and without mental health services and differing role expectations influence treatment and outcomes, especially for women with chronic mental health problems (Morgan 1993).

When researching for this chapter I consulted several key community mental health nursing texts and found that women's mental health needs did not feature, or were given only a cursory mention, that is, a few lines or a paragraph on their specific needs.

Women form 58 per cent of mental health service in-patient admissions (Department of Health 1993) and much more has been written about women's mental health needs in the in-patient setting. Key reports have highlighted how unsafe women often feel when receiving in-patient services and how this impacts on the outcomes of their care. For example, the Mental Health Act Commission visited half the acute mental health units in England and Wales in 1996; one of the focuses of this visit was the care of women patients. They found that 50 per cent of the patients were women; most of the wards were mixed (only 3 per cent were 'women-only'); 27 per cent of the women were sectioned; 35 per cent had access to women-only sleeping areas; 27 per cent had women-only sleeping areas, but patients had to walk past or through parts of the ward used by men in order to get to women-only toilet facilities; a third had access only to toilets used by both men and women; and 3 per cent of women patients used sleeping areas used by men. The Commission also found that the level of sexual harassment of women patients by male patients in mixed-sex acute psychiatric wards was high. Sexual harassment included suggestive or obscene remarks, watching or following women, sexually or explicit gestures or body language, through to sexual exposure or actually touching women. Fifty-six per cent of staff reported sexual harassment of women patients (Warner and Ford 1998). The recommendation was made that there should be women-only wards or 'women-only spaces' within wards, staffed by nurses trained in dealing with sexual harassment and other gender-related issues (Warner and Ford 1998).

England's National Framework for Mental Health (Department of Health 1999) set out seven standards of care delivery. Although women and ethnic minority groups were mentioned in terms of their specific needs, the standards did not set out how the services, including those delivered in the community, might effectively address the mental health needs of these groups. Strategies for preventing social exclusion were set out, but these were fairly generic, aimed at all people affected by a mental health problem. In the document only one specific need of women was addressed; this was that the government wanted to ensure that single-sex accommodation is available and single-sex day space is always provided. Other facilities such as sleeping, toilet and washing must be segregated, to achieve good standards of privacy and dignity for clients and enable women to be cared for safely. No strategies were identified in this document to provide gender-specific services in the community setting (Department of Health 1999).

## GENDER AND DIAGNOSIS

Men and women often receive a different diagnosis when affected by the same symptoms, which has led many writers to look closely at why this occurs. More commonly diagnosed in women are neurotic conditions, including depression and anxiety, anorexia nervosa (though much less common than anxiety/depression) and dementia. Community surveys suggest ratios of anxiety/depression in the order of 2: 1 female to male. Men are more commonly diagnosed with conditions such as substance abuse-related disorders, sexual disorders (e.g. paedophilia) and personality disorders. However, there is no clear distinction in rates of diagnosis of schizophrenia and mania between men and women. However, onset of schizophrenia tends to be later in women than in men (Busfield 1996).

In her classic work on women and madness Chesler (1972) suggested that women show greater help-seeking behaviour than men. Women display 'female psychiatric symptoms' such as depression, frigidity, paranoia, psychoneurosis, suicide attempts and anxiety. Men display 'male diseases' such as alcoholism, personality disorders and brain diseases. Rates of suicide are twice as high in men as in women and the differences are increasing. The fastest growing rates of suicide are amongst young males (Department of Health 1993); it is the leading cause of death among men aged 15–24 (Department of Health 1999). This is largely explained by the successful methods young men choose to kill themselves; 33 per cent of males committing suicide did so through inhaling car exhaust fumes. Self-poisoning is the method chosen by most women (Department of Health 1993).

## WOMEN AND DEPRESSION: THEORIES AND EXPLANATIONS

Since this is where the largest differentials occur between men and women in the prevalence of any mental health problem, depression is the focus for the discussion in this section. The large number of women experiencing depression raises the question 'Is being a woman depressing?' Women and depression is a very well researched area in the sociology of mental health and mental illness, and a vast amount of literature is available. Therefore this section aims to review some of this key literature and the theorists who have researched/commented on this topic over the last few decades.

## Social role theory

In western societies women and men are socialised into gender roles. This is a process which is different for males and females and begins early in life. Primary socialisation occurs within the family: boys and girls are treated differently and sex-appropriate behaviour is encouraged and rewarded and transmitted through vicarious learning; that is, parents act as role models and children imitate them. Secondary socialisation continues this lifelong process; in schools, behaviour is conditioned through reinforcement and attitudes about what constitutes accept-able male and female behaviour (Hargreaves and Colley 1986). Women's roles involve nurturing and supporting the needs of others, which is often to the detriment of their own sense of worth and efficacy (Mowbray *et al.* 1998, ch. 9).

The women's movement during the 1970s identified marital roles as being linked to women's mental health. Feminists applied terms such as the 'trapped housewife' or the 'depressed housewife syndrome' to women's situation (e.g. Johnstone 1989). They argued that the higher rates of depression in women were evidence of their oppression in contemporary society (Busfield 1989). Gove (1978) linked the higher rates of depression in women to their sex and specifically their marital role. Marriage acts as a protective factor for men, who experience lower rates of mental illness than married women do. The evidence suggests that unmarried women have lower rates of mental illness than married women do (Smith 1987).

Women's roles are seen as being more frustrating and less rewarding than men's roles are. Illness results from women's dissatisfaction and conflict with their roles, especially the traditional aspects of them, i.e. housework and childcare (Rosenfield 1980). Rosenfield argued that women's depression was due largely to sex roles. Women who perform traditional roles suffer from more depressive symptoms than women in less traditional roles – those in paid employment, for example. Significantly, it was men who had higher rates of mental illness in non-traditional households. This theory rules out biological explanations for these gender differences. Women also have higher rates of depression across cultures, over time and among different age groups.

Men and women are obviously biologically different, and women are seen as being more emotional. There are also obvious hormonal differences – women do get depressed pre-menstrually, following childbirth and at the menopause (Busfield 1996). It has been estimated that between 10 and 15 per cent of women have postnatal depression after childbirth. Suicide is the second most common form of maternal death in the year after birth (Department of Health 1999). All true, but this does not account for the large differentials in depression between the sexes (see Cochrane 1983). Another study conducted by Kessler and McRae (1981) suggested that 'role-related strain' was a factor. They argued that it is possible that only women in good mental health take up non-traditional roles in the first place. Gove and Tudor (1972–3) supported this view; they suggested that women have more stressful lives than men, especially those who both perform household roles and go out to work. Alternatively one could argue that men and women differ in the types of mental illness they suffer from. In other words, they deviate in different ways. Men, for example, have higher rates of drug abuse, alcoholism, violence and crime. Men also have higher rates of personality disorders (Dohrenwend and Dohrenwend 1975–6).

## Stress and depression in women, life events model

The stress model implies that major life events, particularly those associated with loss, can lead to depression (Brown and Harris 1978). Rather than investigating the effects of major life events, Kandel *et al.* (1985) researched the stressfulness of the daily roles of women, in particular, marital, occupational and household roles. They found that household roles produced the highest levels of stress in women. A combination of roles (marital, household and work), however, reduced stress levels in that they had a buffering effect. It appears that being married does not cause depression in women, unless the marriage is the source of stress.

Women may be more vulnerable to depression than men are. A study conducted by Brown and Harris (1978) found evidence of this. They identified specific 'vulnerability' factors. These included:

- an absence of an intimate, confiding relationship with their partner;
- having three or more children under 14 at home;
- having lost their own mother before the age of 11;
- not being in paid employment outside the home.

The life events theory is linked to the learned helplessness model and depression, developed by Seligman (1975, cited in Cochrane 1983 and Rosenfield 1980). This model states that 'traditional women' have a low capacity to influence their environment and to control their own lives (Cochrane 1983). The traditional role is often associated with a dependent state. Although this is consistent with the accepted behaviour for a woman, it can lead to a condition known as 'learned helplessness' (Seligman 1975, cited in Cochrane 1983 and Rosenfield 1980). Women are not 'trained' to cope with life situations and an inability to effect change in their environment may lead to depression. Helplessness is seen as a salient characteristic of depression. This can lead to a feeling of powerlessness; women as a group lack power in our society and this may more than anything else contribute to women's mental health (Rosenfield 1980).

## Mental health and gender

The stereotype of a neurotic person is a woman. A mentally healthy or 'normal' woman is expected to be economically dependent on a man. A mentally healthy person closely resembles the characteristics of the male stereotype (Jones and Cochrane 1981, cited in Cochrane 1983). In other words, to be seen as being mentally healthy a woman must conform to the set behaviours and characteristics of the male role. In doing so, she risks being labelled as being unfeminine; a 'no win' situation occurs. Mental illness may be a symptom of the oppression women feel in society (Busfield 1989); mental illness becomes a product of a sexist society. Clinicians' judgements are based around these gender stereotypes. Broverman *et al.* (1970) found that healthy women differ from healthy men by being more submissive, less independent, less adventurous, more easily influenced, less aggressive and less competitive. It is hard to see how this description can possibly be seen as one of a healthy, mature adult.

## Societal reaction theory

Social reaction theorists suggest that oppressed people are powerless and are therefore more at risk of being labelled mentally ill. Scheff (1966, cited in Miles 1981) viewed mental illness as rule-breaking behaviour, a violation of society's norms and a social construction. Women are vulnerable to being labelled. This is a form of social control (Schur 1984). In other words, mental illness has no objective reality. If this is true, then we deny the reality that those individual women who suffer from depression need the help and support of mental health nurses.

# DIAGNOSIS, TREATMENT AND PSYCHIATRY

Women may seek help from a general practitioner or a psychiatrist as either an out-patient or an in-patient. The 'help' they are given is often unsatisfactory. Women are more likely to be prescribed drug therapy and electro-convulsive therapy (ECT), and women's admissions to psychiatric hospitals are a third higher than those of men (Graham 1984, Busfield 1996). They receive a different diagnosis to men when presenting with the same symptoms. Women's complaints are seen as having a psychogenic origin, whilst men's complaints are seen as being caused by a physical problem (Penfold and Walker 1983). Can we deduce from this that psychiatrists are treating women in a sexist way, or just treating the 'sickness' which is a product of a sexist society (Busfield 1989)?

Leeson and Gray (1978) argue that doctors' attitudes towards women are based on the general stereotypical views of women in society. The same could be said for other mental health professionals. This is reflected in their diagnosis and treatment of women's depression. Male psychiatrists are more likely to diagnose females with a depressive disorder (Loring and Powell 1988). Treatment often includes role reinforcement; that is, women's roles are seen as 'normal' behaviour – cooking, cleaning, taking care of others, for example. These roles may have been the source of unhappiness which led to a woman becoming depressed in the first place (Johnstone 1989). The medical model tends to treat all illness as having an organic/physical cause. Therefore, depression is treated like any other 'physical' illness. It is treated with drugs and ECT. These treatments are seen as unhelpful for many women because they do not help them to take control of their own lives, make changes and understand the causes of their symptoms.

A form of therapy which enables women to become empowered through challenging the prevailing notions of mental health problems and psychological distress in women, known as 'feminist therapy', may be a much better alternative to the medical model (Segal 1987).

## DISCRIMINATION AND SOCIAL EXCLUSION

Social exclusion can both cause and come from mental health problems. One of the guiding principles and values of England's National Service Framework for Mental Health was to ensure that services to people with mental health problems should be well suited to those who use them and non-discriminatory (Department of Health 1999). One of the aims of the framework is to fight the discrimination and social exclusion associated with mental health problems. Included here are the 50 per cent of women and 25 per cent of men who will be affected by depression at some period in their lives.

People who are abused or affected by domestic violence have higher rates of mental health problems. Women are usually the most frequent victims. The impact of childhood sexual abuse can have long-term consequences for a woman's mental heath in adulthood. Studies have shown that there is a link between abuse and self-harm, severity of 'psychiatric symptoms' and suicide attempts (MIND 1992). People with severe mental illness are also stigmatised and socially excluded; the situation for disadvantaged or oppressed groups, including women, within society is even worse. They encounter difficulties accessing educational opportunities, maintaining employment and sustaining family and other social networks (Department of Health 1999).

The impact of social exclusion and disadvantage means that CMHNs must give long-term support. Perkins and Repper (1996) suggest that the challenge to community mental health services is for everyone to recognise and address the white, heterosexual male assumptions they are making.

## COMMUNITY SERVICES

Mental health professionals have a key role in helping clients to become integrated into communities and tackling the negative impact social exclusion has on a person's mental health. Community mental health nurses can help users, especially women clients, gain access to the full range of community services, and support clients in participating in various social, education and employment activities (Repper 1998, Coyte 2000). Community care services, to be effective in really making an impact on women's lives, must go further than the management and control of symptoms.

Research was conducted recently to examine the existing service provision to women in Nottingham's Rehabilitation and Community Care Service, which provides services to about 500 people with serious and enduring mental health problems. The research team noted that little research has been conducted into the ways in which services are provided for and used by women with severe and enduring mental health problems. In a review of the research evidence available they found significant gaps in what was known about the particular needs of women and little evidence regarding what constituted effective, appropriate and acceptable service provision (Owen and Milburn 2001). Examples of good practice in Nottingham include women-only residential facilities, gender awareness training for staff, women's groups and a choice of sex of keyworker in most areas. Other services offered include: specialist support and counselling to help women cope with loss, sexual abuse, sexuality issues, relationship difficulties, isolation and loneliness; women-only groups; supported access to employment, education, voluntary work, leisure facilities and community activities; a women-only art therapy group; and complementary therapies (Owen and Milburn 2001).

A guiding principle and value of England's National Service Framework for Mental Health was to involve service users and their carers in the planning and delivery of care. Services should be inclusive, equitable and non-discriminatory (Department of Health 1999).

One approach to the delivery of community services, which will enable the recipient to be fully empowered, has been termed 'client-directed' to distinguish it from 'client-centred'. Client-centred delivery of services is undertaken following consultation with women clients, but the final decisions on services are usually made by the provider, in the client's best interest. In contrast 'client-directed' services are implemented after engaging the recipient in defining her service needs and collaboratively designing and implementing services which directly reflect her goals (Kalinowski and Penney 1998, ch. 7).

In the *NHS Plan* (Department of Health 2000) the priority for mental health has been to ensure that people with severe and enduring mental illness receive services that are more responsive to their needs. In this policy document the government acknowledged that mental health services are not always sensitive to the needs of women. Recognising the fact that women are more likely than men to suffer from mental illness, the only planned change in the services to these women is that by 2004 they will be redesigned to ensure that women-only day centres are provided in every health authority.

Women should be consulted about the services that will be most likely to meet their needs, and service provision must be based on what women want. A range of services is needed: primary care and specialist mental health services, employment, education and training, housing and social support (Department of Health 1999). The services identified by MIND (1992) that women want are: crisis houses, information and advocacy, self-help and support groups, housing with flexible support, employment projects, counselling and therapy, telephone crisis services and support for carers. Women must be involved in defining the help they are looking for. The care programme approach introduced into the NHS in April 1991 aimed to provide a network of care in the community. One aspect of this provision is the appointment of a keyworker who will keep in close contact with the patient (Department of Health, 1990). Women clients in theory can choose a female keyworker.

MIND (1992) also suggested that mental health professionals, including post-qualified nurses, need training in gender issues. Specific issues that mental health professionals need to be aware of are: the impact of childhood abuse; the

impact of experiences of loss resulting from miscarriage, hysterectomy, mastec-
tomy and infertility and the impact of domestic violence on mental health. MIND
suggests that women who have experience of these problems have an input into
the training.

## CONCLUSION

Women have different mental health needs from those of men. Currently community services are provided on a generic basis; they are not adapted or tailored
to meet the specific needs of women, especially women with serious mental health
problems. The implication this has for women and practice is that service delivery
will be inappropriate in that it may deal with the mental illness but fail to deliver
what women want from community mental health nurses.

Women's mental health problems have often been linked to loss associated
with adverse life events including childhood sexual abuse, domestic violence and
miscarriage (MIND 1992). These underlying causes of mental illness for women
need to be recognised and addressed. Community mental health nurses when
aware of these issues tend to refer women to other relevant support organisations
such as rape crisis centres and refuges rather than deal with the underlying causes
of the presenting mental illness in an integrated and holistic way.

Effective delivery of services to women by community mental health nurses
will be based on a sound knowledge of gender issues and the specific causes of
mental illness in women. Post-registration courses for community mental health
nurses need to incorporate training in gender issues, drawing on relevant research
in this area; this gender awareness is fundamental to changing care for women
clients.

## REFERENCES

Broverman, I.K., Broverman, D., Clarkson, F., Rosenkrantz, P.S. and Vogel, S.R. (1970)
   'Sex-role stereotypes and clinical judgements of mental health', *Journal of Consulting
   and Clinical Psychology*, 34 (1): 1–7.
Brown, G.W. and Harris, T. (1978) *Social origins of depression: a study of psychiatric
   disorder in women*, London: Tavistock.
Busfield, J. (1989) 'Sexism and psychiatry', *Journal of Sociology*, 23 (3): 343–364.
Busfield, J. (1996) *Men, women and madness: understanding gender and mental disorder*,
   Basingstoke: Macmillan.
Chesler, P. (1972) 'Women and madness: the mental asylum', in Heller, T., Reynolds, T.,
   Gomm, R., Muston, R. and Pattison, S. (1996) *Mental health matters: a reader*,
   Basingstoke: Macmillan.
Cochrane, R. (1983) *The social creation of mental illness*, London: Longman.
Coyte, E. (2000) 'Stepping stones to inclusion', *Mental Health Practice*, 3 (5): 4–5.
Department of Health (1990) *The care programme approach for people with a mental
   illness referred to the specialist psychiatric services.* HC(90)23/LASSL(90)11, London:
   Department of Health.

Department of Health (1993) *The health of the nation key area handbook: mental illness*, London: Department of Health.

Department of Health (1999) *National service framework for mental health: modern standards and service models*, London: Department of Health.

Department of Health (2000) *The NHS Plan: a plan for investment, a plan for reform*, London: The Stationery Office.

Dohrenwend, B.P. and Dohrenwend, B.S. (1975–6) 'Sex differences and psychiatric disorders', *American Journal of Sociology*, 81 (6): 1447–1472.

Gove, W.R. (1978) 'Sex differences in mental illness among adult men and women: an evaluation of four questions raised regarding the evidence on the higher rates in women', *Journal of Social Science and Medicine*, 12B: 187–198.

Gove, W.R. and Tudor, J. (1972–3) 'Adult roles and mental illness', *American Journal of Sociology*, 78 (4–6): 50–73.

Graham, H. (1984) *Women, health and the family*, Brighton: Harvester Wheatsheaf.

Hargreaves, D.J. and Colley, A. (eds) (1986) *The psychology of sex roles*, London: Tavistock.

Johnstone, L. (1989) *Users and abusers of psychiatry: a critical look at traditional psychiatric practice*, London: Routledge.

Kalinowski, C. and Penney, D. (1998) 'Empowerment and women's mental health services', in Levin, B., Blanch, A. and Jennings, A. (eds) *Women's mental health services: a public health perspective*, London: Sage.

Kandel, D., Davies, M. and Raveis, V. (1985) 'The stressfulness of daily roles for women: marital, occupational and household roles', *Journal of Health and Social Behaviour*, 26: 64–78.

Kessler, R. and McRae, J. (1981) 'Trends in the relationship between sex and psychological distress 1957–1976', *American Sociological Review*, 46: 443–452.

Leeson, J. and Gray, J. (1978) *Women and medicine*, London: Tavistock.

Loring, M. and Powell, B. (1988) 'Gender, race, and DSM III: a study of the objectivity of psychiatric diagnostic behaviour', *Journal of Health and Social Behaviour*, 29: 1–22.

Miles, A. (1981) *The mentally ill in contemporary society: a sociological introduction*, Oxford: Martin Robertson.

MIND (1992) *Stress on women: policy paper on women and mental health*, London: MIND.

Morgan, S. (1993) *Community mental health: practical approaches to long-term problems*, London: Chapman and Hall.

Mowbray, C., Oyserman, D., Saunders, D. and Rueda-Riedle, A. (1998) 'Women with severe mental disorders: issues and service needs', in Levin, B., Blanch, A. and Jennings, A. (eds) *Women's mental health services: a public health perspective*, London: Sage.

Owen, S. and Milburn, C. (2001) 'Implementing research findings into practice: improving and developing services for women with serious and enduring mental health problems', *Journal of Psychiatric and Mental Health Nursing*, 8 (3): 221–231.

Penfold, P.S. and Walker, G.A. (1983) *Women and the psychiatric paradox*, Montreal: Eden Press.

Perkins, R.E. and Repper, J. (1996) *Working alongside people with long term mental health problems*, London: Chapman and Hall.

Pilgrim, D. and Rogers, A. (1999) *A sociology of mental health and illness*, 2nd edn, Buckingham: Open University Press.

Repper, J. (1998) 'Social exclusion and mental health problems', *Mental Health Practice*, 1 (8): 4–5.

Rosenfield, S. (1980) 'Sex differences in depression: do women always have higher rates?', *Journal of Health and Social Behaviour*, 21: 33–42.

Schur, E. (1984) *Labelling women deviant: gender, stigma and social control*, New York: Random House.

Segal, L. (1987) *Is the future female?*, London: Virago.

Smith, L. (1987) 'Women and mental health', in Orr, J. (ed.) *Women's health in the community*, Chichester: Wiley.

Warner, L. and Ford, R. (1998) 'Conditions for women in in-patient psychiatric units: the Mental Health Act Commission 1996 national visit', *Mental Health Care*, 1 (7): 225–228.

# FURTHER READING

Brown, G.W. and Harris, T. (1978) *Social origins of depression: a study of psychiatric disorder in women*, London: Tavistock.

This book is now a classic; the authors' work is still regularly referred to in more recent texts. The key finding of the research conducted was that depression in women is caused by social factors.

Busfield, J. (1996) *Men, women and madness: understanding gender and mental disorder*, Basingstoke: Macmillan.

Busfield's work inspired me to write my undergraduate dissertation on 'women and depression'. This book explores from a feminist/sociological perspective the explanations for the differentials between men's and women's mental health. I think it is a 'must read' for all practitioners who work with women or have an interest in gender issues and women's mental health.

Pilgrim, D. and Rogers, A. (1999) *A sociology of mental health and illness*, 2nd edn, Buckingham: Open University Press.

This book gives an excellent overview of the sociological perspectives on mental health and mental illness. The chapter on gender (chapter 3) includes theorising on why women are over-represented in mental health statistics, whether society causes female mental illness and whether women are labelled as mentally ill more often than men.

# CHAPTER 10

# CULTURE AND ETHNICITY

*Suman Fernando*

## SUMMARY OF KEY POINTS

- Mental health needs of black and Asian people in British society are not being met adequately by current mental health services.

- British society is multicultural but the disciplines of psychiatry and psychology that underpin mental health services are unicultural and often institutionally racist.

- Ethnic issues highlighted by black people – being over-represented among people sectioned under the Mental Health Act, diagnosed as 'schizophrenic', etc. – represent fundamental underlying problems in the practice of psychiatry, but these problems can be circumvented.

## INTRODUCTION

The National Service Framework for Mental Health (Department of Health 1999) states, under the heading 'Race and Mental Health': 'Combined evidence suggests that services are not adequately meeting mental health needs, and that black and minority ethnic communities lack confidence in mental health services' (p. 17). The author believes that this is a gross understatement as far as black and minority ethnic people are concerned. In fact, the experience of the mental health services by black and Asian people who access them is often so negative that many tend to avoid the services if at all possible. The unsatisfactory nature of the situation is represented in statistical and 'research' terms by black people being over-represented among people who are compulsorily detained ('sectioned') under the Mental Health Act, diagnosed as 'schizophrenic', admitted to hospital as 'offender patients', etc. The issues are well known (e.g. Fernando 1988, Department of Health and Home Office 1994) and have been discussed elsewhere (e.g. Fernando 1995a, Bhui and Olajide 1999). The need now is for community psychiatric nurses and other professionals in the mental health field to understand the underlying problems involved and move forward to redress the injustices and deficiencies.

This chapter considers briefly the basis for understanding the problems faced by black and Asian people when they access mental health services, and indicates ways in which the practice of psychiatry and psychiatric nursing may be changed so that these problems are minimised. First, it outlines the traditional practice of psychiatry as seen from a transcultural perspective and then considers briefly some of the underlying 'ethnic issues' that may be generating problems for black and minority ethnic communities. Second, the chapter suggests ways in which psychiatry may be practised in community mental health services in a way that is appropriate and just for the needs of a multicultural society.

In order to illustrate some of the points made in this chapter, brief vignettes of some true stories and incidents known to the author are described, but, to avoid any possibility of anyone being recognised, names of individuals mentioned in the case illustrations are fictitious and the case details have been altered, except in the case of a person called John whose details are already in the public domain as a result of a BBC television documentary now available as a video.

The term 'black' is used in this chapter to indicate people of African and black Caribbean backgrounds; the term 'Asian', 'Chinese' or 'minority ethnic' is used as appropriate to denote others who are regarded as, or regard themselves as, not being 'white'. The term 'multicultural society' is used to indicate the diversity in cultural background of people who constitute current British society (for discussion of the topic of 'ethnicity' and ethnic categories see chapter 1 in Fernando 2002; for discussion of 'multiculturalism' see Fernando 1995a).

## TRADITIONAL PSYCHIATRY

Psychiatry is based on the interpretation of mental health problems in terms of illness and, even more importantly from the point of view of a modern multicultural society, it reflects the ethos of a western vision of human experience – a view that emphasises individuality and a self-contained psyche. This means a perception of the human psyche as being more-or-less isolated within an individual who 'lives [primarily] in his [or her] own subjective world, pursuing personal pleasures and private fantasies, constructing a life and fate which will vanish when our time is over' (Kakar 1995, p. 83). Thus, when the western medical model is applied to interpreting problems located within this psyche, anything that interferes with the pursuit of pleasure or the achievement of such an (imagined) fate is seen as an impediment, something that is not required, an abnormality, and therefore gets labelled as 'psychopathology'. Further, this medical model conceptualises 'illness' as an event that 'affects' the individual (as an infection would), and so the psychiatric approach is to *attack* these psychopathological phenomena – 'symptoms' – in an effort to eradicate them or at least control them. Modern psychiatry emphasises the use of drugs as the main line of 'treatment' for attacking illness, but also gives some credence to counselling, psychotherapy and other psychological therapies as necessary adjuncts to (what is called) 'management' of the 'mental illness' that psychiatry diagnoses and locates in the individual psyche.

It is noteworthy that a western worldview that incorporates the idea (represented in psychiatry and psychology) of an individualised psyche that is prone to become 'disordered' or 'ill' is very different from the understandings of the human condition that pervade other cultural systems. In Asian and African traditions, medical belief systems concerned with ideas about health and illness, as well as the conceptualisation of mind and body, are different. In eastern traditions, health is seen as a harmonious balance between various forces in the person and the social context. The Chinese way of thinking sees illness as an imbalance of *yin* and *yang* (two complementary poles of life energy), to be corrected by attempts to re-establish 'balance' (Aakster 1986); the Indian tradition emphasises the harmony between the person and his/her group as indicative of health (Kakar 1982); and the concept of health in African culture is more social than biological (Lambo 1969). In all these non-western cultures, human life is conceptualised as an indivisible 'whole' that includes not just the western 'mind' and 'body' as one but also the spiritual dimension of human life. Further, knowledge generally does not (in non-western cultures) naturally divide up into the fields of study of 'psychology', 'religion', 'philosophy', as defined in the west.

## ETHNIC ISSUES

The understanding of issues concerned with culture and ethnicity developed within the framework of what is called 'transcultural psychiatry' – an interest arising from the encounter between, on the one hand, psychiatry, which developed in western Europe during the eighteenth and nineteenth centuries, and, on the other hand, people living in Africa and Asia and people from these continents who migrated (or were forced to do so) to America and Europe. The earliest transcultural observation is attributable to Kraepelin (1904). When this German psychiatrist noted that Javanese people who became depressed did not exhibit 'guilt', he concluded that they were 'a psychically underdeveloped population' akin to 'immature European youth' (Kraepelin 1921). Thus, transcultural psychiatry began with racist undertones – a tradition that continued when (for example) the apparent rarity of depression among Africans and African-Americans was attributed to their 'irresponsible' and 'unthinking' nature (Green 1914), and when Carl Jung (1930) stated that 'cultural' differences between white Europeans and white Americans were caused by 'racial infection' suffered by the latter from living too close to black people. In modern times the racism inherent in transcultural observations is reflected in the theory propounded by Leff (1973) that people from Africa and Asia and Black Americans (the politically 'Black') have a 'less developed' ability to differentiate emotions when compared with Europeans and white Americans, and the so-called 'finding' by Bebbington *et al.* (1981) that Black West Indians in Camberwell have relatively low rates of depression because they suffer from 'cheery denial'. (For further discussion of racism in psychiatry see Thomas and Sillen (1972) and Fernando (1988). For discussion of wider cultural issues in mental health see Fernando 2002.)

In the 1980s transcultural psychiatry in the UK – at least that version promoted by the Transcultural Psychiatry Society (UK) (TCPS) – shifted its focus from academic 'interest' in recording cultural differences between people looked at from the (ethnocentric) viewpoint of (western) psychiatry, to being a movement that examined the practice of psychiatry as experienced by black people and others whose cultural roots lie in Asia and Africa (Fernando 1988). And so today the confronting of racism in psychiatry is as much an aim of the current British version of 'transcultural psychiatry' as addressing the nature of psychiatry in a culturally diverse society.

Traditional psychiatric practice today is ethnocentric to western culture and often tends to be institutionally racist. The models used are often inappropriate in many respects for many of the clients accessing psychiatric services, mainly because these models fail to address the cultural diversity of society. Further, there is a problem around 'race'. Assessment, diagnosis and therapy are all carried out without much reference to the experiences of people who in society in general are seen as being racially different from the majority 'white' population – and psychiatry fails to allow for racist misperceptions and distortions that affect its practice. So, a significant aspect of the lives of black people in a racist society is discounted and the racist bias of the psychiatric process ignored. The result is that the mental health services are often experienced by black and Asian people as both racist and culturally insensitive. Although overt racial prejudice is occasionally a problem, much of the racism in British society experienced by black and Asian people today stems from institutional attitudes and processes that exist in virtually all systems they encounter, especially education, criminal justice and many employment systems.

Most black and Asian people deal with racism by learning strategies to side-step racism and/or counteract its effects on their psychological and social functioning. Usually, this learning takes place in families and communities. When black people come into contact with the psychiatric system, these strategies may sometimes be interpreted by mental health workers as symptoms of illness. For example, a heightened self-importance (as a strategy to counteract the debasing of self-esteem that racism promotes) may be seen as 'grandiosity'. Or a suspicion or avoidance of white society (as a strategy to protect oneself from being abused) may be seen as 'paranoia'. Once 'illness' is diagnosed, the risk is that the true nature of a situation is ignored and black people presenting to psychiatry get dealt with in an oppressive and damaging manner. Then, psychiatry becomes part of their problem rather than a process through which they can obtain help. The following three vignettes illustrate some of this.

Joseph was a black man in his late twenties when he was diagnosed as 'paranoid' because he was generally suspicious of people, and as 'deluded' because he believed that the police were out to 'get' black people. When he quarrelled with a social worker after the latter failed to keep her promise to get him a grant for further education, Joseph was deemed 'dangerous' and admitted to hospital compulsorily. Joseph isolated himself in hospital and when summoned to ward rounds dressed up in short trousers, a heavy overcoat and no shirt. He made fun of the (white) female nurses by asking them for sexual favours. The diagnosis of schizophrenia was applied on the basis of his alleged bizarre behaviour, inappropriate comments to female staff, withdrawal and paranoid delusions.

Joseph's own explanations for his behaviour were simple. He wore bizarre dress when he wished to show his disrespect. He made fun of people who talked down to him. His attitude to the police was consistent with his own experience as a black man in London and the fact that his brother had died in police custody – 'killed by the police'. Being labelled 'schizophrenic' was seen by him as his main impediment to getting on a course in his chosen career. He saw himself as being out of the ordinary – 'peculiar I suppose'. The only intervention in this instance by the author (as a visiting psychiatrist called upon to provide a second opinion on the need for medication) was to deny permission for the use of compulsory medication to 'control' his 'symptoms'.

Michael was a 34-year-old African-Caribbean man who was apprehended by the police when he attempted to force his attentions on an ex-girlfriend. When he talked of being the King of Barbados he was admitted to hospital compulsorily. Once he got over the initial trauma of admission, he talked calmly about his own importance. While still a young boy Michael had been told by his father, 'whatever white people do to you remember that you are of royal ancestry'; and his father gave him an ivory-headed walking stick to prove this background. It was this knowledge that had carried Michael through many adverse circumstances and he believed that he was destined to be an example to black youth in London. Once this man's beliefs were accepted as valid, he agreed to compromise with society by keeping them to himself even when he got excited under stress. He managed to do this, although with occasional lapses.

Jane was a 30-year-old black woman who was admitted after she set fire to some furniture in her flat. In the course of therapy she talked about her anger towards her (black) parents for 'pretending to be white' by living in a middle-class white area and denying the existence of racism. She had sought to destroy whatever she identified as property owned by white society, but eventually accepted a compromise of living in peace with society far away from her parents and the 'white society' of London that she had grown up in.

The brief vignettes described above represent people who survived abuse inflicted on them by the psychiatric system and were partly rescued through intervention that took them seriously as black people. However, there are a vast number of black people like them who have succumbed; many live destitute lives as 'chronic schizophrenics' heavily medicated – often to a zombie-like state – lost to society and themselves.

## PROMOTING MULTICULTURAL PRACTICE

The long-term answer to problems of race and culture in mental health services and psychiatry – represented above by 'ethnic issues' – lies in fundamental changes in psychiatry and psychology in conjunction with changes in society at large. These should include opening up the discipline to concepts of mental health from all cultures, getting away from the illness approach in mental health care, and reforming psychiatry within an anti-racist movement in society as a whole (Fernando 1995b). However, in the short term, we can aim to enable services to be 'culture-sensitive' and minimise the effects of institutional racism, taking note of the Macpherson definition of institutional racism:

> The collective failure of an organisation to provide an appropriate and professional service to people because of their colour, culture or ethnic origin. It can be seen or detected in processes, attitudes and behaviour which amount to discrimination through unwitting prejudice, igno-rance, thoughtlessness and racist stereotyping which disadvantages minority ethnic people.
>
> (Home Department 1999, p. 28)

Addressing race and culture problems boils down to two simple matters: counter-acting racism (including institutional racism in psychiatry and psychology); and enabling mental health services to encompass a wide cultural diversity both in theory and in practice. So, it may seem that strategies to address the problems should be fairly simple to devise. However, the reality is very different. The field of cultural diversity itself has many ramifications when one tries to apply it in ser-vice provision; and counteracting racism is far from simple. Traditional psychiatry is rooted in the era of institutional care epitomised by the asylums. The movement into community care provides an opportunity to change many of the dis-advantages suffered by clients of institutional care – and foremost among these must be the problems referred to above as 'ethnic issues'.

The primary basis for a mental health service in the statutory sector is a clear framework of policies that are set out and understood by everyone working in the service. In the case of a community service for a multicultural population these policies must address issues of culture and ethnicity, based on knowledge of the problems outlined above. Ongoing training in culture and ethnicity should be established within this framework. However, training should not be seen as a circumscribed event or process. In this field, training is a matter of continuous reappraisal and practice. Thus, there is a need for policies that enable profes-sionals to both challenge racism and promote cultural sensitivity actively by observing practice and checking out the need for changes. If racism is detected, it needs to be challenged, and lessons learned from incidents need to be fed back into the system – especially in the case of institutionalised racism. When cultural insensitivity is seen, there must be means of obtaining help and guidance and, again, feeding back the lessons learned from incidents. These matters have been discussed in some detail elsewhere (e.g. Ferns and Madden 1995).

Psychiatry is based on a system of diagnosing, looking for causes, and finding cures. The current Mental Health Act is based on this approach and what goes for 'normal practice' is judged by it. So anyone working in the community mental health field has to keep to this model as much as possible. However, even while keeping to this approach, it is possible – indeed essential – to be mindful of the multicultural nature of society, and the limitations of applying an essentially unicultural body of knowledge from psychiatry and psychology. The first thing is to be sensitive to culturally diverse ways of feeling and expressing distress and to various explanatory models (for distress) held by people of different cultures – some of which the professionals may be unaware of and few of which are accepted by traditional psychiatry. Secondly, the professional, be they white, black or Asian, has to make a definite attempt to be anti-racist in their work with service users. It should be obligatory on all professionals to understand the nature of institutional racism as well as the nature of their own prejudices. They would then be in a position to correct their own – and other people's – behaviour and to set up services that address racism. The most important element in achieving all this is vigilance; one needs to examine oneself continuously and consistently for signs of racist practice and cultural insensitivity. And one needs to examine the practice of other people around –the rest of the multidisciplinary team – and the service users. This topic is addressed in greater depth elsewhere (Fernando 2002).

# DIAGNOSIS AND THERAPY

It is now well established that the cross-cultural validity of current diagnostic categories is often dubious (see Fernando 2002). Indeed, some diagnoses, such as 'schizophrenia', may have a racist bias in the way they are used (Fernando 1998). Yet diagnoses are so much a part of the system that procures resources for people in need that the option *not* to make diagnoses in an NHS psychiatric setting (if one wants to use resources) is sometimes not available. Therefore professionals in community care practice need to be sceptical about making *any* diagnosis, and, if a diagnosis has to be made, the extent to which racist stereotypes affect diagnoses must be foremost in their mind. At all times it is necessary to be mindful of the *meaning* of making a diagnosis in a multicultural and multiracial setting. Ideally, diagnosis must be marginal to the main assessment – and that must be geared to what is best in the circumstances, taking note of all aspects of a person's life. If a diagnosis is made, its meaning must be discussed with the client concerned and (if possible) with his or her family. The diagnosis should never be seen as a fixed entity; the professional must be prepared to alter the diagnosis whenever the 'clinical picture' changes, since it merely reflects the nature of (what are seen as) 'symptoms'. Most importantly, diagnosis must be separated from therapy as much as possible.

Great care in listening to clients with respect is the bedrock of good psychiatric practice in a multicultural society. Thus all 'symptoms' must be explored as to their meaning, be they (psychiatrically speaking) delusions, hallucinations or any other so-called 'psychopathology'. The following vignette of a person dealt with by the author, when called in as an 'independent psychiatrist' to provide a report for a Mental Health Review Tribunal, illustrates some aspects of the approach that is being suggested.

The case of John was depicted in a documentary film (BBC 1995) made at a hospital in South London. John was a young black man from Ghana who claimed that he was born white and was related to the (English) Queen. The consultant psychiatrist in charge of John's case, the 'responsible medical officer' (RMO), argued that John required treatment under a compulsory order ('sectioning') of the Mental Health Act, while the independent psychiatrist (IP) argued that this was not necessary. Both psychiatrists agreed that a diagnosis of 'mental disorder' was appropriate. The RMO considered John's beliefs to be delusions that required treatment with medication, while the IP argued that his 'delusions' needed to be dealt with by analysing their meaning for John – a meaning that emanated from his childhood background in a colonial country and his experiences in a racist Britain. The IP foresaw a situation whereby John's beliefs might be suppressed and his personality destroyed by heavy medication if sectioning and committal to a traditional psychiatric hospital were allowed. In the circumstances (as the film shows so clearly) this is exactly what happened.

In a multicultural setting there would be (culturally determined) diversity in the meaning and aims of therapy. The professionals concerned may not always understand the nature or extent of this diversity. Therefore, an open exploration of therapeutic possibilities must be undertaken with the service user before any decisions are made about therapy. And the degree to which family members of the client are involved in decision-making about therapy needs to be investigated, taking on the cultural diversity of service users' views and feelings on the subject. However, great care is necessary to avoid falling into assumptions based on stereotypes of family relationships. On the whole, therapy must be geared to problems identified by the service user and his or her family, rather than diagnosis made by professionals. However, the balance of the influence of each (i.e. diagnosis vs. problems) may vary and careful assessment may be needed, taking on a variety of dimensions of a person's life. The following vignette illustrates some aspects of the approach suggested here.

Abdul was about 19 when he first presented at a psychiatric unit because he had assaulted his father. Abdul had arrived in the UK a few weeks earlier from Bangladesh to join his father and his stepmother. In hospital, although he could not communicate very well in English, Abdul claimed that he was a doctor. At times he took other people's possessions saying he owned them, and became very agitated when frustrated in this. No diagnosis was made but a small dose of a tranquilliser calmed him considerably and he returned home. The conclusion was that Abdul's problems resulted from conflicts in the family. Abdul assaulted his father again and was then arrested by the police because the hospital stated that he had no mental illness. A few days later, his father brought him to the hospital because he had been physically injured while in the custody of the police. A decision was then made that he did have a diagnosis of 'psychotic state' and that any further incidents should be dealt with by mental health staff as 'illness' rather than being reported to the police. Abdul gradually worked through his family problems and finally left to live in a hostel where there were several other Bangladeshi people.

## CONCLUSION

Traditional psychiatry is ethnocentric and racist in practice. The shift from institution-based psychiatry to community mental health care provides an opportunity for community psychiatric nurses and other professionals to move away from some of the traditional practices in order to create services that are culturally sensitive and minimise the effects of institutional racism. This involves careful planning, enlightened policies and well-constructed and facilitated ongoing training of staff, based on a full understanding of both cultural diversity and racism.

## REFERENCES

Aakster, C.W. (1986) 'Concepts in alternative medicine', *Social Science and Medicine*, 22: 265–273.

BBC (1995) *Minders (States of Mind): whose mind is it anyway?* Video for education and training, London: British Broadcasting Corporation.

Bebbington, P. E., Hurry, J. and Tennant, C. (1981) 'Psychiatric disorders in selected immigrant groups in Camberwell', *Social Psychiatry*, 16: 43–51.

Bhui, K. and Olajide, D. (1999) *Mental health service provision for a multi-cultural society*, London: Saunders.

Department of Health (1999) *National service framework for mental health: modern standards and service models*, London: Department of Health.

Department of Health and Home Office (1994) *Review of health and social services for mentally disordered offenders and others requiring similar services* (Chairman, Dr John Reed), vol. 6, *Race, gender and equal opportunities*, London: HMSO.

Fernando, S. (1988) *Race and culture in psychiatry*, London: Croom Helm; reprinted as paperback 1989, London: Routledge.

Fernando, S. (1995a) 'Social realities and mental health', in Fernando, S. (ed.) *Mental health in a multi-ethnic society*, London: Routledge.

Fernando, S. (1995b) 'The way forward', in Fernando, S. (ed.) *Mental health in a multi-ethnic society*, London: Routledge.

Fernando, S. (1998) 'Modern schizophrenia and racism', in Fernando, S., Ndegwa, D. and Wilson, M. (eds) *Forensic psychiatry, race and culture*, London: Routledge.

Fernando, S. (2002) *Mental health, race and culture*, 2nd edn, London: Palgrave.

Ferns, P. and Madden, M. (1995) 'Training to promote racial equality', in Fernando, S. (ed.) *Mental health in a multi-ethnic society*, London: Routledge.

Green, E.M. (1914) 'Psychoses among negroes – a comparative study', *Journal of Nervous and Mental Disorder*, 41: 697–708.

Home Department (1999) *The Stephen Lawrence inquiry. Report of an inquiry by Sir William Macpherson of Cluny*, London: The Stationery Office.

Jung, C.G. (1930) 'Your Negroid and Indian behaviour', *Forum*, 83 (4): 193–199.

Kakar, S. (1982) *Shamans, mystics and doctors. A psychological inquiry into India and its healing tradition*, New York: Knopf; republished 1984, London: Unwin Paperbacks; and 1991, Chicago: University of Chicago Press.

Kakar, S. (1995) 'Modern psychotherapies in traditional cultures: India, China, and Japan', in Kang, S. (ed.) *Psychotherapy east and west. Integration of psychotherapies*, Seoul: Korean Academy of Psychotherapy.

Kraepelin, E. (1904) 'Vergleichende Psychiatrie', *Zentralblatt Nervenheilkunde und Psychiatrie*, 27: 433–437; trans. Marshall, H., in Hirsch, S.R. and Shepherd, M. (eds) (1974) *Themes and variations in European psychiatry*, Bristol: Wright.

Kraepelin, E. (1921) *Manic-depressive insanity and paranoia*, trans. and ed. Barclay, R.M. and Robertson, G.M., Edinburgh: Livingstone.

Lambo, A. (1969) 'Traditional African cultures and Western medicine', in Poynter, F.N.L. (ed.) *Medicine and culture*, London: Wellcome Institute of History of Medicine.

Leff, J. (1973) 'Culture and the differentiation of emotional states', *British Journal of Psychiatry*, 123: 299–306.

Thomas, A. and Sillen, S. (1972) *Racism and psychiatry*, New York: Brunner/Mazel.

## FURTHER READING

Dutt, R. and Ferns, P. (1999) *Letting through light*, London: Department of Health and Race Equality Unit (available from Department of Health, London).
A workbook for multidisciplinary training in mental health, but it is essential that whoever leads this training is familiar with the book beforehand and is trained themselves.

D'Ardenne, P. and Mahtani, A. (1999) *Transcultural counselling in action*, 2nd edn, London: Sage.
The best available practical guide for professionals (who may be from any of the disciplines that comprise mental health teams) who wish to undertake counselling in a multicultural setting.

Fernando, S. (2002) *Mental health, race and culture*, 2nd edn, London: Palgrave.
A general text that covers a wide range of topics presented in fairly simple language.

# CHAPTER 11

# STRESS, BURNOUT AND COPING

*Deborah Edwards*

---

## SUMMARY OF KEY POINTS

- Community mental health nurses' responses to stressful situations are dependent on a variety of factors, including type of client group worked with, encouragement and support that they receive from their line managers, and security of the working environment.

- Burnout may be the end result, which represents the outcome of a prolonged process of attempting to cope with the demands of stress.

- Intervention strategies should be aimed at both the primary and secondary levels of stress management, thereby attempting to prevent stress from occurring as well as treating the consequences.

---

## INTRODUCTION

There is a growing body of evidence that suggests that community mental health nurses (CMHNs) experience considerable stress and burnout. The first part of the chapter aims to bring together the research evidence in this area for CMHNs working within the United Kingdom. The second part of the chapter focuses on coping strategies and management support issues.

## BACKGROUND

In the mental health field, care is increasingly being provided in community settings, involving workers representing a range of agencies and professions. In 1996, in the most recent quinquennial community mental health nursing survey, the total community mental health nursing workforce in England and Wales was estimated at just under 7,000 (Brooker and White 1997). Community mental health nurses play a key role in providing and co-ordinating a variety of services to people experiencing mental health problems including those suffering from severe and enduring mental illness such as schizophrenia.

In recent years there has been much concern over the job-related satisfactions and difficulties of mental health nurses working in the community setting (Kipping and Hickey 1998). Rees and Smith (1991) identified mental health nurses as one of the professional groups with the highest sources of stress, along with speech therapists. Increasing workloads, increasing administration and lack of resources have been indicated as sources of increasing stress and burnout for health professionals working as part of community mental health teams (Edwards et al. 2000).

This chapter first seeks to review the literature for CMHNs in relation to stress and burnout and will then move on to explore the issue of coping and stress management interventions.

## STRESS AND BURNOUT

Carson et al. (1991) conducted preliminary investigations of stress in community mental health nursing. The findings gathered from open-ended interviews suggested that the most stressful aspects of the CMHN's job were lack of facilities for referral, potential violence from clients, and too many interruptions when trying to work in the office (Carson and Bartlett 1993). This preliminary investigation led to the development of the community psychiatric nursing (CPN) stress questionnaire (Brown et al. 1995), which was demonstrated to be a reliable and valid measure of occupational stress in community mental health nurses. This tool revealed areas of stress to include professional isolation and ineffective communication channels as well as inadequate support, supervision and training (Leary et al. 1995). The finalised questionnaire was utilised to determine levels and sources of stress in the Claybury CPN stress study for 245 community mental health nurses and 323 ward-based nurses in the Northeast Thames Regional Health Authority. The results for CMHNs revealed that the greatest stressors were: not having enough facilities in the community to refer your clients on to; knowing that there were long waiting lists; and having to deal with suicidal clients. Other findings were that 41 per cent of CMHNs were vulnerable to psychological distress. With regard to burnout, 1 in 2 reported being seriously emotionally drained, 1 in 4 had lost the ability to feel for clients, and 1 in 5 reported not achieving personal fulfilment from their work (Carson et al. 1995, Fagin et al. 1995).

The authors reported that the Claybury study was carried out during a time of transition and major change. This was revealed as CMHNs who were under the most stress were taking more sick leave, had higher caseloads and lower self-esteem, felt unfulfilled in their work and generally felt unhappy about their lives. This in turn affected their relationships with clients and their ability to empathise. Despite this the CMHNs were committed to and satisfied with their direct work with clients. However, they reported dissatisfaction with their working conditions and environment, the resources available, the support they received from line managers and the reward they got for their labours (Carson *et al.* 1995, 1996a).

Four further studies have utilised the CPN stress questionnaire. The first was conducted by Schafer (1992) to assess the effect of organisational change as one cohesive unit of CMHNs split into three functional units, in west Essex. Results from the research indicated that reorganisation into functional units was associated with greater levels of stress. However, the results did not reach statistical significance, which was probably due to the small sample size. Drake and Brimblecombe (1999) found that working in a team providing rapid assessment and intensive home treatment for those with severe acute mental health problems was not necessarily more stressful than working in a generic team.

Research conducted by Coffey (1999) using the CPN stress questionnaire revealed that concerns of forensic community mental health nurses (FCMHNs) were similar to findings for generic CMHNs from other studies, i.e. lack of facilities and interruptions in the office. Dealing with violent patients did not feature in the top ten stressors, although dealing with suicidal patients did. Burnout was also investigated, with just over 1 in 2 being emotionally drained.

The all Wales community mental health nurse (CMHN) stress study is the largest study undertaken in the UK to date to investigate stress, burnout and coping amongst the CMHN workforce (Burnard *et al.* 2000, Coyle *et al.* 2000, Edwards *et al.* 2000, Fothergill *et al.* 2000, Hannigan *et al.* 2000). Questionnaires were sent out to 614 CMHNs from ten NHS trusts throughout Wales, with 49 per cent responding. Community mental health nurses indicated that trying to maintain a good-quality service in the midst of long waiting lists, poor resources, and having too many interruptions while trying to work in the office were particularly stressful items, as identified by the CPN stress questionnaire. Forty per cent of CMHNs tended to view themselves negatively, feeling that others did not hold much respect for them. Thirty-five per cent of CMHNs were vulnerable to psychological distress. Measured against a normative sample of mental health workers, 51 per cent of CMHNs were experiencing high levels of long-term emotional exhaustion. Twenty-four per cent were suffering from high levels of depersonalisation burnout and were not relating well to clients, whilst 14 per cent were experiencing severe long-term feelings of lack of personal accomplishment.

Other studies on CMHNs and stress have utilised their own questionnaires to determine a number of issues. McLeod (1997) conducted a small study to determine whether stress levels of CMHNs varied with type of clients catered for. The results indicated that CMHNs working with long-term mentally ill clients reported higher caseloads, less training, lack of respect and understanding of their role, and the need for more supervision and support. However, the sample size was too small for any inferences to be made and there was no statistical evidence presented to support the findings.

In a study conducted in Northern Ireland, Parahoo (1991) identified 30 factors that contributed to CMHNs' job satisfaction, and 36 factors that contributed to their dissatisfaction. The most frequently identified factors contributing to job satisfaction were 'working independently', 'being one's own manager' and 'being an independent practitioner'. The respondents indicated that working in a team can be both satisfying and frustrating. Seventy per cent of CMHNs rated their job satisfaction as 'high' or 'very high'.

Snelgrove (1998) compared stress levels of CMHNs and other community nurses. The study showed that there were significant differences in stress levels between health visitors, community psychiatric nurses and district nurses, and this was found to be a function of occupation. It was suggested that these differences could be attributed to differences in caseloads, with health visitors seeing a larger proportion of children. Community mental health nurses reported lower stress than both health visitors and district nurses.

Parry-Jones and Grant (1998) looked at the impact of care management practice in Wales amongst social workers, community nurses and CMHNs, two years after the implementation of the NHS and Community Care Act 1990. This research was undertaken using a postal questionnaire that the authors had developed themselves based on the work of Nolan et al. (1995). The research indicated increases in stress and decreases in job satisfaction, which were associated with increased workload and administrative duties combined with reduced time for service user and family contact. However, the generalisability of these findings is limited due to the low response rate (30.8 per cent) and small number of CMHNs (15 per cent) included in the study.

The greater autonomy of CMHNs and the nature of their role in the community suggest that the work might be more stressful than that of mental health nurses working in large hospitals (Carson and Bartlett 1993). However, there is a lack of consensus on this issue. Fagin et al. (1995) indicated that although it appeared to be more stressful to work in the community, CMHNs found their jobs more rewarding than hospital-based nurses and had better therapeutic relationships with their clients (Carson et al. 1995). However, work conducted by the same research team a few years later, on a nationwide level, provided conflicting results, with CMHNs and their hospital counterparts having experienced similar levels of stress (Carson et al. 1997). Research carried out by Fielding and Weaver (1994) confirmed this finding, with no differences detected between the two groups with regard to levels of stress and burnout. However, community-based nurses described their work environment more positively, reported higher levels of concern and commitment to their jobs and had more supportive supervisors than their hospital-based colleagues. Results from both these studies have limited generalisability, however, due to the small sample size (Fielding and Weaver 1994) and poor response (Carson et al. 1997).

The studies presented here are all cross-sectional and there is a need for more longitudinal research to look at the longer-term effects of stress and burnout on work performance, job satisfaction and absenteeism over time. Only one such study has been conducted to date for community and hospital mental health based staff (Prosser et al. 1999). There was no evidence to suggest that levels of stress or burnout were increasing over time. In this study, however, high turnover of staff meant that few workers from the original phase of the research were still employed at the study's end.

Other work in this area has looked at all members of community mental health teams. Prosser *et al.* (1996, 1997) looked at the differences between hospital and community mental health staff (n=121, response rate 76 per cent), in an inner city team in London, in relation to perceived sources of work stress and job satisfaction. Community staff were more emotionally drained and vulnerable to psychological distress than hospital in-patient, day-care and out-patient staff. Job satisfaction, however, did not vary between the settings. Important sources of stress for community workers were perceived to be increased workload and administration.

In 1993, two large-scale national surveys by the Sainsbury Centre for Mental Health attempted to capture data on the current organisation and operation of CMHTs (Onyett *et al.* 1994, 1995, 1996). A total of 517 teams in 144 district health authorities were identified. Data were obtained from a sample of 60 individuals from 302 teams to examine burnout, job satisfaction, team role clarity, personal role clarity, team and professional identification, sources of pressure and reward, and features of practice (e.g. caseload size and composition). The major concerns of team members were threats to their efficacy arising from lack of resources, work overload and bureaucracy. Team members cited contact with team colleagues and multidisciplinary working as being the most rewarding part of their job, along with working directly with clients and being clinically effective (Onyett *et al.* 1995). Generally job satisfaction was high among team members, particularly where they had a positive sense of belonging to the team and were clear about its role. However, 45 per cent of CMHNs fell into the 'high' burnout category for emotional exhaustion.

In 1994, the Sainsbury Mental Health Initiative awarded a total of £3 million to eight projects in England and Wales to set up innovative services in the community. Seven of these sites included some sort of community team. The study aimed to examine the impact on practitioners involved in working in the new community teams with the most severely ill clients (Harper and Minghella 1997). Burnout levels were low, and this is to be expected, given that these were new services to which most CMHT members had been especially recruited within the previous year. There were no differences in burnout between the different members of the CMHTs. Community mental health teams reported high job satisfaction. The 'intrinsic' aspects of their work were described as being the most rewarding, along with seeing the patients and service improve, and working within teams. Working structures, lack of resources and, above all, management problems were the main sources of pressure.

Wykes *et al.* (1997) asked the question 'is community care sustainable?' by examining the levels of stress and burnout that affect community mental health staff. Results indicated that community care staff experienced high levels of burnout as a result of work stressors. Levels were higher than those found in any published study of health professionals within hospitals, but similar to those found in community teams.

## COPING

Studies into coping are many, with some focusing on coping strategies within the workplace. However, many of these seem to be of limited use when attempting to focus on the working world of health care professionals. Occupational stress studies that do exist for psychiatric nurses have used a variety of methods to evaluate coping skills. These include:

- the use of a coping scale (Sullivan 1993, Fagin *et al* 1995, Ryan and Quayle 1999);
- open-ended questions, such as 'what helps you best to cope with the pressures of a job', on a questionnaire (Kipping and Hickey 1998, Coffey 1999, Burnard *et al*. 2000);
- focus groups and semi-structured interviews (Trygstad 1986, Hopkinson *et al*. 1998);
- stress management intervention studies (Milne *et al*. 1986, Watson 1986, Kunkler and Whittick 1991, Carson and Kuipers 1998, Lemma 2000).

Even less literature exists when narrowing the search to the experience of coping within community psychiatric nursing. In the Claybury community psychiatric nursing (CPN) stress study, researchers using a generic coping skills scale found that nurses scored high on involvement (the level and degree to which an individual identifies with the tasks within work) and task strategies (dealing with stress by reorganising workload) (Fagin *et al*. 1995).

Carson *et al*. (1996b) questioned the use of a generic coping questionnaire applied to mental health nurses. The generic scale used in the Claybury study was designed for use within industry and may not be sensitive or robust enough to measure the inherent work-related stress of mental health nurses. It has been well established that the stressors encountered by mental health nurses are different from those that affect general nurses and that a specific set of coping strategies may be required to deal with them. A pilot study was therefore conducted to develop a new measure of coping skills for mental health nurses, the Psychnurse Methods of Coping Questionnaire. This is a 35-item scale, which was based on the work of Moos (Moos *et al*. 1984) and previous research conducted by the team (Carson *et al*. 1996b). This new measure was demonstrated to be a more suitable measure for mental health nurses than a generic coping skills scale (McElfatrick *et al*. 2000).

Further work was conducted using the Psychnurse tool by the all Wales CPN stress survey (Coyle *et al*. 2000). In terms of the validity of the tool, the results almost mirrored those previously reported by the authors. Of the five subscales the two strategies that were utilised the most were diverting one's attention away from work and having a positive attitude towards one's role at work. By viewing their role at work positively the CMHNs managed to overcome the kinds of stress created by working in often difficult situations and sometimes with challenging and difficult clients.

Studies that have asked CMHNs to report what they consider helps them to cope with stress in the workplace (Carson *et al*. 1999, Carroll 2000, Coffey 2000, Coyle *et al*. 2000) have reported the following:

- use of social support;
- having stable relationships;
- ability to recognise own limitations;
- ability to deal with problems immediately they occur;
- peer support;
- good, content home life/family/partner;
- interests outside of work.

Some coping strategies build upon structures available within the workplace such as supervision and staff support groups. This suggests that the organisation can play a role in helping with stress. The evidence from the literature is inconsistent. Kipping and Hickey (1998) found that the majority of respondents did not mention such structures. Reid *et al*. (1999) found that supervision was the most frequently mentioned as an important way of coping with difficult or stressful situations. Staff reported supervision to be supportive and educational, and helpful in managing caseloads and as a forum for training and development of their careers. However, only a third of staff mentioned supervision spontaneously when asked more open questions about important sources of support and coping.

# CONCLUSION

Community mental health nurses' responses to stressful situations are dependent on a variety of factors, including type of client group worked with, encouragement and support that they receive from their line managers, and security of the working environment. Burnout may be the end result, and represents the outcome of a prolonged process of attempting to cope with the demands of stress.

The consequences of stress and burnout in the workplace impact both on the individual and on the organisation. This affects not only the level of performance and success of interventions, but also job satisfaction and ultimately mental and physical health (Carson and Fagin 1996), and can lead to absenteeism and labour turnover (Sutherland and Cooper 1990).

It has been reported that many nurses leave the profession because they find the job stressful and feel unsupported (Thomas 1997). Prosser *et al*. (1999) found that high turnover of staff meant that few workers from the original phase of his research were employed at the study's end. A similar high rate of turnover was reported by Wykes *et al*. (1997), who found that only 28 per cent of those working in community teams had been in the same post for over five years.

In order to prevent large numbers of CMHNs from taking time off sick due to stress, or leaving the profession altogether, intervention strategies should be aimed at both the primary and secondary levels of stress management, thereby attempting to prevent stress from occurring as well as treating the consequences. The literature indicates that the most helpful strategies are those that combine individual strategies (relaxation, exercise, time management, etc.) and changes in the organisational environment. Further research is needed in order to evaluate the effectiveness of such strategies. As this chapter has demonstrated, we know a great deal about the sources of stress at work, about how to measure them, and about their impact on a range of outcome indicators. What is lacking is a translation of these results into practice, into research that assesses the impact of interventions that attempt to moderate, minimise or eliminate some of these stressors.

# REFERENCES

Brooker, C. and White, E. (1997) *The fourth quinquennial national community mental health nursing census of England and Wales*, Manchester and Keele: Universities of Manchester and Keele.

Brown, D., Leary, J., Carson, J., Bartlett, H. and Fagin, L. (1995) 'Stress and the community mental health nurse: the development of a measure', *Journal of Psychiatric and Mental Health Nursing*, 2: 9–12.

Burnard, P., Edwards, D., Fothergill, A., Hannigan, B. and Coyle, D. (2000) 'Community mental health nurses in Wales: self reported stressors and coping strategies', *Journal of Psychiatric and Mental Health Nursing*, 7: 523–528.

Carroll, L. (2000) 'Community psychiatric nursing within a climate of change: a study to identify perceptions of stress and coping strategies' (personal communication).

Carson, J. and Bartlett, H. (1993) 'Stress and the CPN (community psychiatric nurse)', *Nursing Times*, 89 (3): 38–40.

Carson, J. and Fagin, L. (1996) 'Editorial: Stress in mental health professionals: a cause for concern or an inevitable part of the job?' *International Journal of Social Psychiatry*, 42: 79–81.

Carson, J. and Kuipers, E. (1998) 'Stress management interventions', in Hardy, S., Carson, J. and Thomas, B. (eds) *Occupational stress: personal and professional approaches*, London: Stanley Thornes.

Carson, J., Bartlett, H. and Croucher, P. (1991) 'Stress in community psychiatric nursing: a preliminary investigation', *Community Psychiatric Nursing Journal*, 12 (2): 8–12.

Carson, J., Leary, J., De Villiers, N., Fagin, L. and Radmall, J. (1995) 'Stress in mental health nurses: comparison of ward and community staff', *British Journal of Nursing*, 4 (10): 579–582.

Carson, J., Brown, D., Fagin, L., Leary, J. and Bartlett, H. (1996a) 'Do larger caseloads cause greater stress in community mental health nurses?', *Journal of Clinical Nursing*, 5 (2): 133–134.

Carson, J., Cooper, C., Fagin, L., West, M., McElfatrick, S., De Villiers, N., O'Malley, P. and Holloway, F. (1996b) 'Coping skills in mental health nursing: do they make a difference?', *Journal of Psychiatric and Mental Health Nursing*, 3: 201–202.

Carson, J., Wood, M., White, H. and Thomas, B. (1997) 'Stress in mental health nursing: findings from the Mental Health Care survey', *Mental Health Care*, 1 (1): 11–14.

Carson, J., Maal, S., Roche, S., Fagin, L., De Villiers, N., O'Malley, P., Brown, D., Leary, J. and Holloway, F. (1999) 'Burnout in mental health nurses: much ado about nothing?', *Stress Medicine*, 15 (2): 127–134.

Coffey, M. (1999) 'Stress and burnout in forensic community mental health nurses: an investigation of its causes and effects', *Journal of Psychiatric and Mental Health Nursing*, 6: 433–443.

Coffey, M. (2000) 'Stress and coping in forensic community mental health nurses: demographic information and qualitative findings', *NT Research* 5 (2): 100–114.

Coyle, D., Edwards, D., Hannigan, B., Burnard, P. and Fothergill, A. (2000) 'An explanation of coping strategies used by community psychiatric nurses in Wales', *Nursing and Health Sciences*, 2: 59–67.

Drake, M. and Brimblecombe, N. (1999) 'Stress in community mental health nursing: comparing teams', *Mental Health Nursing*, 19 (1): 14–15.

Edwards, D., Burnard, P., Coyle, D., Fothergill, A. and Hannigan, B. (2000) 'Stressors, moderators and stress outcomes: findings from the all Wales community mental health nurse study', *Journal of Psychiatric and Mental Health Nursing*, 7: 529–538.

Fagin, L., Brown, D., Bartlett, H., Leary, J. and Carson, J. (1995) 'The Claybury community psychiatric nurse stress study: is it more stressful to work in hospital or the community?', *Journal of Advanced Nursing* , 22 (2): 347–358.

Fielding, J. and Weaver, S.M. (1994) 'A comparison of hospital and community based mental health nurses: perceptions of their work environment and psychological health', *Journal of Advanced Nursing*, 19 (6): 1196–1204.

Fothergill, A., Edwards, D., Hannigan, B., Burnard, P. and Coyle, D. (2000) 'Self esteem in community mental health nurses: findings from the all-Wales stress study', *Journal of Psychiatric and Mental Health Nursing*, 7: 315–322.

Hannigan, B., Edwards, D., Coyle, D., Fothergill, A. and Burnard, P. (2000) 'Burnout in community mental health nurses: findings from all Wales stress study', *Journal of Psychiatric and Mental Health Nursing*, 7: 127–134.

Harper, H. and Minghella, E. (1997) 'Pressures and rewards of working in community mental health teams', *Mental Health Care*, 1 (1): 18–21.

Hopkinson, P.J., Carson, J., Brown, D., Fagin, L., Bartlett, H. and Leary, J. (1998) 'Occupational stress and community mental health nursing: what CPNs really said', *Journal of Advanced Nursing*, 27 (4): 707–712.

Kipping, C.J. and Hickey, G. (1998) 'Exploring mental health nurses' expectations and experiences of working in the community', *Journal of Clinical Nursing*, 7 (6): 531–538.

Kunkler, J. and Whittick, J. (1991) 'Stress-management groups for nurses: practical problems and possible solutions', *Journal of Advanced Nursing*, 16: 172–176.

Leary, J., Gallagher, T., Carson, J., Fagin, L., Bartlett, H. and Brown, D. (1995) 'Stress and coping strategies in community psychiatric nurses: a Q-methodological study', *Journal of Advanced Nursing*, 21 (2): 230–237.

Lemma, A. (2000) 'Containing the containers. The effects of training and support on burnout in psychiatric nurses', Surrey University, unpublished Psychol.D. thesis.

McElfatrick, S., Carson, J., Annett, J., Cooper, C.L., Holloway, F. and Kuipers, E. (2000) 'Assessing coping skills in mental health nurses: is an occupation specific measure better than a generic coping skills scale?', *Personality and Individual Differences*, 28: 965–976.

McLeod, T. (1997) 'Work stress among community psychiatric nurses', *British Journal of Nursing*, 6 (10): 569–574.

Milne, D., Burdett, C. and Beckett, J. (1986) 'Assessing and reducing the stress and strain of psychiatric nursing', *Nursing Times*, 82 (19): 59–62.

Moos, R.H., Cronkite, R.C., Billings, A.G. and Finney, J.W. (1984) *Health and daily living form manual*, Palo Alto, CA: Consulting Psychologist Press.

Nolan, P., Cushway, D. and Tyler, P. (1995) 'A measurement tool for assessing stress among mental health nurses', *Nursing Standard*, 9 (46): 36–39.

Onyett, S., Pillinger, T. and Bushnell, D. (1994) 'A national survey of community mental health teams', *Journal of Mental Health*, 3: 175–194.

Onyett, S., Pillinger, T. and Muijen, M. (1995) *Making community mental health teams work*, London: Sainsbury Centre for Mental Health.

Onyett, S., Pillinger, T. and Muijen, M. (1996) 'Job satisfaction and burnout among members of community mental health teams', *Journal of Mental Health*, 6 (1): 55–66.

Parahoo, K. (1991) 'Job satisfaction of community psychiatric nurses in Northern Ireland', *Journal of Advanced Nursing*, 16 (3): 317–324.

Parry-Jones, B. and Grant, G. (1998) 'Stress and job satisfaction among social workers, community nurses and community psychiatric nurses: implications for the care management model', *Health and Social Care in the Community*, 6 (4): 271–285.

Prosser, D., Johnson, S., Kuipers, E., Szmukler, G., Bebbington, P. and Thornicroft, G. (1996) 'Mental health, "burnout" and job satisfaction among hospital and community-based mental health staff', *British Journal of Psychiatry*, 169 (3): 334–337.

Prosser, D., Johnson, S., Kuipers, E., Szmukler, G., Bebbington, P. and Thornicroft, G. (1997) 'Perceived sources of work stress and satisfaction among hospital and community mental health staff, and their relation to mental health, burnout and job satisfaction', *Journal of Psychosomatic Research*, 43 (1): 51–59.

Prosser, D., Johnson, S., Kuipers, E., Dunn, G., Szmukler, G., Reid, Y., Bebbington, P. and Thornicroft, G. (1999) 'Mental health, "burnout" and job satisfaction in a longitudinal study of mental health staff', *Social Psychiatry and Psychiatric Epidemiology*, 34 (6): 295–300.

Rees, D.W. and Smith, S.D. (1991) 'Work stress in occupational therapists assessed by the occupational stress indicator', *British Journal of Occupational Therapy*, 54 (8): 289–294.

Reid, Y., Johnson, S., Morant, N., Kuipers, E., Szmukler, G., Bebbington, P., Thornicroft, G. and Prosser, D. (1999) 'Improving support for mental health staff: a qualitative study', *Social Psychiatry and Psychiatric Epidemiology*, 34 (6): 309–315.

Ryan, D. and Quayle, E. (1999) 'Stress in psychiatric nursing: fact or fiction?' *Nursing Standard*, 14 (8): 32–35.

Schafer, T. (1992) 'CPN stress and organisational change', *Community Psychiatric Nursing Journal*, 13: 16–24.

Snelgrove, S.R. (1998) 'Occupational stress and job satisfaction: a comparative study of health visitors, district nurses and community psychiatric nurses', *Journal of Nursing Management*, 6 (2): 97–104.

Sullivan, P.J. (1993) 'Occupational stress in psychiatric nursing', *Journal of Advanced Nursing*, 18 (4): 591–601.

Sutherland, V.J. and Cooper, C.L. (1990) *Understanding stress. A psychological perspective for health professionals*, London: Chapman and Hall.

Thomas, B. (1997) 'Management strategies to tackle stress in mental health nursing', *Mental Health Care*, 1 (1): 15–16.

Trygstad, L.N. (1986) 'Stress and coping in psychiatric nursing', *Journal of Psychosocial and Mental Health Nursing Services*, 24 (10): 23–27.

Watson, J. (1986) 'A step in the right direction . . . relaxation training for psychiatric staff', *Senior Nurse*, 5 (4): 12–13.

Wykes, T., Stevens, W. and Everitt, B. (1997) 'Stress in community care teams: will it affect the sustainability of community care', *Social Psychiatry and Psychiatric Epidemiology*, 32: 398–407.

## FURTHER READING

Carson, J., Fagin, L. and Ritter, S. (1995) *Stress and coping in mental health nursing*, London: Chapman and Hall.

The areas of discussion in this book include the background to studies of stress in mental health nursing, the examination of coping skills and the practical implications of present and future research.

Hardy, S., Carson, J. and Thomas, B. (1998) *Occupational stress: personal and professional approaches*, London: Stanley Thornes.
This book represents a theoretical and practical overview of the issues relating to stress and burnout among health care professionals.

# CHAPTER 12

# CLINICAL SUPERVISION AND REFLECTIVE PRACTICE

*John Cutcliffe*

---

## SUMMARY OF KEY POINTS

- The work of community psychiatric nurses is often isolating. CPNs need structured opportunities for support, and to reflect on and learn from their practice.

- It is likely that the majority of CPNs regularly participate in clinical supervision, and research evidence indicates that many report benefits from this.

- Education and training for participation in clinical supervision are important. However, preparation for supervision is patchy, delivered by a wide variety of individuals and organisations.

---

## INTRODUCTION

It is rare these days for any nursing education or practice publication not to include some reference to 'reflection' and/or clinical supervision. The prominence of both practices in nursing has grown exponentially over the last decade or two, to the extent that contemporary curricula for nursing courses now make frequent reference to both practices. Indeed, recent reviews by the English National Board for Nurses, Midwives, and Health Visitors and policy documents (e.g. ENB 1997) emphasise the importance of reflective practice. Similarly, the largest review of mental health nursing to date, *Working in partnership* (Department of Health 1994), stressed the need for all practitioners to receive regular clinical supervision.

More recent policy documents, such as *The new NHS* (Department of Health 1997), *A first class service* (Department of Health 1998) and the UKCC's (1996) position statement on clinical supervision, make reference to the need for mental health nurses to engage in lifelong learning, reflection and clinical supervision. Furthermore, they link such practices to increased quality of care. Additional quality initiatives, e.g. clinical governance (Department of Health 1998), have been linked to the practice of clinical supervision so much that, according to Butterworth (2001, p. 317), 'there is an obvious relationship between clinical governance and clinical supervision', and, he continues, 'we have thus for perhaps the first time a formal link between the individual and the organisation in a framework for ensuring the quality of clinical services'.

Consequently, as Kelly *et al.* (2001) point out, it might be prudent to accept that clinical supervision is here to stay, and that mental health nurses need to engage in reflection if they are to remain as viable and effective practitioners. However, having established these practices as fundamental to the contemporary mental health nurse, it is worth examining if the same can be said of the contemporary community psychiatric nurse (CPN).

Rather than relying on the simplistic, though cogent, argument that because community psychiatric nurses are also mental health nurses, they *ipso facto* need to engage in reflective practice and clinical supervision, additional arguments can be made that indicate that these practices are even more necessary and important to CPNs. This argument centres on the major differences in care delivery and access to formal/informal support systems that exist between CPNs and hospital-based mental health nurses.

It is widely accepted, and there is ample evidence to support this position, that CPNs have a more 'isolated' position than mental health nurses who work in a hospital setting. This point needs clarifying. This is not to proffer an image of the community psychiatric nurse as some form of independent, wilderness-based 'maverick', who rarely comes into contact with any of his/her peers. But what needs to be understood is that, in the large majority of cases, the CPN will spend more time working alone, more time working without immediate recourse to the support of their peers, and, arguably, more time making independent judgements and decisions than would a hospital-based mental health nurse. Additionally, these differences in practice do not make community-based nurses better or worse than their hospital-based colleagues. But they do make them different and this needs to be acknowledged.

Accepting the premise that the community psychiatric nurse works in a more 'isolated' position thus begs questions about the nature of the support for such practitioners, and how decisions made in a more 'independent manner' are examined and evaluated. There can be little doubt that while working on their own CPNs do not have access to informal support from their peers. They do not have the opportunity to check their decisions with another colleague as they are making them. Neither do they have the physical 'back up' and additional sense of security that can arise from knowing that help and support are close by.

Consequently, the need for formal support structures that additionally provide the opportunity and environment for reflection becomes abundantly clear. Whilst acknowledging that some informal support structures may exist for CPNs, this in no way negates the need for more formal support structures. Neither do informal support structures allow (or create) the permissive, reflective, yet challenging interpersonal environment that is created in clinical supervision, where the CPN's clinical decisions, success, stresses, strengths and dilemmas can be examined, and learned from.

Thus, there is a cogent case for CPNs to engage in clinical supervision and reflective practice. Having established this case, it is necessary to examine the rudiments of clinical supervision and, similarly, the nature of reflective practice.

# THE RUDIMENTS OF CLINICAL SUPERVISION

An examination of the theoretical and empirical literature indicates that there is a wealth of material that focuses on clinical supervision. Furthermore, many of these texts attempt to provide definitions or concise descriptions of the nature of clinical supervision. Along with Professor Butterworth and Brigid Proctor, who are two of the key figures in the development of clinical supervision within nursing in the UK, the author of this chapter would suggest that there is no one single correct way to carry out clinical supervision. However, any activity is based on certain implicit or explicit assumptions. Rather than give yet another definition of clinical supervision, I will spell out some of those assumptions, and in so doing draw on Cutcliffe *et al.*'s (2001) view of what they think clinical supervision is and is not. In no particular order of priority, these parameters are described in Box 12.1.

---

**Box 12.1   Cutcliffe, Butterworth and Proctor's (2001) view of the central rudiments of clinical supervision**

Clinical supervision is:

- supportive
- safe, because of clear, negotiated agreements by all parties with regard to the extent and limits of confidentiality
- centred on developing best practice for service users
- brave, because practitioners are encouraged to talk about the realities of their practice
- a chance to talk about difficult areas of work in an environment where the person attempts to understand
- an opportunity to ventilate emotion without comeback
- the opportunity to deal with material and issues that practitioners may have been carrying for many years (the chance to talk about issues which cannot easily be talked about elsewhere and which may have been previously unexplored)
- not to be confused with or amalgamated with managerial supervision
- not to be confused with or amalgamated with personal therapy/ counselling
- regular
- protected time

---

- offered equally to all practitioners
- something that involves a committed relationship (from both parties)
- separate and distinct from preceptorship or mentorship
- a facilitative relationship
- challenging
- an invitation to be self-monitoring and self-accountable
- at times hard work and at others enjoyable
- something that involves learning to be reflective and becoming a reflective practitioner
- an activity that continues throughout one's working life

# THE NATURE OF REFLECTIVE PRACTICE

As with the preceding section, there is a wealth of theoretical material, and a smaller empirical literature, that focuses on reflective practice. Within this literature there exist a range of models (e.g. Schön 1983) and, similarly, a range of descriptions of reflective practice. Therefore, rather than give yet another definition of reflective practice, the author will spell out some of the implicit assumptions, and, in so doing, draw on Ghaye and Lillyman's (2000) twelve key principles of reflective practice (see Box 12.2). These provide a useful framework for highlighting the rudiments of reflective practice.

---

**Box 12.2   Ghaye and Lillyman's (2000) twelve key principles of reflective practice**

Principle 1.   Reflective practice is about you (the practitioner) and your practice.

Principle 2.   Reflective practice is about learning from experience.

Principle 3.   Reflective practice is about valuing what we do and why we do it.

Principle 4.   Reflective practice is about learning how to account positively for ourselves and our work.

Principle 5.   Reflective practice does not separate practice from theory.

Principle 6.   Reflective practice can help us make sense of our thoughts and our actions.

Principle 7.   Reflective practice generates locally owned knowledge.

Principle 8.   The reflective conversation is at the heart of the process of reflecting on practice.

Principle 9.   Reflection emphasises the links between values and actions.

Principle 10.   Reflection can improve practice.

Principle 11.   Reflective practitioners develop themselves and their work systematically and rigorously.

Principle 12.   Reflection involves respecting and working with evidence.

# ISSUES AND CHALLENGES IN CLINICAL SUPERVISION AND REFLECTION PRACTICE FOR COMMUNITY PSYCHIATRIC NURSES

Having highlighted the rudiments and principles of clinical supervision and reflective practice, it is now necessary to consider some of the issues and challenges facing CPNs as they embark on such practice. Five key issues have been chosen for closer examination and these are:

1    How common is clinical supervision in community psychiatric nursing?
2    How useful is clinical supervision for community psychiatric nurses?
3    How much training in clinical supervision do community psychiatric nurses receive or need?
4    Who should community psychiatric nurses receive clinical supervision from?
5    How can reflective practice be utilised within clinical supervision?

These five issues are by no means the only issues facing CPNs as they consider clinical supervision and reflective practice. Other issues that should be considered include: what are legitimate topics for discussion within clinical supervision, issues of record keeping, ethical issues, and confidentiality. There is not enough room in this chapter to do justice to all these issues. However, a substantial literature exists which can inform the CPN on these matters and it might be prudent for the CPN to familiarise himself/herself with this literature, some of which is included in the 'References' and 'Further reading' below.

## How common is clinical supervision in community psychiatric nursing?

When compared to other specialist groups of nurses (e.g. practice nurses, paediatric nurses), the empirical evidence is consistent in suggesting that a high proportion of CPNs engage in clinical supervision. Brooker and White's (1997) survey of community mental health nursing in Northern Ireland, for example, indicated that 80 per cent of the total population were receiving clinical supervision, and that this supervision incorporated purposeful reflection on practice. Similar levels of activity and associated positive outcomes from engaging in clinical supervision were also found in other UK studies (see Bulmer 1997, Butterworth 1997). Indeed, Bishop's (1998) nationwide survey determined that, of all the nursing specialities that responded, CPNs showed the highest level of engagement in clinical supervision. These results were echoed in Brocklehurst's regional surveys (see, for example, Brocklehurst 1997).

More recent studies continue to verify that a very high proportion of community psychiatric nurses engage in clinical supervision (see, for example, Kelly *et al.* 2001). From this body of evidence we can see that the large majority of CPNs in the UK appear to engage in clinical supervision. This is perhaps not altogether surprising given the arguments highlighted in the 'Introduction'. Thus, perhaps the most pertinent question to ask is: why are 20 per cent of CPNs in the

UK apparently reluctant to engage in clinical supervision? Clearly, this is an area that is under-researched, and much-needed research needs to be undertaken to explore the reasons for this reluctance. Without this evidence, one can only speculate. However, possible reasons can be categorised into two broad groups, namely: organisational and individual.

### Organisational

- Inappropriate 'top-down' implementation of clinical supervision systems.
- No opportunity for choosing one's supervisor.
- Shortage of appropriately trained supervisors.

### Individual

- Inaccurate perceptions of clinical supervision (e.g. viewing supervision as a form of management monitoring or personal therapy).
- A lack of clarity and understanding of the nature and purpose of supervision.
- A personal reluctance to engage in reflecting on uncomfortable, difficult or awkward intra- and interpersonal issues.

Consequently, if these reasons are correct, there is a requirement for organisations to rethink their clinical supervision infrastructure, and a concomitant need for practitioners to re-examine their perceptions of clinical supervision.

## How useful is clinical supervision for community psychiatric nurses?

The evidence is consistent in suggesting that the majority of CPNs who engage in clinical supervision find the experience to be beneficial. The extent and degree of benefit, and, indeed, in what domains the benefit is experienced, appear to vary from individual to individual. Additionally, there appear to be certain key practices that enhance the benefits experienced.

In their recent survey of CPNs' perceptions of clinical supervision, Kelly *et al.* (2001) found an overall support for clinical supervision, a wide range of reported benefits and, interestingly, a degree of uncertainty around how these benefits were actualised. Writing in depth of his personal experience of engaging in clinical supervision as a CPN, Smith (2001) makes some powerful statements. He states:

> but I have experienced how, when done adequately, clinical super-vision is about growth and development, not about censure. As importantly it has enabled me to improve my service to patients and they have directly benefited by changes in my clinical practice.
>
> (Smith 2001, p. 167)

Perhaps some of the most illuminating research findings in this area are provided by Winstanley's (2001) Ph.D. research. In developing the 'Manchester Clinical Supervision Scale' she sampled 1,027 nurses, divided equally (roughly) between hospital- and community-based staff. The major findings from the study were:

- CPNs engaged in longer and more frequent supervision sessions than their hospital-based counterparts.
- CPNs engaged in more reflection within their supervision if they had chosen their supervisor, rather than had a supervisor allocated to them.
- More significant (both statistically and clinically significant) benefits were encountered by the CPNs when they held their clinical supervision sessions away from their workplace.
- CPNs experienced greater benefits when they engaged in group supervision rather than one-to-one supervision sessions.

Whilst it needs to be acknowledged that the large majority of CPNs report significant benefits from engaging in supervision, such a perception is not universal. There are some CPNs who do not appear to receive much benefit from engaging in supervision (see Kelly *et al.* 2001). Interestingly, low levels of benefit appear to be inextricably linked to the following: lack of adequate preparation (Cutcliffe 1997); confusion regarding the purpose and nature of clinical supervision (Cutcliffe and Proctor 1998); the inappropriate amalgamation (and resulting confusion) of managerial supervision and clinical supervision (Epling and Cassedy 2001). Consequently, in order to maximise the benefits for CPNs who engage in clinical supervision, it is vital that their employers access and provide adequate training that can eradicate confusion. Furthermore, in place of pyramidal, top-down systems of clinical supervision delivery, wherein line managers provide the supervision, alternative (and perhaps more imaginative) systems should be put in place.

## How much training in clinical supervision do community psychiatric nurses receive or need?

This issue of adequate training in clinical supervision is not exclusive to CPNs. In the largest study yet undertaken in the UK on clinical supervision, Butterworth *et al.* (1997) found that the participants received a wide range of training, ranging from no training at all to one full week. Unfortunately, the data collected in this study were not scrutinised for a direct correlation between the extent of training and the degree of positive outcomes. However, Cutcliffe (1997) reasoned that if supervisors receive inadequate training, then it is unlikely that supervisors will produce (or facilitate) positive outcomes in their supervisees. Kelly *et al.* (2001) reported similar findings, in that only 37.3 per cent of their sample of CPNs had received formal training in clinical supervision. Unfortunately, this study did not describe the length or content of the training.

As yet, there is no standardised minimum specification for how long clinical supervision training should last. Similarly, there exists no standardised curriculum, no guidelines for training content, and no regulatory body to monitor the quality of the training. Training in clinical supervision is provided by a wide range of individuals, from 'in-house' NHS trust training and development staff, to individuals who offer private consultancy training, to validated courses provided by university departments. As a result, it is fair to say that these variations in training produce practitioners who demonstrate a wide range in the overall quality of clinical supervision provided.

Whilst it would be impracticable, and inappropriate, to insist that all CPNs should undergo the same extent of preparation for supervision, it is not unrealistic to argue that all CPNs should receive the same *minimum level of preparation* for clinical supervision. However, it is difficult to see this development being actualised since current CPN education is not standardised throughout the UK. In a survey which was designed to measure aspects of CPN education in the UK, Hannigan (1999) found that, overall, courses for CPNs appeared to be characterised by considerable variation in specialist content, including clinical supervision.

This disparity in preparation produces a situation where, at least in part, the individual CPN is responsible for determining the extent of training in clinical supervision. This is less the case for those practitioners who intend to become CPNs in the future. Over a decade ago, Butterworth argued that clinical supervision preparation should be an integral aspect of pre-registration training. He stated: 'Introduction to a process of clinical supervision should begin in professional training and education, and continue thereafter as an integral part of professional development' (Butterworth 1992, p. 15). Furthermore, similar arguments were constructed by Cutcliffe and Proctor (1998). One can hope, therefore, that future cohorts of CPNs would be introduced to the processes of clinical supervision during pre-registration training. If they don't receive this introduction in their pre-registration training, the option remains that CPN preparation courses could (and most probably already do) provide some introduction to clinical supervision. It is important to note that these preparations are not mutually exclusive, and should be regarded as complementing one another.

Even if CPNs have received an introduction to clinical supervision, the author would recommend that they still engage in post-graduate clinical supervision training, provided it is of high quality. Additionally, training should not be regarded as a 'one off'. Since, according to Butterworth (1992) and Cutcliffe *et al.* (2001), clinical supervision is a practice that is regarded as a lifelong activity, it follows that, from time to time, a 'top up' course is necessary.

In conclusion, it is clearly down to the individual CPN how much training is adequate. The intensity and duration of this training may well vary from person to person, and it is not my place to dictate how much training is sufficient. However, I would argue that *some* preparation/training is required for all CPNs.

## Who should community psychiatric nurses receive clinical supervision from?

As stated above, I would suggest that there is no one single correct way to carry out clinical supervision. Likewise, there is no one single professional group that the CPN should seek out to receive supervision from. Given the nature of the work undertaken in clinical supervision, it is axiomatic that the CPN should be able to choose his/her supervisor rather than having one dictated. However, accepting this axiom, there is a body of evidence accumulating that attests that some choices of supervisor appear to be more facilitative than others.

Perhaps the situation that appears to create more difficulty than any other is when supervisees receive supervision from the person who is also their direct line manager. The evidence on this substantive issue, such as it is, is consistent in suggesting that this position is impracticable, if not untenable.

Epling and Cassedy (2001) collected data from over 120 clinical supervision trainees. Students were asked to rank a range of statements relating to issues in supervision. The statement 'The supervisor should be a manager' was consistently ranked as the least important aspect of clinical supervision. Nurses undertaking the training provided by the Epling and Cassedy (2001) course frequently report that the development of their clinical supervision structures has been imposed from the top down rather than growing 'organically' out of practice. Whatever the framework in which supervision takes place – group, individual or peer, or hierarchically structured with higher-grade nurses supervising lower-grade nurses – the discussions in many areas of clinical practice have been few or the options have not been considered. Epling and Cassedy go on to point out that nurses may resist entering into a supervisory relationship if they perceive it to be a management-led initiative, imposed on them with little regard for 'ownership'.

Within Kelly et al.'s (2001) survey, they discovered that whilst some NHS trusts maintained a clear distinction between managerial and clinical supervision, there were also examples of policy and procedure that were implicitly managerially focused. Yegdich's (1999) insightful paper drew attention to the significant difficulties that can arise when supervision is provided by direct line managers. Cutcliffe et al. (2001) declared that this theme (and research finding) recurs throughout their book. Both practices are legitimate and valuable. However, the overlap of boundaries leads to confusion regarding power issues in supervision and concerns regarding confidentiality; it may inappropriately emphasise the normative aspects of supervision, and focus on the needs of the organisation rather than the individual.

Drawing on a range of authors who have commented on the difficulties of having one's line manager as a supervisor, here is a summary:

- There is a tendency for those in senior roles to focus on performance and action rather than exploring the subtleties of process.
- There is the potential for material offered during supervision to be used in a disciplinary manner.
- There is a tendency to focus on management issues as the major agenda.
- Confusion is caused by the duality of supervisory and managerial roles.

Therefore, the author would strongly recommend that the practices of clinical and managerial supervision remain separate yet complementary to one another, and that CPNs might benefit from receiving supervision from someone other than their line manager.

The second issue to consider within this discussion point is: should CPNs receive supervision only from other CPNs? It is the author's experience from running training courses in clinical supervision that when first embracing the concept, supervisees, including CPNs, often initially want someone from the same discipline and background to supervise them. Cassedy *et al.* (2001) argue that there is probably an element of safety here, in that potential supervisees don't want to feel vulnerable and exposed and they have always previously gone to a colleague for support. There may also be an element of confusion regarding the purpose of supervision underpinning such a view.

If clinical supervision is (incorrectly) conceptualised as an opportunity for a more experienced colleague to monitor, educate and support a less experienced nurse in practical skills, then this creates the need for all supervisors to be more 'expert' in the particular speciality of nursing than the supervisee. However, a more accurate conceptualisation of clinical supervision sees it as an opportunity to help and support practitioners in reflecting on their dilemmas, difficulties and successes, and exploring how they reacted to, solved or achieved them. This situation creates the need for supervisors to be effective at supporting practitioners in self-monitoring, identifying difficulties in practice and finding the proper place to make good the deficit, not necessarily to be more expert in the particular nursing speciality. Consequently, as supervisees gain knowledge and experience of the purpose of supervision, they gradually realise there is a greater opportunity for development in choosing someone, irrespective of their background, who will stretch them and be more challenging.

## How can reflective practice be utilised within clinical supervision?

Several authors have written that reflection-on-practice is an integral aspect of clinical supervision (e.g. Ghaye and Lillyman 2000). However, there is less con-sensus on how this reflection is operationalised. One school of thought posits the supervisor as the person who directs the focus of the reflection. Topics and issues raised in previous sessions are subsequently followed up in later sessions. In this view, the power and control reside with the supervisor, and such approaches are commonly termed 'supervisor-led'.

An alternative approach, and an approach more in keeping with the original conceptualisation of clinical supervision, posits the supervisee as the person who directs the focus of the reflection. The supervisee sets the agenda and the supervisor responds. In this view, the power and control reside with the supervisee, and such approaches are commonly termed 'supervisee-led'. This is the approach to supervision and associated reflection that Butterworth (1992) described, and the approach that I subscribe to. Thus, if the supervisee is responsible for directing the reflection, the question to be asked is: how does the supervisee decide what to reflect on? What would be a valuable and appropriate topic for reflection?

There are parallels here with deciding on what are legitimate topics to discuss in supervision. Clearly, one cannot reflect on every aspect of practice (and our reaction to that practice). Furthermore, since there is usually a finite time for supervision (usually one to one and a half hours per month), it is important that this time for reflection is used constructively. Inexperienced 'reflectors' sometimes mistakenly focus on 'extra-ordinary' or 'dramatic' events. Whilst there is clearly merit in such reflection, it would not be prudent to exclude the huge value of reflecting on, and 'un-picking', the routine, the everyday work, the taken for granted and the ordinary. Psychiatric nursing has often been described as working in ordinary ways with extra-ordinary people. Accepting this axiom, it follows that there resides great merit in exploring, and thus gaining a deeper understanding of, the processes of ordinary ways of working.

So, in conclusion, in deciding what to discuss in supervision, and thus what to reflect on, the supervisee needs to maintain an open mind. Critical incidents, any event within one's practice that causes a 'moment of pause', an event that ushers the supervisee into questioning themselves, are often keys to effective reflection. In addition to this, CPNs in particular may find great value in reflecting on the subtle, unobtrusive processes of everyday practice: the ordinary. Finally, if the supervisee still needs guidance on what to reflect on, he/she may find additional help by examining some of the models for choosing a topic for reflection that exist in the literature (e.g. Bond and Holland 1998).

# REFERENCES

Bishop, V. (1998) 'Clinical supervision: what is going on? Results of a questionnaire', *NT Research*, 3 (2): 141–149.

Bond, M. and Holland, S. (1998) *The skills of clinical supervision*, Buckingham: Open University Press.

Brocklehurst, N. (1997) *Developing clinical supervision in Anglia and Oxford: a regional survey*, Report prepared for the NHS Executive, Anglia and Oxford, University of Birmingham.

Brooker, C. and White, E. (1997) *The fourth quinquennial national community mental health nursing census of England and Wales*, Manchester and Keele: Universities of Manchester and Keele.

Bulmer, C. (1997) 'Supervision: how it works', *Nursing Times*, 93 (48): 53–54.

Butterworth, T. (1992) 'Clinical supervision as an emerging idea in nursing', in Butterworth, T. and Faugier, J. (eds) *Clinical supervision and mentorship in nursing*, London: Chapman and Hall.

Butterworth, T. (1997) 'Clinical supervision . . . or a honey pot', *Nursing Times*, 93 (44): 27–29.

Butterworth, T. (2001) 'Clinical supervision and clinical governance for the 21st century: an end or just the beginning?', in Cutcliffe, J.R., Butterworth, T. and Proctor, B. (eds) *Fundamental themes in clinical supervision*, London: Routledge.

Butterworth, T., Carson, J., White, E., Jeacock, J., Clements, A. and Bishop, V. (1997) *It is good to talk. Clinical supervision and mentorship: an evaluation study in England and Scotland*, Manchester: School of Nursing, Midwifery and Health Visiting, University of Manchester.

Cassedy, P., Epling, M., Williamson, L. and Harvey, G. (2001) 'Providing cross discipline group supervision to new supervisees: challenging some common apprehensions and myths?', in Cutcliffe, J.R., Butterworth, T. and Proctor, B. (eds) *Fundamental themes in clinical supervision*, London: Routledge.

Cutcliffe, J. (1997) 'Evaluating the success of clinical supervision', *British Journal of Nursing*, 6 (13): 725.

Cutcliffe, J.R. and Proctor, B. (1998) 'An alternative training approach in clinical supervision. Part one', *British Journal of Nursing*, 7 (5): 280–285.

Cutcliffe, J.R., Butterworth, T. and Proctor, B. (2001) 'Introduction. Fundamental themes in clinical supervision: national and international perspectives of education, policy, research and practice', in Cutcliffe, J.R., Butterworth, T. and Proctor, B. (eds) *Fundamental themes in clinical supervision*, London: Routledge.

Department of Health (1994) *Working in partnership: a collaborative approach to care. Report of the Mental Health Nursing Review Team*, London: HMSO.

Department of Health (1997) *The new NHS: modern, dependable*, London: Department of Health.

Department of Health (1998) *A first class service: quality in the new NHS*, London: Department of Health.

English National Board for Nurses, Midwives, and Health Visitors (ENB) (1997) *Standards for approval of higher education institutions and programmes*, London: ENB.

Epling, M. and Cassedy, P. (2001) 'Clinical supervision: visions from the classroom', in Cutcliffe, J.R., Butterworth, T. and Proctor, B. (eds) *Fundamental themes in clinical supervision*, London: Routledge.

Ghaye, T. and Lillyman, S. (2000) *Reflection: principles and practices for healthcare professionals*, Salisbury: Quay Books.

Hannigan, B. (1999) 'Education for community psychiatric nurses: content, structure and trends in recruitment', *Journal of Psychiatric and Mental Health Nursing*, 6: 137–145.

Kelly, B., Long, A. and McKenna, H.P. (2001) 'A survey of community mental health nurses' perceptions of clinical supervision in Northern Ireland', *Journal of Psychiatric and Mental Health Nursing*, 8: 33–44.

Schön, D. (1983) *The reflective practitioner: how professionals think in action*, New York: Basic Books.

Smith, P. (2001) 'Clinical supervision: my path towards clinical excellence in mental health nursing', in Cutcliffe, J.R., Butterworth, T. and Proctor, B. (eds) *Fundamental themes in clinical supervision*, London: Routledge.

United Kingdom Central Council for Nursing, Midwifery and Health Visiting (UKCC) (1996) *Proposed position statement on clinical supervision for nursing and health visiting*, London: UKCC.

Winstanley, J. (2001) 'Developing methods for evaluating clinical supervision', in Cutcliffe, J.R., Butterworth, T. and Proctor, B. (eds) *Fundamental themes in clinical supervision*, London: Routledge.

Yegdich, T. (1999) 'Clinical supervision and managerial supervision: some historical and conceptual considerations', *Journal of Advanced Nursing*, 30 (5): 1195–1204.

# FURTHER READING

Cutcliffe, J.R., Butterworth, T. and Proctor, B. (eds) (2001) *Fundamental themes in clinical supervision*, London: Routledge.

A comprehensive and inclusive text that looks at the areas of education/training in supervision, the introduction/policy of supervision, and the practice/research of supervision, from both a national and an international perspective.

Ghaye, T. and Lillyman, S. (2000) *Reflection: principles and practices for healthcare professionals*, Salisbury: Quay Books.

A good introduction to the main principles and practices of reflective practice.

Bond, M. and Holland, S. (1998) *The skills of clinical supervision*, Buckingham: Open
    University Press.
A text that focuses on the specific skills of clinical supervision, using the conceptual
framework of John Heron's 'Six Category Intervention Analysis'.

# PART 2

## PRACTICE

## INTRODUCTION

Mirroring the increase in the size of the community mental health nursing workforce over the years has been an increase in the number and variety of specialist areas that CMHNs work in, and in the therapeutic approaches that they employ. The chapters which follow in this section of the book attest to the diversity of community mental health nursing practice.

The first chapter addresses the area of mental health promotion. As Judy Boxer suggests, promoting the mental health of individuals and communities is a job for more than CMHNs – and even the health service – alone. Judy emphasises the importance of health-promoting activities which cross organisational and professional boundaries, and which tackle the causes of poor health.

In his chapter, Rob Newell turns his attention to the use of evidence to inform practice. Rob makes the point that much of what goes on in health care delivery lacks a sound evidence base. Moreover, Rob observes that what little research there is in mental health nursing tends not to focus on clinical care, but on professional and educational issues.

All practising community mental health nurses, whatever their particular area of specialism, are involved in the assessment of needs. This is the focus of Mike Slade's chapter. Mike argues for a structured and comprehensive approach to assessment, and points to the value of using standardised measures in everyday practice.

In his chapter, Andy Alaszewski takes issue with the concept of 'risk'. Risk, Andy argues, is a powerful word, and can be used to the disadvantage of people with mental health problems. A challenge for community mental health nurses is to exercise professional judgement in ways which meet the twin aims of empowering service users, and minimising harm.

Reducing the incidence of suicide has been a public and professional concern for many years. Steve Wood makes the point that, by definition, the population of people who use the services of community mental health nurses are at an increased risk of suicide. As Steve suggests, developing specific knowledge and skills in the assessment of suicide risk remains a priority area for mental health nurses.

In the first of two chapters which focus on approaches to working with families, Billy Hardy writes about the application of systemic family therapy to community mental health nursing. Despite sustained interest in systemic work in some areas of mental health nursing, Billy observes that in many quarters approaches to working with families are often limited to behavioural interventions. Billy identifies areas in which the work of CMHNs might be enriched by the use of systemic techniques.

In the second 'Working with families' chapter, Geoff Brennan provides an overview of the use of psychosocial interventions. As Geoff writes, this approach to working with families is derived from research into 'expressed emotion'. The value of family interventions of this type lies in reducing the stress that carers of people with severe mental health problems can experience, and in reducing rates of relapse.

Another clinical intervention which has proven its value in helping people with severe mental health problems is the use of cognitive behavioural therapy (CBT). Norman Young begins his chapter with an overview of cognitive psychology, and then provides an account of the theory and practice of CBT with people experiencing psychosis.

In his chapter on early interventions and relapse prevention, Michael Coffey shows how community mental health nurses can assist people towards recovery from severe mental health problems. Michael notes that relapse prevention has its roots in the emergence of service user-led self-management approaches. Now, as Michael adds, early warning signs work conducted in a spirit of collaboration can be a valuable way to reduce the impact of recurrent mental illness.

There is much confusion over the terminology used to describe approaches to the care of people with complex needs. In his chapter, Steve Morgan tackles the meaning and application of 'case management' and 'assertive outreach'. Steve stresses the importance of a team approach in the delivery of assertive care, and also makes an important distinction between care which is 'assertive' and care which is 'aggressive'.

Medication remains a major component in mental health care and treatment. In their chapter, Richard Gray, Elizabeth Brewin and Daniel Bressington describe the actions of the most commonly-used groups of medications, and their side effects. Richard and colleagues also address important issues in the management of medication, including the use of standardised assessment measures.

In his chapter, Tony Gillam shows how 'being creative', in the sense of 'being daring' or 'challenging assumptions', can be used to enhance community mental health nursing care. Drawing on the experience of leading the Music Workshop Project, Tony also demonstrates the value of integrating creative art and music therapies into mental health nursing care.

The final five chapters in this section all address approaches to working with particular groups of service users. Mentally disordered offenders are a high-profile group, and Michael Coffey's chapter points to the importance of engaging with both service users and their carers. Michael also looks towards the importance of liaison, and the need for the further development of services – such as 'assertive inreach' – for this group of people.

People with combined mental health and substance misuse problems are another high-profile, and often challenging, group. Jeff Champney-Smith begins his chapter by unravelling the meaning of the term 'dual diagnosis', before arguing for the development of integrated services for this group. Jeff points out that evidence for the effectiveness of different approaches to care is sparse, but that brief, motivational interventions delivered by community mental health nurses have value.

In his chapter, John Keady notes how, in recent years, care for older people with dementia and their families has started to shake off its over-medicalised roots. However, John also draws attention to criticisms that community mental health nurses working in this area lack role clarity, and lack clear models of practice. John argues that a major challenge for CMHNs caring for older people is to more clearly evaluate and articulate their contribution.

People with learning disabilities and mental health problems are a neglected group, and services to meet their particular needs are often poorly integrated. In his chapter, Dave Coyle looks at assessment strategies and models of care delivery, and argues that many community mental health nurses could do more to help with the delivery of services to this group of people.

In the final chapter in this 'Practice' section, Richard Williams and Fiona Gale focus on current approaches to working with children and young people with mental health problems, and their families. This is an expanding area of community mental health practice, but is one which – until recently – has been relatively neglected by policy-makers and service planners. Richard and Fiona strike an optimistic note, and see exciting opportunities for nurses as the new emphasis on promoting the mental health of young people takes shape.

# CHAPTER 13

# PROMOTING MENTAL HEALTH

*Judy Boxer*

---

## SUMMARY OF KEY POINTS

- Mental health promotion, supported by a sound theoretical and evidence base, is high on the agenda of current mental health policy.

- Mental health promotion is now embedded in community regeneration agendas throughout the UK, and is a real opportunity to promote mental health for individuals and neighbourhoods.

- It is vital that mental health practitioners become familiar with, and competent in, mental health promotion at the levels of the individual and the community, and in reducing structural barriers to accessing services and treatment because of factors such as discrimination.

---

## INTRODUCTION

In this chapter I intend to outline more clearly the key aspects of mental health promotion and how it relates to our practice. It is hoped that this will provide students and practitioners with a useful basis for incorporating mental health promotion (MHP) as a core activity and skill. A framework has been identified and is also now clearly evidenced by the Department of Health (2001a) publication *Making it happen*. In the book I co-wrote on mental health promotion, a pragmatic approach was taken in that it seemed important to state a very clear value base to this aspect of our practice, in terms of it being anti-oppressive (McCulloch and Boxer 1997).

It is also important for practitioners to increase their understanding of the complexity of modernisation agendas in health and social care. To do this it is necessary to understand why strategic planning, policy, service development and clinical governance are the foundation of our day-to-day practice, however far removed people can feel from them at times. A main focus of mental health promotion is the development of services that are user-led. User-led services are characterised by real partnership working, and by the existence of user representation at different levels of NHS and local authority services. The recent rationalisation of trusts and the increasing numbers of integrated mental health trusts can only enhance this approach. Mental health promotion is also something that has to be addressed throughout the life cycle. Activities that highlight the needs of children, those with a disability and older adults are crucial to all aspects of community nursing practice (Department of Health 2001b). Although this chapter concentrates on mental health practice, it has relevance to other health and social care professionals and is a desired focus for multidisciplinary and inter-agency working. It is a required skill in health visiting, district, school and practice nursing and spans both primary and secondary care (Boxer and McCulloch 1996).

Recent government approaches such as the 'New Deal for Communities' and European funding opportunities such as the Single Regeneration Budget provide the chance to concentrate on areas of the country with high levels of deprivation, unemployment and poverty. The fact that a high percentage of black and minority ethnic groups live in such areas means that race and culture are an integral part of modern British society and the impact of these has different outcomes for different people (Alexander 1999, Keating and Robertson 2002). A clear example of the negative side of this is the perceptions held by many people of refugees and asylum seekers; mental health promotion is probably the icing on the cake for someone faced with such basic human rights issues. For mental health practitioners there are many conflicting priorities. For those who work in community settings the opportunities to link with community projects, such as Sure Start, or to play an active role in addressing mental health promotion as envisaged by those who have researched and written about it, are much easier than they were a few years ago. The priority, for those working in NHS-led mental health services, is currently undergoing a paradigm shift. An example of this is in the way that in-patient care is a high priority for change and development, as supported by projects such as 'Acute Solutions' (Sainsbury Centre for Mental Health 1999). Another example is in the development of specific community teams for those with severe and enduring illness, with the introduction of early intervention, home treatment and assertive outreach services.

## WHAT IS MENTAL HEALTH PROMOTION?

The benefits of mental health promotion are considered to be to:

- improve physical health and well-being;
- prevent or reduce the risk of some mental health problems, notably behaviour disorders, depression and anxiety, substance misuse;
- assist recovery from mental health problems;

- improve mental health services and the quality of life for people experiencing mental health problems;
- strengthen the capacity of communities to support social inclusion, tolerance and participation, and reduce vulnerability to socioeconomic stressors;
- increase the 'mental health literacy' of individuals, organisations and communities;
- improve health at work, increasing productivity and reducing sickness absence.

(Department of Health 2001a, p. 33)

# DEFINITIONS OF MENTAL HEALTH PROMOTION

Finding a suitable definition of mental health promotion as a basis for identifying values and approaches in community mental health practice is not easy. Previous definitions have tended to adopt a broad health promotion focus, and this also applies to how the World Health Organization has addressed the issue of mental health at a global level, as Box 13.1 shows.

---

**Box 13.1    Health for all**

*Health for all* is concerned with creating structures and mechanisms that empower and support individuals in developing and using their own capabilities to the fullest extent possible. It aims to enable them to realise their potential for health and thereby enhances the quality of their lives.

(World Health Organization 1991)

---

One of the first mental health promotion projects to be developed in this country was in Sheffield and my involvement with this project has helped both in clarifying definitions that assist practice and in developing a framework for that practice (Box 13.2).

---

**Box 13.2    The concept of mental health promotion**

Mental health promotion is developing positive mental health both for and with the community in general and individuals who may have mental health problems. It includes self-help, service provision and organisational skills. The concept of mental health promotion recognises that an individual's mental health is inextricably linked with their relationship to others, their lifestyle and the environmental factors that affect this, and the degree of power they can exert over their lives to change their situation if they want or need to.

(adapted from Sheffield Mental Health Promotion Group definition 1996)

---

The Department of Health has supported a definition of mental health promotion that clearly links to the definition in Box 13.2 and is a more refined approach than attempted by key policy documents such as *The health of the nation* (Department of Health 1992). This attempted to tackle a typology of health promotion still very limited in the way it could address social exclusion and the politics of health, and steeped in traditional views of disease management and prevention (Naidoo and Wills 1994).

In *Making it happen* the definition is very brief: 'Mental health promotion involves any action to enhance the mental well-being of individuals, families, organisations or communities' (Department of Health 2001a, p. 27). Those interested in developing their knowledge base about this subject need to read this document, as it clearly outlines a wide range of theoretical perspectives and a number of different models to be the basis for a strategic mental health promotion framework. There are useful discussion points raised, and clear ideas about how negative factors could be overcome by being organised at a number of different levels at the same time. This sits well with the move towards collaborative working across NHS trusts and other organisations.

It is necessary to consider mental health promotion at three key levels of analysis, the magical trick being to find a way to incorporate all aspects in health and social policy agendas (Box 13.3). It is clear that for those who are identified as being vulnerable through mental illness or who face additional problems in terms of race, ethnicity, gender, disability and age, targeted policies and specific funded projects, such as those mentioned below, are an essential element.

---

**Box 13.3   Three levels of mental health promotion analysis**

*Strengthening individuals*: or increasing emotional resilience through interventions designed to promote self-esteem, life and coping skills, e.g. communicating, negotiating, relationship and parenting skills.

*Strengthening communities*: this involves increasing social inclusion and participation, improving neighbourhood environments, developing health and social services which support mental health, anti-bullying strategies at school, workplace health, community safety, childcare and self-help networks.

*Reducing structural barriers to mental health*: through initiatives to reduce discrimination and inequalities and to promote access to education, meaningful employment, housing, services and support for those who are vulnerable.

(Department of Health 2001a, p. 30)

---

'Mentality', which was responsible for writing *Making it happen*, is an organisation at the forefront of campaigning to raise the profile of mental health promotion. Mentality has provided useful outlines of what constitutes positive and negative mental health promotion factors at an individual level, especially in terms of addressing the needs of children in trying to avoid the progression from problems in childhood to mental illness in adult life.

# ANTI-OPPRESSIVE PRACTICE

In the book I co-wrote on mental health promotion (McCulloch and Boxer 1997), the link to the promotion of good mental health was not a realistic one without examining our competence in anti-oppressive practice (Box 13.4). This is at the heart of social work practice, however difficult the role, and would seem to be an area of community mental health nursing that needs addressing. It is not usually taught as a core subject on mental health nursing courses and it is clear from service users' accounts that many psychiatrists probably have not even heard of the term or do not subscribe to needing to engage with service users in this way.

---

**Box 13.4   Anti-oppressive practice**

Anti-oppressive practice aims to provide more appropriate and sensitive services by responding to people's needs regardless of their social status. AOP embodies a person centred philosophy; an egalitarian value system concerned with reducing the deleterious effects of structural inequalities upon people's lives; a methodology focusing on both process and outcome; and a way of structuring relationships between individuals that aim to empower users by reducing the negative effects of hierarchy on their interactions and the work they do together.

(Dominelli 1997, p. 24)

---

There are also other necessary elements to the theory and practice of mental health promotion that help identify a personal framework for work in this field:

- anti-oppressive practice;
- empowerment of self and others;
- self-awareness and reflection at the level of the personal and professional commitment given to the above;
- holistic interpretation;
- co-operative and social practice;
- therapeutic, culturally sensitive and feminist practice;
- ethical practice;
- developing knowledge base;
- experiential and person-centred approaches to learning;
- lifelong learning and refinement of knowledge and skills.

(adapted from McCulloch and Boxer 1997)

# PROMOTING MENTAL HEALTH GLOBALLY AND LOCALLY

Because good health depends on so many different factors, many sectors need to be involved in health promotion. The World Health Organization has identified five objectives, which form the basis for improving health. These are:

- to build healthy public policy;
- to create supportive environments;
- to strengthen community action;
- to develop personal skills;
- to reorient health services.

To achieve these objectives and effectively improve the health of the population, many organisations need to work together. While health and social services have an important role to play, their work is most effective when complemented by other sectors such as education, recreation, environment, central and local government, commerce, industry and the non-statutory and voluntary sectors. Social integration and support are also important, so the involvement of community organisations and individual members of local communities is vital.

The WHO Health Report on Mental Health (WHO 2001) sees the community as a resource to stimulate change and deliver public health policy. WHO places great importance on the community as an important resource and setting for tackling the causes and effects of mental health problems. This includes self-help and mutual aid, lobbying for changes in mental health care and resources, carrying out educational activities, participating in the monitoring and evaluation of care, and advocacy to change attitudes and reduce stigma. Local communities are also more sensitive to local realities and are usually strongly committed to innovation and change. Consumer groups have also emerged as a powerful, vocal and active force, often dissatisfied with the established provision of care and treatment.

WHO places mental health in as much a social as a medical context and recognises that successful health and mental health promotion generally involves change at a number of levels. This includes individuals and the family, organisations, communities and society. This should be translated at the macro governmental level to policy and action designed to actively support the right of all citizens to good health. More recently, health promoters have come to perceive health in socio-ecological terms, recognising the fundamental link between health and conditions in economic, physical, social and cultural environments. Policy-makers are beginning to look beyond the traditional health care (illness-oriented) system to improve population health, in recognition that, in addition to biological factors, health is also determined by external factors such as poverty, housing, environment and social support.

Given the social context of mental health it is useful to examine the range of new social regeneration initiatives currently being implemented. These can contribute significantly to mental health promotion. They also offer practitioners new cross-discipline resources, models and methodologies, and, as part of this, a whole new partnership approach with local people and mental health service users. This new 'regeneration' context will be explored further.

# HEALTH AND MENTAL HEALTH POLICY

Repper (2000) offers a comprehensive summary of mental health policy development from the 1950s to the present in an analysis of social inclusion and mental health. She defines a pattern of deinstitutionalisation in the 1960s to the current 'plethora of policy and recommendations' in response to the community care agenda of the 1970s and 1980s. In the last decade health policy has shifted from experimentation with market forces for service improvement back to a rediscovery of inequalities and poverty (Acheson 1998). The last Conservative administration set up a contractual framework of purchasers and providers to secure health improvement. With it came a national health strategy, *The health of the nation*, with long-term targets for key illness areas including mental health (Department of Health 1994). The present Labour administration has reaffirmed the principles of the NHS, seeking to increase investment and structural change. Recognising that the root causes of ill health are multi-factorial, they have seen health service provision as one of many services and interventions for public health improvement. This has culminated in a range of regeneration and urban renewal policies relevant to mental health.

Over the last several years the government has launched a range of area-based initiatives to help tackle social exclusion and reduce inequalities. Each initiative has specific objectives relating to education, health, employment, crime prevention, urban regeneration and wider social well-being. They also contain other common characteristics. These include: a focus on areas and communities where there is a need for priority action, support for innovative approaches, strong local involvement, new partnerships, flexibility and responsiveness in public programmes.

For example, the three main regeneration policies using an Action Zone approach – focusing on a specific geographical area – aim to intervene at several levels. At the individual level in terms of Employment Action Zones, at the community or organisation level for Health Action Zones, and at a service or strategic level for Health Action Zones. The New Deal for Communities initiative includes many of the aims of the specific Action Zones to deliver improvements at a neighbourhood level. This is directly comparable with a mental health promotion strategy that aims to promote public mental health at all levels in society.

# SIGNIFICANT CONTEMPORARY HEALTH AND REGENERATION POLICIES

The government White Paper on the public's health, *Saving lives: our healthier nation* (Department of Health 1999a) went further than its predecessor, *The health of the nation* (Department of Health 1992), with its recognition of inequalities in health. It has four priority areas including mental health, with specific targets on suicide prevention and the promotion of mental health. An operational arm of this policy was the establishment of Health Action Zones to tackle health inequalities.

Health Action Zones (HAZs) were one of the first area-based initiatives established by the New Labour government in 1997. Areas were invited to develop bids for HAZ status by bringing together a range of organisations that would develop proposals for local projects and programmes to tackle issues of health and social exclusion in their communities.

*Making it happen* (Department of Health 2001a) places MHP within a broad health and social improvement model. The document also reaffirms government policy identifying the promotion of health as not the sole reserve of the NHS (Box 13.5).

---

**Box 13.5   Effective mental health promotion**

Many of the factors which influence mental health lie outside health and social care, so mental health promotion is relevant to the implementation of a wide range of policy initiatives, including social inclusion, neighbourhood renewal and health at work. Effective mental health promotion depends on harnessing expertise, resources and partnerships across all sectors and disciplines.

(Department of Health 2001a, p. 5)

---

*The NHS Plan* (Department of Health 2000) sees the establishment of primary care trusts (PCTs). Covering population sizes of between 100,000 and 150,000 people, these new organisations aim to achieve the government's vision of a modern, patient-centred health service. PCTs have several core responsibilities including: improving health and reducing health inequality, developing primary care and community health services, and commissioning hospital services. Cross-organisational work to meet these responsibilities is at the forefront of the Department of Health's approach (Box 13.6).

---

**Box 13.6   Primary care trusts**

PCTs will engage in improving the health of the local community through community development, health promotion and education and occupational health services. They will be the lead NHS organisation for partnership working with local authorities and other partners to improve the health of local communities and to deliver wider objectives for social and economic regeneration. PCTs will work as part of Local Strategic Partnerships to ensure co-ordination of planning and community engagement, integration of service delivery and input to the wider government agenda including Modernising Social Services, Sure Start, Community Safety, Quality Protects, Youth Offending Teams and Regeneration Initiatives.

(Department of Health 2001c, p. 13)

This mandate for partnership working makes explicit the need for health improvement through social and economic regeneration. If this is to be achieved, a greater onus on voluntary and user sector activity is required.

# REGENERATION POLICY CONTEXT

Urban policy in the United Kingdom has long been sustained by a tradition of analysis that has demonstrated the impact of structural economic change upon cities and the socioeconomic consequences of that change. Industrialisation and urbanisation occurred earlier in Britain than in most countries, as has a process of deindustrialisation. The legacy of vacant land, derelict buildings, outdated infrastructure and poor or unwanted housing has posed a major renewal problem. In the post-war period this was compounded by the need to repair war-damaged towns and cities and to renew the housing stock. The increased concentration of people suffering from the effects of poverty, ill health and inadequate housing led in the 1960s to recognition of the need for a renewal policy to complement the hitherto successful dispersal policies of the new towns. The 1970s and 1980s saw a range of policies targeted at the physical structure of cities and improving local economies. These policies assumed that local residents would benefit from a large-scale redevelopment.

However, residents were frequently spectators to external experts improving the physical infrastructure of an area, with little legacy of skills, training or raised aspiration. To tackle this, a new approach to social capital building has been to the fore of policy. This 'bottom-up' approach envisages a partnership arrangement between government policy and its local implementation by agencies and locally inspired solutions to problems. Much of this calls for a community development approach to tackling deep-rooted problems in the social environment. Contemporary policy seeks to reduce inequalities in health status and to look beyond health services to address equity issues. The vehicle to achieve this is the various 'zone' programmes and neighbourhood regeneration initiatives.

One aspect of community living recognised as a root cause of problems is the experience of black and minority ethnic groups. Initiatives such as the New Deal for Communities are attempting to tackle racism and prejudice at all levels. This is a great ideal to strive for, and involves linking key elements that have to be addressed at the same time: health, crime, housing, employment and education. Whether it is a viable solution remains to be seen, but the government has at least adopted a logical approach in its attempt to provide 'joined-up solutions' to complex social problems.

# MENTAL HEALTH AND REGENERATION

There is some significant analysis and identification of the importance of mental health for regeneration policy expounded in the King's Fund report, *Urban regeneration and mental health* (Hoggett *et al.* 1999). Although focusing on the

London population, there are significant implications for other urban environments. The report identified the strengths of the Single Regeneration Budget (SRB) in providing a more integrated approach to regeneration by bringing together a range of partners in the private, public and community sectors. It also identified some of the problems of these initiatives including bureaucracy, a contract focus, top-down nature and a lack of key input from the community and voluntary sectors. Hoggett *et al.* (1999) defined strategies to promote the well-being of communities as including the promotion of community safety, anti-poverty campaigns and bottom-up forms of community economic regeneration, as well as preventive initiatives. These fit with the raft of new health and social care policies with their focus on neighbourhoods, joined-up working across departments and agencies, and, most crucially of all, being community led.

Some other key programmes and reports include:

- The Social Exclusion Unit's report, *Bringing Britain together: a national strategy for neighbourhood renewal* (Social Exclusion Unit 1998). This set out a range of interventions to reduce poor housing, crime, social division and exclusion. The policy is an 'area-based' agenda to improve opportunities in neighbourhoods of deprivation, ill health and social and economic inequality. It describes some key 'structural tasks' including investing in people, involving communities and avoiding 'parachuting in' solutions.

- The Neighbourhood Renewal Fund (NRF) (Neighbourhood Renewal Unit 2002a) is worth £800 million over three years. It is designed to help local authorities in the eighty-eight most deprived areas to improve local services. The main purpose is to narrow the gap between the most deprived areas and the rest of the country, in line with the National Strategy for Neighbourhood Renewal.

- New Deal for Communities (Neighbourhood Renewal Unit 2002b) is a key programme in the government's strategy to tackle multiple deprivation in the most deprived neighbourhoods in the country. It aims to equip communities with high indices of poverty with the resources to tackle problems in an intensive and co-ordinated way. The problems partnerships must address are fivefold: poor job prospects, high levels of crime, educational under-achievement, poor health, and problems with housing and the physical environment. Seventeen pathfinder partnerships were announced in 1998, followed by a second round of twenty-two partnerships in 1999.

Neighbourhood renewal can have a direct impact on the mental health of the general population and at-risk and vulnerable groups. Strategic programmes such as the Health and Education Action Zones, Single Regeneration Budget, Sure Start and New Deal for Communities will make significant contributions to promoting mental health as well as addressing key public health issues.

# GOOD PRACTICE AND MENTAL HEALTH PROMOTION

There are an increasing number of committed people and groups who have 'made a difference' in terms of the approaches they have taken to tackling mental health problems and illness. Some of these are identified in *Making it happen*, through the work of 'Mentality' and in the mental health promotion newsletters published by the Department of Health as part of its mental health promotion project. These are available to download from the Department's website (http: //www.doh. gov.uk/mentalhealth), and provide very useful and relevant material about mental health promotion. However, as Berry has put it:

> Whilst I think we have made a reasonable start in the 20 months or so that our team has been in place in establishing a voice for mental health promotion within the Department of Health at long last and in beginning to establish a sense of community amongst colleagues out in the field, many of whom have been advocating locally for mental health promotion for many years, there is still clearly much work to be done.
>
> (Berry 2002, p. 1)

What is important is that practitioners feel that mental health promotion has something to do with them, first in terms of their own personal needs and development, and second as an integral part of upholding the value base of community mental health practice and its foundation in empowerment, therapeutic alliance and ethical and reflective decision-making.

Having worked in the mental health field since the early 1970s and having experienced the conflict inherent in the role, I have come to a stage in my practice that I think upholds these values and is the most meaningful aspect of my work. I have provided an outline of what I and others feel is a successful project that fits the requirements of both the National Service Framework for Mental Health (Department of Health 1999b) and *Making it happen* (Department of Health 2001a).

*Making it happen* provides pro formas that can be used to send in details of the projects people are engaged in, and also identifies a clear problem-solving approach to project development and evaluation. I have used these headings to provide an example of the work being undertaken in Derbyshire, involving a mental health service user-focused monitoring project as one of a number of initiatives to establish service user involvement across all levels of this mental health trust (Rose 2000) (Box 13.7).

This is obviously just an outline of one project and further details of existing groups working at national level can be obtained from the Sainsbury Centre for Mental Health (http: //www.scmh.org.uk).

Using the problem tree approach includes consideration of the following:

- What are the objectives?
- What are the key elements?

**Box 13.7   An example of a user-focused monitoring project**

*Problem*: service users need to be more involved in monitoring services and having a voice in what these services are.

*The causes of this problem*: many factors based on previous work undertaken by the Sainsbury Centre for Mental Health (Rose 2000).

*The effects of this problem*: service users feel their experience is undervalued, and they have a contribution that cannot be recognised unless they are engaged with trust staff in a different way and at all levels.

*A solution to this problem is*: a service-user focused monitoring project funded by the trust and supported by a steering group made up of service users and staff, including in-patient and community services.

*The objective would be achieved by*:

- training and supporting service users in research and interviewing skills;
- providing evidence for change by undertaking two monitoring projects a year, with agreement that recommendations from the findings will be acted upon by the trust;
- a strategy for service user involvement written collaboratively and including key issues such as payment for work undertaken and support systems in place for individuals and groups.

*The results of these actions*:

- service user involvement in line with government policy and as an example of Standard 1 of the NSF;
- enhanced knowledge, satisfaction and inclusion in the process of change taking place in all aspects of mental health services;
- effective service user-led initiatives with secured yearly funding;
- a clear link to a national group of service users who can help avoid some of the problems by being at the forefront of these changes;
- to avoid replication and increase sample size for more valid and reliable evidence.

- What evidence is available to support action?
- Which policy initiatives support the action?
- Who should be the key stakeholders?
- What are the chosen interventions – individual, community and organisation?
- What indicators will show progress?

It is also important to redefine the problem, and if a yearly action plan is used then it would be useful to consider:

•    What has been achieved by the end of the first year?
•    Have any new issues emerged during this time?
•    Have problems been considered in another way because of the mental health strategy?
•    How would a problem tree be defined now?

## SUMMARY

One brief chapter on mental health promotion cannot do much more than give an overview of the key elements and issues for further study and debate. As this is a book about community mental health practice the emphasis has been on identifying a framework best suited to community work, in the context of strategic and service development (McCulloch and Boxer 1997). The emphasis on community practitioners working within the framework outlined by the Department of Health is crucial and is not something that can be avoided any longer if the long-awaited changes to mental health service development are to be effective. Finding ways of working collaboratively with service users is at the core of mental health promotion from the perspective I have taken. I have not dwelt on what constitutes mental health or what is 'good' mental health because that has been addressed elsewhere (Department of Health 2001a).

The days when community nurses saw their role only in therapeutic person-centred terms, whatever the theoretical psychological position adopted, are over. There are many factors that have always impacted on this anyway. I am aware that, as is discussed in other chapters in this book, defensive practice and risk assessment as driven by statutory requirements dominate the agenda. However, considering anti-oppressive practice as a way of redefining our professional position as nurses is also essential, and has only been touched on in this chapter. It is hoped that in the future this will be a focus for debate when discussing mental health promotion in educational and community settings. It is also essential that students and practitioners have a good understanding of how strategies, service developments and policies inform our practice at all levels. It is not unusual these days to have mental health service users as members of trust and commissioning boards or in other clinical and non-clinical reference groups such as strategic development, clinical governance and local service delivery implementation teams. There is evidence supporting service user involvement at a wide level and with mental health promotion as a core focus of this process; the future of mental health provision in this country does not have to be steeped in negative connotations.

# REFERENCES

Acheson, D. (1998) *Independent inquiry into inequalities in health*, London: The Stationery Office.

Alexander, Z. (1999) *Study of black, Asian and ethnic minority issues*, London: Department of Health.

Berry, R. (2002) 'Editorial', *Mental Health Promotion Update*, issue 4, London: Department of Health.

Boxer, J. and McCulloch, G. (1996) 'Mental health: policy and practice', in Gastrell, P. and Edwards, J. (eds) *Community health nursing: frameworks for practice*, London: Baillière Tindall.

Department of Health (1992) *The health of the nation: a strategy for health in England*, London: HMSO.

Department of Health (1994) *The health of the nation key area handbook: mental illness*, 2nd edn, London: HMSO.

Department of Health (1999a) *Saving lives: our healthier nation*, London: Department of Health.

Department of Health (1999b) *National service framework for mental health: modern standards and service models*, London: Department of Health.

Department of Health (2000) *The NHS Plan: a plan for investment, a plan for reform*, London: The Stationery Office.

Department of Health (2001a) *Making it happen: a guide to delivering mental health promotion*, London: Department of Health.

Department of Health (2001b) *National service framework for older people: modern standards and service models*, London: Department of Health.

Department of Health (2001c) *Shifting the balance of power within the NHS: securing delivery*, London: Department of Health.

Dominelli, L. (1997) *Anti-racist social work*, 2nd edn, Basingstoke: Macmillan.

Hoggett, P., Stewart, M., Razzaque, K. and Barker, I. (1999) *Urban regeneration and mental health in London*, London: King's Fund.

Keating, F. and Robertson, D. (2002) 'Breaking the circle of fear: a review of mental health services to African and Caribbean communities', in *Mental Health Promotion Update*, issue 4, London: Department of Health.

McCulloch, G. and Boxer, J. (1997) *Mental health promotion: policy, practice and partnerships*, London: Baillière Tindall.

Naidoo, J. and Wills, J. (1994) *Health promotion: foundations for practice*, London: Baillière Tindall.

Neighbourhood Renewal Unit (2002a) *Our programmes*. Online. http://www.neighbourhood.gov.uk/ourprogs.asp?pageid=4

Neighbourhood Renewal Unit (2002b) *New deal for communities*. Online. http://www.neighbourhood.gov.uk/ndcomms.asp?pageid=34

Repper, J. (2000) 'Interventions in mental health practice', in Thompson, A. and Mathias, P. (eds) *Lyttle's Mental Disorder*, 3rd edn, London: Baillière Tindall.

Rose, D. (2000) *Users' voices*, London: Sainsbury Centre for Mental Health.

Sainsbury Centre for Mental Health (1999) *Acute solutions*, London: Sainsbury Centre for Mental Health.

Social Exclusion Unit (1998) *Bringing Britain together: a national strategy for neighbourhood renewal*, London: Social Exclusion Unit.

World Health Organization (WHO) (1991) *Health for all targets: European health for all series, no. 4, The health policy for Europe*, Geneva: World Health Organization.

World Health Organization (WHO) (2001) *Mental health: new understanding, new hope*, Geneva: World Health Organization.

# FURTHER READING

Department of Health (2001) *Making it happen: a guide to delivering mental health promotion*, London: Department of Health.

*Journal of Mental Health Promotion*, edited by 'Mentality'.

McCulloch, G. and Boxer, J. (1997) *Mental health promotion: policy, practice and partnerships*, London: Baillière Tindall.

# CHAPTER 14

# USING EVIDENCE TO INFORM PRACTICE

*Rob Newell*

---

## SUMMARY OF KEY POINTS

- Evidence to support mental health practice is scarce.
- Comparatively little nursing research is concerned with clinical work.
- Reliance on 'expert' opinion is detrimental to service user needs.

---

## INTRODUCTION – WHY EVIDENCE? WHY NOW?

Mental health nursing has, through most of its recent history, been a discipline subject to changes in its knowledge base and to the ways in which care is organised. In recent years, government policy has impacted upon our profession in such ways that the level and pace of change have grown considerably (see Chapter 3). It may be argued that nurses, as the largest NHS workforce, have seen more of the effect of such changes than any other group of health professionals. In particular, mental health nurses working in the community might be expected to be greatly affected, since the move to care of people with mental illness in the community is now firmly established as the major way in which care is organised. Indeed, community mental health nurses have seen successive changes to the ways in which they are expected to work with clients. Currently, they are expected to span the spectrum from primary prevention initiatives through to highly specific targeted interventions with hard-to-engage groups.

Many of these initiatives are supported by evidence of some kind, and much of this evidence was created and gathered by groups other than nurses. Yet nursing is the largest element within the NHS workforce (Department of Health 2000), and accounts for most of the professional contact experienced by patients and clients. Given this level of contact, plus the long tradition nurses have in working alongside service users to ensure that their voice is heard, we might expect nurses to have a strong voice in deciding on the selection of interventions and organisation of care. In order to possess such a voice, we must be able to speak authoritatively. This chapter argues that such authority comes best from an ability to understand, evaluate and marshal what evidence there is for practice, and to create such evidence where it is lacking. In the course of this argument, we shall examine the nature of evidence, explore why it is often lacking in mental health nursing and suggest how current government policies concerning NHS research and development (R&D) might help or hinder the aspirations of mental health nurses in the community to build or use the evidence base for their practice.

## WHAT IS EVIDENCE-BASED PRACTICE?

Evidence-based practice has been described as:

> a process of lifelong self directed learning in which caring for our patients creates the need for clinically important information about diagnosis, prognosis, therapy and other clinical and health care issues.
> (Batstone and Edwards 1996, p. 19)

The notion of basing clinical practice on evidence is relatively recent, and it has been suggested that only a tiny minority of our interventions are based on evidence from methodologically strong research studies such as randomised controlled trials. Estimates of the percentage of care which is evidence based vary between 5 and 15 per cent for medical interventions in general, and are likely to be at least as low in nursing. Muir Gray (1997) identifies three broad stages in the practice of evidence-based health care: production of evidence, making evidence available, and using evidence (getting research into practice). The lack of available evidence represents an important handicap to the first of these three stages, but also affects our ability to disseminate and utilise evidence. Moreover, there are deficits associated with these latter stages even where evidence exists. For example, DiCenso et al. (1998) noted that only 35 per cent of small hospitals in Canada had nursing research journals available to staff, only 38 per cent of health agencies based changes in practice on the research process, and only 15 per cent had implementation programmes for staff. This is worrying, since we often regard the USA and Canada as being at the forefront of nursing practice and research.

Evidence-based practice is a continuous educational *process*, not an end. Whilst the practice of evidence-based care is certainly the responsibility of institutions, and one which is increasingly being policed by government via such organisations as the National Institute for Clinical Excellence (NICE) and the Commission for Health Improvement (CHI), it is also the responsibility of individual clinicians, who are expected to take responsibility for their learning

(Sackett *et al.* 1997). In nursing, such ongoing learning is a requirement for continuing registration (UKCC 2001).

In many ways, for the clinician, involvement with evidence-based care begins at the third of Muir Gray's stages. Clients are perceived as presenting clinical challenges which the clinician seeks to respond to through a five-stage process of educational investigation (Sackett *et al.* 1997), involving: defining an answerable question to the challenge presented by the client; finding the best available evidence; appraising this evidence; applying the results in practice; and evaluating performance. This process can operate at a variety of levels, from individual involvement with a service user, through service and practice development, to the clinician's own learning and training needs and the identification of such needs for an entire service. An example from my own field of practice, behavioural medicine, at the level of the individual and the institution, is given in Box 14.1.

---

**Box 14.1   Introducing an evidence-based care initiative**

*Individual client*

*Client with uncontrolled eczema with persistent excoriation not responding to topical medication*

*Question*: What factors might be maintaining this person's problem? What psychological techniques might assist?

*Evidence sources*: *British Journal of Dermatology*; *British Journal of Dermatology Nursing*; *Cognitive and Behavioural Psychotherapy*.

*Appraisal*: Habit reversal has been used in small studies to address the problem of continual scratching. Scratching is known to be important in the maintenance of eczema.

*Application and evaluation*: Negotiate with patient to use habit reversal. Use single-case experimental methodology to assess effectiveness.

*Training needs*: Minimal – habit reversal is a recognised technique in cognitive behavioural therapy (CBT) in other contexts.

*Institution*

*Dermatology ward*

*Question*: Does cognitive behavioural therapy have anything to offer nursing staff working in this setting?

*Evidence sources*: As above, plus: *British Journal of Psychology*; etc.

*Appraisal*: Structured review of cognitive behavioural interventions across a broad range of dermatological complaints.

*Application and evaluation*: Structured training in application of the best verified techniques from the literature review. Audit of patient outcomes at six months after initiation.

*Training needs*: Information searching and appraisal skills; training in specific interventions identified; training in assessment for suitability.

# THE CONTEXT FOR EVIDENCE-BASED CARE

Whilst we tend to think of evidence predominantly in terms of evidence of effectiveness available from the research literature, its definition is, from the viewpoint of the clinical practitioner, much broader than this, and includes results from medical tests, impressions gained from the patient at interview, and so on. The clinician is expected to use all such data in a holistic way.

Evidence-based care has often been criticised for taking individual choice away from clinicians – for being a 'cookbook' approach, which applies a recipe of a well-validated treatment to client groups (Sackett *et al.* 1997). However, there is no logical reason why using the best available evidence should lead to a disregard for individualised patient care. On the contrary, reliance on care which has no basis other than custom and practice is easily the best way of ensuring ritualised care which assaults patient individuality. By contrast, as I suggested in the previous paragraph, clinical expertise and judgement are seen as crucial to evidence-based care, providing awareness of the whole context within which specific evidence-based initiatives might be introduced. Evidence-based practice (EBP) and research findings enrich and inform that expertise and individual client and clinician choice, by enhancing the information upon which they are based, rather than impoverishing it by introducing meaningless standardisation.

# THE NATURE OF EVIDENCE

A further criticism of evidence-based practice, and one which has been applied (often with considerable heat) in mental health, is the notion that the definitions of evidence employed by proponents of evidence-based care are too narrow and mechanistic. The National Service Framework for Mental Health (NSF) (Department of Health 1999) has been a major driver for future change in mental health care, and has adopted an accepted definition of levels of evidence (Harris *et al.* 1998) and tied this definition to the actions it recommends for the future of mental health care. However, if we were to consider that this definition was too rigid, it might provide an unfair constraint upon innovation in clinical practice. Let us examine the definitions of levels of evidence it uses.

The most reliable form of evidence is regarded as the systematic review. In this process, reviewers use recognised criteria for searching for relevant literature, which they then evaluate in terms of its methodological strength and relevance to practice, again often using robust agreed criteria. Typically, such reviews contain studies which report randomised controlled trials (RCTs). Where insufficient evidence exists to mount a systematic review, evidence from a single robust RCT is regarded as the next most reliable level of evidence, followed by evidence from one or more non-randomised trials (quasi-experimental study). For proponents of evidence-based practice, this third level of reliability represents a considerable step down, since the possibility of unwanted bias is materially increased where randomisation is not used. Within mental health care, randomisation is often difficult to undertake because of service constraints, the difficulty of 'blinding' raters, and the assumed complexity of the treatments being tested. Further down the hierarchy, observational studies are regarded as providing some evidence of effectiveness, whilst where no research evidence exists, clinicians may regard expert opinion as appropriate evidence on which to base practice. Importantly, the NSF broadens the definition of expert opinion to include the opinions of users and carers.

It might be thought that requiring the use of good evidence is an important contribution to the organisation of mental health care. However, it has given rise to some controversy within mental health nursing, perhaps in part because of the identification of the RCT with medical models of care and research. Nurse behaviour therapists in particular have been characterised as 'nurse brutalists' (Clarke 1999), in part because of their assumed espousal of care based on the results of RCTs. This is surprising given, on the one hand, the considerable amount of hostility faced by nurse behaviour therapists from medically oriented psychiatrists, and, on the other, the insistence of behaviour therapy in general and nurse behaviour therapy in particular on a denial of the idea of pathology in mental ill health, and the necessity of individualised care and the primacy of the patient in defining the process of such care. Indeed, it could be argued that, sensitively applied, the results of RCTs offer the most client-centred form of care imaginable, since they represent the choice of care which is offered *least* according to the personal preference of clinicians and *most* according to the previous responses of service users who share key characteristics with the client being offered treatment based on such evidence.

Nevertheless, it seems that those who espouse the use of evidence based primarily on RCTs have come to be identified with an inflexible attitude to care, and an artificial division within mental health nursing may be a consequence of this. However, as noted earlier, there is no reason to regard the use of evidence as a constraint on practice. Rather it should facilitate the clinician's decisions and allow fuller discussion with clients about the best course of action. By contrast, each time we offer clients a rationale for the interventions we intend to offer them, without adequate knowledge of the evidence base, we take choice away from them. This is because, if we fail to be aware of the evidence base (or lack of it) underlying our practice, we are denying patients the right to adequate information. In effect, we are asking them to take *our* word for it, and this is the ultimate denial of patient-centred care. I find the debate over evidence as a basis of care regrettable in a discipline which has all too often seen the introduction of ineffective interventions, usually at considerable personal (and sometimes monetary) cost to service users, their relatives and the health service.

## EVIDENCE AND POWER

Part of the reasoning behind the distrust of evidence-based care is the notion that the definition of evidence is too narrow. For example, although the NSF recognises the value of user testimony, this is at the bottom of the evidence hierarchy, whilst we might not unreasonably consider it to belong near the top. This is an instance of how the definition of evidence may be constructed by those with the power to make, disseminate and implement such constructions. I have argued elsewhere

(Newell 1997) that those in positions of power decide what counts as evidence, and, as a result, I want to argue that, paradoxically, the definitions of evidence enshrined in the NSF are, if anything, too *broad* rather than too narrow. Most particularly, reliance on expert testimony is an inadequate safeguard of appropriate standards of care. Similarly, it is a potential contributor to the persistence of outmoded forms of care. In health care, since the majority of our care is *not* underpinned by evidence, it follows that much of it is based on professional opinion. Traditionally, this opinion has come from medical practitioners, who have occupied and protected positions of professional and administrative power within health care. Nowhere is this more inappropriate than in mental health, where the roles of medicine and medication are equivocal at best. Yet it has been suggested that, in mental health, the shortage of research evidence for practice is particularly acute. In consequence, it might be within mental health that the potential for domination of care by 'expert' opinion might be most encountered, since other sources of evidence are often not available. I want to argue that nurses, by virtue of the amount of contact they have with patients, and their readiness to adopt a variety of approaches to care, are the best sources of potential support that service users have, other than other users. More than this, we are well placed to use our influence for the good or ill of our client, whether this be by virtue of the increasing policy-making role which nurses have been expected to adopt, particularly in community and primary care, or by virtue of the large amount of clinical work we perform. If we are unable or unwilling to take responsibility for the organisation, content and delivery of the care we give, we risk having others take this responsibility instead, and, in consequence, risk a diminution of our voice in support of clients.

## THE CONSTRUCTION OF EVIDENCE

In the introduction, I argued that we should be able to speak authoritatively. There is no doubt that other professions in health care are able to do this, at least in large part, as a result of their traditional and continuing professional power. Given that we do not have this tradition, evidence can be our strongest ally. However, there is not, as yet, an overpowering level of such evidence for the effectiveness of mental health nursing initiatives. We *have* made use of supporting evidence from other disciplines, and nurses have often taken a leading role in the implementation of important research findings from other disciplines as well as contributing to the original generation of such research. We need to increase our contribution to such work in order to ensure that future research reflects and enhances the clinical contribution of nurses. However, there is not, as yet, room for us to be confident in our performance in the field of clinical research. In exploring research and development in nurse education (Newell 2002), I examined the publishing records of the leading UK psychiatric journal (the *British Journal of Psychiatry*) and its mental health nursing counterpart (*Journal of Psychiatric and Mental Health Nursing*) over the past two years. A rough division of its published papers into four categories – outcome studies, clinical papers, educational and professional matters, and general papers (position papers, policy papers, historical papers) – revealed several issues. First, the overall level of out-come studies was low (11.4 per cent in *BJPsych* and 6.2 per cent in *J Psych and-MH Nursing*). More worrying, however, were two key differences between the journals. *BJPsych* carried 80.5 per cent clinical papers, whilst *J Psych and-MH Nursing* carried only 30.2 per cent. By contrast, *J Psych and MH Nursing* carried 43.3 per cent educational and professional papers, whilst *BJPsych* carried 1.3 per cent. The conclusions from this are easily drawn – nursing is, as yet, insufficiently concerned with sharing practice or researching on topics directly related to issues of care of patients and clients, and is still emphasising, in its scholarly activity, matters concerned with nurses themselves and their preparation for practice. Nor is this exclusively a UK phenomenon. In Australia and New Zealand, the major mental health journals are the *Australia and New Zealand Journal of Psychiatry* and the *Australia and New Zealand Journal of Mental Health Nursing*. Once again, there were sharp contrasts between the proportions of the two journals devoted to clinical versus educational and professional papers. The *AandNZJPsych* carried 70.2 per cent clinical papers and 4.8 per cent educational and professional papers, whilst the *A and NZ J MH Nursing* carried 36.2 per cent clinical papers and 41.4 per cent educational and professional (Newell 2001). In the UK, it is well known that nursing research is poorly developed, with deficits at all levels in our ability to support or undertake research. Moreover, it is recognised that the university sector, from which we should expect scholarship in the profession to be led, suffers from a shortage of research leaders and is insufficiently engaged with the examination of research into clinical practice. These factors, combined with the low amount of clinical research currently being undertaken and published in nursing journals, suggest that, in the practice of evidence-based care, there is considerable work to be done at Sackett *et al.*'s (1997) first level of evidence-based practice – generating evidence – without which little practice of evidence-based care can be possible. This offers a considerable challenge to people in clinical practice, since it leads us to question, for example, how far our current care is likely to be evidence-based and where we can look for support, how we can ourselves create evidence where it is lacking, and how far we can look to innovate in clinical practice without recourse to robust evaluation strategies.

## RESOURCES FOR THE PRACTICE OF EVIDENCE-BASED CARE

If, as I have suggested, the amount of research into nursing care in general, and community psychiatric nursing care in particular, is slight, does this then mean that we are inevitably faced with recourse to tradition and ritual? The most immediate alternative is to recognise that much work of relevance to nursing is published in non-nursing journals and textbooks, and is, indeed, published by non-nurses. In the long term, there is no doubt that, as a profession, we will want to take responsibility for the care we give, not only in practice, but in generating the evidence base to underpin that practice. In the meantime, we will be well served if we do not emulate the apparent introspection of the profession in its own research in the way we search for and examine evidence. If our interventions are to be client-centred, it is logical that our literature searching should be based on clinical topics (including 'diagnosis') rather than the professional group responsible for the intervention.

Adopting this policy, we are in a position to use findings from a wide raft of national initiatives around evidence-based practice. The Cochrane collaboration has been described as a health initiative to rival the human genome project in terms of its potential importance (Naylor 1995). Its principal activity is organisation and publication of systematic reviews, and to date over 1,300 such reviews have been published. Members of Cochrane groups who carry out the reviews also agree to continue to keep the reviews updated. This is a considerable, unpaid voluntary activity which demonstrates the importance that group members assign to the endeavour. Abstracts of Cochrane reviews are freely available through the Web (http: //www.cochrane.org) and full copies of reviews can be ordered. Many NHS trusts and an increasing number of primary care trusts are subscribers.

The following Cochrane groups are highly relevant to nurses working in community mental health:

- Cochrane Consumers and Communication Group
- Cochrane Dementia and Cognitive Improvement Group
- Cochrane Depression, Anxiety and Neurosis Group
- Cochrane Developmental, Psychosocial and Learning Problems Group
- Cochrane Drugs and Alcohol Group
- Cochrane Schizophrenia Group.

Between them, these groups currently comprise eighty-three reviews, which range in topic matter from biologically oriented projects to studies of psychosocial interventions.

The NHS Centre for Reviews and Dissemination (CRD), based at the University of York, has a similar role to the Cochrane collaboration, although it examines evidence from a wider range of sources than randomised controlled trials. Again, this group has a considerable Web presence (http: //www.york.ac.uk/inst/crd/). It also publishes evidence-based practice materials on a wide variety of issues in three different paper-based formats:

- *CRD Reports* – This is the most detailed of CRD's publications, but executive summaries of many issues are available via the Web.
- *Effectiveness Matters* – This is a more succinct publication in brief magazine format. Most issues are available in electronic form. For the community mental health nurse, it is worth looking at a recent issue (CRD 2001) which examines evidence for the effectiveness of counselling in primary care. Also of considerable importance for hard-pressed clinicians is an issue examining the effectiveness of numerous different methods of accessing evidence for clinical effectiveness. As well as assessing the relative merits of different access methods, the report is an excellent catalogue of such methods.
- *Effective Health Care Bulletin* is a lengthier, journal-style publication. Once again, many issues are available via the Web. Perhaps the most relevant for

community mental health nurses are the issues which examine psychosocial interventions for schizophrenia, drug treatment in schizophrenia, deliberate self-harm and mental health promotion in high-risk groups. Nurses with more of a primary care and primary prevention/health promotion role may also be interested in examining issues which deal with preventing uptake of smoking in young people, prevention and reduction of adverse affects of teenage pregnancy, and prevention and treatment of obesity. As with *Effectiveness Matters*, there is also an issue of *Effective Health Care Bulletin* which is relevant to the process of evidence-based practice itself, and deals with getting evidence into practice. This document contains evidence-based information about how most effectively to implement evidence-based initiatives and support an evidence-based culture within an institution. Its findings are discussed in more detail below. All the above publications can be found through the CRD website.

# ADOPTING AN EVIDENCE-BASED INITIATIVE

In deciding whether to adopt a particular intervention, Sackett *et al*. (1997) draw attention to the need to examine three simple questions: is the evidence reliable, is the evidence important and is the evidence applicable? The first of these criteria, if we are thinking about evidence from the literature (rather than evidence from, for example, clinical tests), requires an ability to critically evaluate the available literature or, if we lack the time in clinical practice, or lack these often scarce skills, access to a reputable source of such skill. Many clinicians, particularly from a medical background, along with many health service managers, have come to regard Cochrane reviews, CRD publications and – perhaps to a lesser degree and perhaps quite rightly – national service frameworks as such reputable sources. Regardless of whether one evaluates the evidence oneself or trusts the evaluation of another, the principle is the same – that the evidence will be sufficiently methodologically strong to give us confidence in its findings. The notion of importance is related to this. Given that we can accept that the findings show that a certain treatment has an effect on patient well-being, is that effect likely to be of sufficient size and sufficient duration (and sufficient safety or absence of negative side effects) to offer the patient an appreciable improvement in their health and broader life status? Finally, if both these criteria are met, is the intervention likely to be applicable in my clinical setting? This is a difficult criterion to meet in, for example, cases where expensive equipment is needed, or considerable further training required by the clinicians concerned, or where some other practical constraints apply (such as unavailability of the intervention outside certain distant centres of excellence). When these three questions have been answered we may attempt to implement an evidence-based initiative.

This is not, however, the end of the story, particularly when implementation is required across an entire service. At this point, a whole series of change management initiatives which are outside the scope of this chapter are required. In their examination of factors likely to facilitate the uptake of evidence-based initiatives, the NHS Centre for Reviews and Dissemination (CRD 1999) reported factors likely to aid in successfully getting research into practice. As well as individual beliefs and attitudes, environmental constraints such as economics and organisational environment should be considered. In this context, an examination of likely impediments and facilitating factors (a 'diagnostic analysis') should be conducted, and its findings used to inform choice of how dissemination will be carried out. The analysis should include: identification of all groups affected by the proposed change; assessment of those elements of the change that might affect its likely adoption; assessment of preparedness for change of involved parties; identification of barriers; identification of enabling factors. Effective introduction of change will involve a strategic plan related to implementation, and dissemination of information alone is unlikely to be effective. Finally, there should be an appropriate monitoring strategy associated with the introduction of change.

# THE EVIDENCE BASE AND INNOVATIVE PRACTICE DEVELOPMENTS: BUILDING EVIDENCE FOR THE FUTURE

At the beginning of this chapter, we noted that only a small proportion of health care is evidence-based. It was also reported that higher education has often been seen as remote from clinical practice, and that nurse academics may not necessarily share the same research agendas as their clinical colleagues. However, there are some signs that government is beginning to recognise the gap between the clinical work nurses do and the evidence base needed to support it. It is important that nurse researchers remain in contact with their clinical colleagues in order to ensure that innovative practice has an adequate research strategy attached to it. Without evaluation, the most exciting clinical or educational innovation is severely limited, since we will have no evidence upon which to recommend its continuation or adoption as mainstream mental health nursing practice. Many of the best ideas for research come from clinical practice and the clinical questions that practice generates. During the last universities research assessment exercise, there was some indication that members of the review panel took particular account of the ability of university departments to engage with clinical practice, a view which has been regarded as important at least since the 1993 report of the Department of Health taskforce on research in nursing, midwifery and health visiting, which stated that:

> The fundamental research task is to evaluate the effectiveness of clinical procedures, practices and interventions.
>
> (Department of Health 1993, p.8)

If this trend continues into the future, it will be healthy both for research and for clinical practice, and, ultimately, for service users. Given the scarcity of evidence for mental health nursing practice, researchers and clinicians have a joint responsibility to build that evidence base, working together to ensure that innovative practice is sufficiently supported by robust evaluation to allow it eventually to become part of mainstream, evidence-based care.

# REFERENCES

Batstone, G. and Edwards, M. (1996) 'Achieving clinical effectiveness: just another initiative or a real change in working practice?', *Journal of Clinical Effectiveness*, 1 (1): 19–21.

Centre for Reviews and Dissemination (CRD) (1999) 'Getting evidence into practice', *Effective Health Care*, 5, 1, York: University of York.

Centre for Reviews and Dissemination (CRD) (2001) 'Counselling in primary care', *Effectiveness Matters*, 5, 2, York: University of York.

Clarke, L. (1999) 'Nursing in search of a science: the rise and rise of the new nurse brutalism', *Mental Health Care*, 2 (8): 270–272.

Department of Health (1993) *Report of the taskforce on the strategy for research in nursing, midwifery and health visiting*, London: Department of Health.

Department of Health (1999) *National service framework for mental health: modern standards and service models*, London: Department of Health.

Department of Health (2000) *Towards a strategy for nursing research and development: proposals for action*, London: Department of Health.

DiCenso, A., Cullum, N. and Donna Ciliska, D. (1998) 'Implementing evidence-based nursing: some misconceptions', *Evidence Based Nursing*, 1: 38–39.

Harris, L., Davidson, L. and Evans, I. (1998) *Health evidence bulletin Wales: mental health*, Cardiff: Welsh Office.

Muir Gray, J.A. (1997) *Evidence-based healthcare: how to make health policy and management decisions*, New York: Churchill Livingstone.

Naylor, C.D. (1995) 'Grey zones of clinical practice: some limits to evidence-based medicine', *Lancet*, 345: 840–842.

Newell, R. (1997) 'Editorial: Towards clinical effectiveness in nursing', *Clinical Effectiveness in Nursing*, 1 (1): 1–2.

Newell, R. (2001) 'Keynote address: evidence based practice in mental health nursing: securing the evidence', *27th Annual Conference of the Australia and New Zealand College of Psychiatric and Mental Nurses*, Melbourne, November.

Newell, R. (2002) 'Research and its relationship to nurse education', *Nurse Education Today*, 22 (4): 278–284.

Sackett, D.L., Richardson, W.S., Rosenberg, W. and Haynes, R.B. (1997) *Evidence-based medicine: how to practice and teach EBM*, New York: Churchill Livingstone.

UKCC (2001) *The PREP handbook*, London: UKCC.

# FURTHER READING

Muir Gray, J.A. (1997) *Evidence-based healthcare: how to make health policy and management decisions*, New York: Churchill Livingstone.
An excellent general introduction to the practice of evidence-based health care. Although the book is written mainly from a medical perspective, its general recommendations are relevant across the disciplines.

Centre for Reviews and Dissemination (1999) 'Getting evidence into practice', *Effective Health Care*, 5, 1, York: University of York.
A good review, but also a great guide to getting evidence into practice. Reads almost like a primer of 'dos and don'ts'.

# CHAPTER 15

# ASSESSING NEEDS IN COMMUNITY MENTAL HEALTH CARE

*Mike Slade*

---

## SUMMARY OF KEY POINTS

- Assessment of need facilitates individualised care planning.
- Needs assessment should be standard practice for community mental health nurses.
- The Camberwell Assessment of Need Short Appraisal Schedule (CANSAS) is suitable for routine clinical use.

---

## INTRODUCTION

A *needs-led* approach to the provision of mental health care has been one of the most consistent themes to emerge from the evolution of community mental health services. The requirement to base the provision of services on level of need was first made explicit in the National Health Service and Community Care Act (House of Commons 1990), and is retained in the National Service Framework for Mental Health (Department of Health 1999).

A needs-led approach has two components. First, patients with the most wide-ranging and severe health and social needs should receive the most specialist mental health care. In practice, this means that the caseload of nurses working in a primary care context with patients experiencing mental health problems should consist predominantly of people with a small number of relatively simple needs. By contrast, the caseload of nurses working in a specialist mental health service should mainly comprise people whose needs are more multiple and complex.

Second, the process of assessment and care planning for patients should consider their individual circumstances, problems and personal goals. Assessment should not be undertaken in terms of or on the basis of existing services, i.e. assessment should not be *service-based*. This means that assessment of need is a separate process from decisions about what care or treatment to provide. Needs-led assessment means, for example, that a nursing assessment should look at whether the person has access to enough activities which are meaningful (to them) each day, rather than whether they need to attend a day centre. If the assessment indicates that there is a problem with daytime activities, one response might be to arrange a place at a day centre. Other responses, however, might be to offer support in undertaking voluntary work or to refer the patient to a befriending scheme.

The needs-led approach offers two benefits. It gives guidance about the most appropriate form of service response, both in terms of *where* the patient is offered treatment (e.g. primary care, mental health service), and in terms of *what* treatment or care to offer. It also facilitates individualised care, by closely matching the patient's needs to the help offered. This may involve identifying needs for which there is currently no service provision, which a service-based assessment by definition would not identify.

The ongoing assessment of needs is good practice and is compulsory, not optional. This has particular relevance to community mental health nurses, who will often have long-term relationships with patients. Nurses should be completing a high-quality initial assessment of the needs of the patient, providing or arranging for care to meet the identified needs, and monitoring the impact of interventions over time.

This chapter is organised to provide different types of information. Section 1 gives a conceptual introduction to needs. Section 2 provides a discussion of specific measures which have been developed for assessing needs. Section 3 describes how to use one particular approach – the Camberwell Assessment of Need Short Appraisal Schedule (CANSAS). Section 4 provides a step-by-step guide to making an assessment of needs using CANSAS to plan treatment. Each section is self-contained. For the nurse simply wanting to use a well-developed approach, Sections 3 and 4 can be read as a guide to assessing needs.

# SECTION 1: INDIVIDUAL AND POPULATION NEEDS

So, what is a need? Despite the wide recognition that people with severe mental health problems usually have a range of health and social needs, there is continuing debate about how such needs should be defined and assessed (Holloway 1993). Part of the confusion arises because the term is used to mean both the needs of an individual and the needs of populations. The majority of community mental health nurses will only be concerned with assessing the needs of patients rather than populations, so the remainder of this chapter will mainly consider individual needs assessment. Further information about approaches to population-based needs assessment can be found elsewhere (Slade and Glover 2000).

## Individual needs

Before considering specific proposals for a definition of what constitutes a need, one issue needs to be highlighted: the importance of perspective. The sociologist Bradshaw (1972) proposed a taxonomy of four types of need: that which is either 'felt' (experienced) or 'expressed' (reported) by the patient, 'normative' need which is assessed by an expert, and 'comparative' need which arises from comparison with other groups or individuals. Patients may feel but not express needs, for a variety of reasons – they may not report suicidal feelings because they do not want help, or they may not report command hallucinations because they fear compulsory detention. Furthermore the patient's expressed need may – and frequently does – differ from the normative staff view. Finally, the assessment of a need will be affected by the chosen reference group – do mental health patients need a car, or a telephone, or meaningful daytime activities? Probably, the answer partly depends on whether their needs are considered in relation to other patients (many of whom will unfortunately not have any of these), or to other members of the general public.

Similarly, from a health economics perspective, Stevens and Gabbay (1991) distinguished need (which they defined as the ability to benefit in some way from health care), demand (wish expressed by the service patient) and supply of services. For instance, mental health services for homeless mentally ill people are rarely demanded by homeless people, but most professionals would agree that a need exists. In contrast, the demand for counselling services frequently outstrips supply. These frameworks highlight that need is a subjective concept, and that the judgement of whether a need is present or not may in part depend on whose viewpoint is being taken. This point will be returned to later.

## Definitions of need

Many definitions of need have been proposed. Brewin (1992) categorises definitions of need within mental health care into three types: a lack of health, a lack of access to services or institutions, and a lack of action by lay or professional mental health workers. For completeness, definitions of need from all three categories will be reviewed.

### 1  Needs for improved health

The American psychologist Maslow established probably the most well-known hierarchy of need, when he formulated a theory of human motivation (Maslow 1954). In Maslow's model, fundamental physiological needs (such as the need for food) underpin the higher needs of safety, love, self-esteem and self-actualisation. He proposed that people are motivated by the requirement to meet these needs, and that higher needs could only be met once the lower and more fundamental needs were met.

The National Health Service and Community Care Act (1990) states that needs are 'the requirements of individuals to enable them to achieve, maintain or restore an acceptable level of social independence or quality of life' (Department of Health Social Services Inspectorate 1991, p. 10). This definition equates need with social disablement, which occurs when a person experiences lowered psychological, social and physical functioning in comparison with the norms of society (Wing 1986).

## 2 Needs for services

The second category of definition suggested by Brewin relates to access to psychiatric services. The assumption here is that an unmet need arises due to a lack of access to some form of psychiatric service. For example, the Mini Finland Health Survey equated unmet need with an inadequate level of service response for the severity of problem (Lehtinen *et al.* 1990). The National Institute of Mental Health Epidemiologic Catchment Area Program collected data on psychiatric disorder prevalence, which were used to infer the population level of need (Regier *et al.* 1984). This category is oriented towards population-level needs, and may be most suitable for informing the development of mental health services. It is less appropriate at an individual level, since it assesses needs through the filter of existing psychiatric services.

## 3 Needs for action

The final category of needs assessment schedules measures the need for action by professional or lay mental health workers. The MRC Needs for Care Assessment originally defined need as present when the person's functioning falls below a specified level *due to a potentially remediable cause* (Brewin *et al.* 1987). This was criticised for failing to identify needs which could not be met, and so a new category of 'no meetable need' was introduced (Mangen and Brewin 1991). This definition reduces the extent to which assessment can be needs-led, since intervention effectiveness rather than need is being assessed.

# SECTION 2: NEEDS ASSESSMENT MEASURES

What measure should nurses use for assessing needs? Current practice often involves the use of locally developed assessments. Although widespread, this type of assessment is susceptible to bias in what it asks about, and in how questions are phrased. In particular, it will inevitably focus on areas of particular interest to the people – or more commonly the person – who developed it. Home-grown assessments will also not have had their psychometric properties established. Important properties to investigate are shown in Table 15.1.

Constructing a 'standardised' assessment, which is systematically developed and has established psychometric properties, is a complex and time-consuming endeavour. However, patients are poorly served if their care is provided on the basis of non-standardised assessments – a standardised assessment of need should be used.

*Table 15.1* Psychometric properties of needs assessment measures

| Psychometric property | Description |
| --- | --- |
| Inter-rater reliability | The assessment yields the same information irrespective of which team member completes it |
| Test–retest reliability | Providing nothing has changed for the patient, the assessment yields the same information on repeat administration |
| Internal validity | The assessment information is internally consistent and does actually assess needs, rather than something else, such as satisfaction with care |
| External validity | The assessment is usable outside the context in which it was developed |
| Sensitivity to change | The assessment can detect changes in the needs of the patient |
| Feasibility | The assessment is suitable for use in routine clinical practice |

Social role performance measures are the most important for community mental health nurses undertaking assessment of need. These measures assess a person's performance in their major roles of work, relationships, home and self-care. The Camberwell Assessment of Need (CAN) assesses twenty-two domains of health and social need, recording staff and patient views separately (Phelan *et al.* 1995). It is specifically intended to meet the requirements of the National Health Service and Community Care Act (1990), and is described in more detail later in the chapter. The AVON Mental Health Measure was developed by service users, and assesses physical, social, behaviour, access and mental health domains (Lelliott 2000). It can take up to twenty minutes for completion by the patient and five minutes by the staff, and there are no published data on its psychometric properties. The Carers' and Users' Expectations of Services (CUES) was developed by service users and staff, and assesses sixteen domains: the place you live, money situation, the help you get, the way you spend time, your relationships, social life, information/advice, access to services, choice of mental health services, relationship with mental health workers, consultation and contact, advocacy, stigma, any treatment, access to physical health services, and relationship with physical health workers (Lelliott *et al.* 2001). Completion can take up to thirty minutes.

Finally, the Medical Research Council Needs for Care Assessment (NFCAS) (Brewin *et al.* 1987) assesses whether further action by health care professionals is indicated. There are difficulties in assessing when there is an available intervention which would be at least partly effective, since deciding that a treatment has not worked is seldom easy. However, as Bebbington notes, 'the inevitable value judgements inherent in the procedure have the virtue of being public and consequently accessible to argument' (Bebbington 1992, p. 106). Training is needed for using the NFCAS, which is primarily used for research purposes.

The most widely used assessment is the Camberwell Assessment of Need (CAN), which is described in the next section.

# SECTION 3: ASSESSING NEEDS WITH THE CAMBERWELL ASSESSMENT OF NEED

The Camberwell Assessment of Need (CAN) assesses the health and social needs of patients with severe mental health problems. Four principles governed the development of the CAN. First, everyone has needs, and although people with mental health problems have some specific needs, the majority of their needs are similar to those of people who do not have a mental illness. Second, the majority of people with a severe mental illness have multiple needs, and it is vital that all of them are identified by those caring for them. Therefore a priority of the CAN is to identify, rather than describe in detail, serious needs. Third, needs assessment should be both an integral part of routine clinical practice and a component of service evaluation. Therefore the CAN should be usable by a wide range of staff. Fourth, need is a subjective concept, and there will frequently be differing but equally valid perceptions about the presence or absence of a specific need. The CAN therefore records the views of staff and patients separately.

The first version of the CAN was the CAN-R, a research version for use with adults of working age with mental health problems (Phelan *et al.* 1995). Two variants of the adult CAN have since been developed: a long clinical version providing a more detailed assessment and care plan, called the CAN-C; and a single-page version called the Camberwell Assessment of Need Short Appraisal Schedule (CANSAS). The CANSAS has emerged as the most appropriate version for most clinical and research uses with adults of working age. The CAN book (Slade *et al.* 1999) provides comprehensive guidance on training in and use of the CANSAS, CAN-C and CAN-R, along with copyright permission to use the assessments. Each assessment is given in a form designed for photocopying.

Versions of the CAN have also been developed for use with the elderly, people with mental health problems and learning disabilities, and mentally disordered offenders. Further information on all English and translated versions can be found at www.iop.kcl.ac.uk/prism/can

## Using the CANSAS

The CANSAS assesses needs over the last month in twenty-two health and social domains: accommodation, food, looking after the home, self-care, daytime activities, physical health, psychotic symptoms, information, psychological distress, safety to self, safety to others, alcohol, drugs, company, intimate relationships, sexual expression, childcare, basic education, telephone, transport, money and benefits.

For each domain, the goal is to identify whether the patient has any difficulties, and, if they do, then to establish whether they are getting sufficient help so that the difficulties are manageable. The terminology used is that the *need rating* for each domain is: *no need* (meaning they have no problems at all in the domain), *met need* (they have no or moderate problems in the domain *because* of help they are given), or *unmet need* (a serious problem, irrespective of any help given).

Patients can either be shown how to complete the CANSAS or the nurse can ask questions about each domain and make the need rating on the basis of the patient's responses. After the patient assessment, the nurse records their own assessment. The views of staff and patient are given equal weight in the way the CANSAS is designed, which is intended to maximise user involvement in the assessment process (Slade and Thornicroft 1999).

The patient and the nurse may disagree about whether a problem exists. For example, a smelly and oddly-dressed patient may report that they have no self-care needs. Similarly, there may be disagreement about whether the help being given is sufficient, since the difference between a met and an unmet need is a matter of judgement. The goal is to differentiate between problems which are current and severe and those which have been ameliorated by help, but there may still be a blurred boundary where the patient is receiving help which only partly addresses their difficulties. Hence the views of patients and staff are recorded in separate columns in the CANSAS. The CANSAS also allows the recording of the views of the carer, where appropriate.

# SECTION 4: NEEDS ASSESSMENT – A STEP-BY-STEP GUIDE

A framework for nursing assessment has been proposed by Barker (1997), comprising five steps: choose the method, gather the information, analyse the information, develop a picture, and make a judgement. Undertaking these five steps will lead to high-quality assessment and care planning. Needs assessment can be undertaken within this framework.

## Step 1: Method

Decide what methods for assessing the patient's needs will be employed. Barker (1997) suggests there are six questions to consider:

1    Why am I doing this assessment?
2    What is the aim of the assessment?
3    When should I assess – what level of urgency?
4    How will I get the information?
5    How will I judge what this information means (problem formulation)?
6    How might the person function differently if their problems are resolved?

Assessment is normally not a one-off procedure, but an ongoing process of gathering information and reviewing the client's progress. However, these questions highlight a number of choices which need to be made, such as whether a joint assessment is needed, whether the perspective of an informal carer is to be considered, and what methods to employ for assessment. For most community nurses, meeting and talking to the patient will be a central source of information. This assessment meeting will now be considered.

## Step 2: Information

Nursing assessment may involve learning about the patient's past history, present situation and future plans. Knowing the history of the patient will help to make sense of their current problems and will guide treatment plans. Understanding the patient's current situation involves identifying and contextualising their needs. Future plans are important motivators for patients, and care goals should be consistent with the patient's goals for their life. Clearly the balance between these three aspects will vary, and these assessment issues are explored further by Maphosa and colleagues (2000). Here the focus will be on assessment of current needs.

The assessment meeting can be structured using the CANSAS, but this does not necessarily mean having a copy of the CANSAS on show during the assessment. Especially at the initial meeting with patients, visible paperwork is best kept to a minimum. A focus on listening and attending skills will help the patient feel that they are being treated as an individual (rather than being 'processed'), and will best facilitate the development of a therapeutic relationship. A good approach is often an open-ended beginning, such as 'Could you tell me about the difficulties you've been having?' or 'How can I help you?' Overly structured questioning can appear impersonal and threatening, and may impede full disclosure of the patient's difficulties.

The challenge is to undertake a comprehensive assessment of need whilst maintaining the focus on the patient and their story. The clinical skill is to weave discussion of a wide range of areas into the flow of the conversation. One approach is for the nurse to use the CAN domains as a mental checklist of areas to cover in the assessment. Some topics will be brought up by the patient, and others will need to be introduced at appropriate times by the nurse. Judgement is needed about whether all domains need to be covered. For example, intimate relationships and sexual expression can be awkward to introduce, but if done with a light touch this provides a chance for patients to talk about areas they might find too embarrassing to bring up themselves. It is worth remembering that sexual dysfunction as a medication side effect is often not reported by patients unless asked. Similarly, risk of violence and suicide should be assessed with sensitivity, using questions such as 'Do you ever have problems with your temper?' and 'Do you ever feel you can't cope with all your problems?' Some domains may not relate to the previous conversation. These should be assessed after the patient has outlined all their current difficulties, with a statement such as 'To help me get a fuller picture, can I also ask you about . . .'.

## Step 3: Analysis

All available information should then be analysed. Information normally comes from a number of sources, including the initial referral letter, case-notes, the patient, other health professionals, and other agencies. After analysing the assessment information, the nurse should be able to make a need rating for each of the twenty-two CANSAS domains, both from the patient's perspective and their own perspective. The patient's perspective on their needs should be based solely on what they have said, whereas the nurse's perspective will be based on all available information – not just the assessment meeting.

The CANSAS form is designed to be a summary recording sheet, on which the need rating from each perspective is recorded. Completing the CANSAS after the assessment simply involves recording the need rating for each domain, with one column used for the patient and one for the nurse. Alternatively, the CANSAS can be completed during the assessment. The CANSAS need rating is not of course a complete assessment, and the full assessment information (the patient's 'story') should be recorded in the clinical case-notes as normal.

The merit of completing the CANSAS is that it helps the nurse to consider the key questions of what needs the person has, and which are currently unmet. The number of unmet needs is the best predictor of the patient's quality of life (UK700 Group 1999), and treatment should be intended to turn unmet needs into met needs. The CANSAS also provides a written summary of the patient's needs at a particular point in time, which is helpful information when treatment is reviewed.

## Step 4: Picture

The next stage is to use this analysis to create an overall formulation of the patient's needs. This will involve the nurse coming to a view about the needs the patient has, what has caused them, and what maintains them. In other words, using all of the assessment information to make sense of the patient's needs. The skill in developing this picture is in separating the relevant assessment information from all that has been found out, and developing a formulation which is brief and specific to the patient. It can be a helpful discipline to write the formulation down. A sample formulation is:

> Ian was brought up with traditional views about the man's role as a breadwinner in the family, and he has always provided for his wife and two children (now aged 8 and 10). He has become increasingly depressed since his unexpected redundancy 8 months ago, resulting in low mood, social withdrawal, feelings of hopelessness and recent suicidal ideation. His low energy levels make it difficult for him to seek new employment, and his increased irritability and alcohol consumption have put strains on the marriage. Ian is keen to find a new job, but unsure how to start.

A good formulation makes sense of the patient's needs in terms of their history and current coping strategies. Ian's redundancy meant he was no longer able to meet what he perceives as his obligations to his family, and his coping strategies of drinking and social isolation may be maintaining his depression. A formulation also gives indicators about how to improve the situation. For Ian, counselling to look at developing other roles in the family might reduce his depression, and antidepressants or behavioural therapy to reduce the impact of his depression may help him to find a new job.

## Step 5: Judgement

In the above formulation, Ian has several areas of need. It is therefore important to decide which area(s) to focus treatment on, and what type of help to provide. Where possible, this is best done through an explicit discussion leading to agreement with the patient. The discussion may be facilitated by comparing the CANSAS assessments, to identify those domains which are seen by both staff and patient as a need, and those about which there is disagreement.

It is helpful to acknowledge disagreement, since negotiating care goals improves the working alliance and adherence to the treatment plan (Fenton *et al.* 1997). Not acknowledging differences often results in a care plan which over-emphasises the staff perspective, and for which the patient is less motivated. In the example formulation the nurse may assess Ian's alcohol consumption as a maintaining factor for his depression (i.e. an unmet need in the alcohol domain), whereas he may view it as a coping strategy (i.e. no need). A care plan directly aimed at reducing alcohol consumption is unlikely to be adhered to by Ian, and may in fact damage the working alliance and be counter-therapeutic. However, negotiation might lead to the identification of the primary care goal as getting a new job. This offers the possibility of discussing whether Ian's alcohol consumption is helping him towards that goal.

Similarly, the treatment options should be openly discussed. Many patients will express preferences for particular types of treatment. These preferences are important to consider, partly to maximise adherence to treatment and partly because patients are more likely to benefit from their preferred treatment (e.g. Chilvers *et al.* 2001). Patients will want to know the full range of treatment options, what the costs (e.g. side effects, personal effort) and likely benefits are, how long the treatment takes to work, and whether there is any waiting time before receiving the treatment.

# CONCLUSION

Needs assessment is here to stay. People using primary and specialist mental health services should receive a comprehensive assessment of their mental health needs. Nurse education should therefore be providing training in the use of standardised needs assessment measures, and community mental health nurses must be competent in assessing needs, and planning care on the basis of the assessment. Using the CANSAS within a framework for nursing assessment provides one method of meeting the obligation to assess needs.

# REFERENCES

Barker, P.J. (1997) *Assessment in psychiatric and mental health nursing*, Cheltenham: Stanley Thornes.
Bebbington, P. (1992) 'Assessing the need for psychiatric treatment at the district level: the

role of surveys', in Thornicroft, G., Brewin, C. and Wing, J. (eds) *Measuring mental health needs*, London: Royal College of Psychiatrists.

Bradshaw, J. (1972) 'A taxonomy of social need', in McLachlan, G. (ed.) *Problems and progress in medical care: essays on current research* (7th series), London: Oxford University Press.

Brewin, C. (1992) 'Measuring individual needs for care and services', in Thornicroft, G., Brewin, C. and Wing, J. (eds) *Measuring mental health needs*, London: Royal College of Psychiatrists.

Brewin, C., Wing, J., Mangen, S., Brugha, T. and MacCarthy, B. (1987) 'Principles and practice of measuring needs in the long-term mentally ill: the MRC Needs for Care Assessment', *Psychological Medicine*, 17: 971–981.

Chilvers, C., Dewey, M., Fielding, K., Gretton, V., Miller, P., Palmer, B., Weller, D., Churchill, R., Williams, I., Bedi, N., Duggan, C., Lee, A. and Harrison, G. (2001) 'Antidepressant drugs and generic counselling for treatment of major depression in primary care: randomised trial with patient preference arms', *British Medical Journal*, 322 (7289): 772–775.

Department of Health (1999) *National service framework for mental health: modern standards and service models*, London: Department of Health.

Department of Health Social Services Inspectorate (1991) *Care management and assessment: practitioners' guide*, London: HMSO.

Fenton, W.S., Blyler, C.R. and Heinssen, R.K. (1997) 'Determinants of medication compliance in schizophrenia', *Schizophrenia Bulletin*, 23: 637–651.

Holloway, F. (1993) 'Need in community psychiatry: a consensus is required', *Psychiatric Bulletin*, 18: 321–323.

House of Commons (1990) National Health Service and Community Care Act, London: HMSO.

Lehtinen, V., Joukamaa, M., Jyrkinen, E., Lahtela, K., Raitasala, R., Maatela, J. and Aromaa, A. (1990) 'Need for mental health services of the adult population in Finland: results from the Mini Finland Health Survey', *Acta Psychiatrica Scandinavica*, 81: 426–431.

Lelliott, P. (2000) 'What do people want from specialist mental health services and can this be routinely measured in routine service settings?' *Behavioural and Cognitive Psychotherapy*, 28: 361–368.

Lelliott, P., Beevor, A., Hogman, J., Hogman, G., Hyslop, J., Lathlean, J. and Ward, M. (2001) 'Carers' and users' expectations of services – user version (CUES-U): a new instrument to measure the experience of users of mental health services', *British Journal of Psychiatry*, 179: 67–72.

Mangen, S. and Brewin, C. (1991) 'The measurement of need', in Bebbington, P. (ed.) *Social psychiatry: theory, methodology, and practice*, New Brunswick, NJ: Transaction Press.

Maphosa, W., Slade, M. and Thornicroft, G. (2000) 'Principles of assessment', in Newell, R. and Gournay, K. (eds) *Mental health nursing: an evidence-based approach*, Edinburgh: Churchill Livingstone.

Maslow, A. (1954) *Motivation and personality*, New York: Harper and Row.

Phelan, M., Slade, M., Thornicroft, G., Dunn, G., Holloway, F., Wykes, T., Strathdee, G., Loftus, L., McCrone, P. and Hayward, P. (1995) 'The Camberwell Assessment of Need: the validity and reliability of an instrument to assess the needs of people with severe mental illness', *British Journal of Psychiatry*, 167: 589–595.

Regier, D., Myers, J., Kramer, M., Robins, L., Blazer, D., Hough, R., Eaton, W. and Locke, B. (1984) 'The NIMH Epidemiologic Catchment Area Program: historical context, major objectives and study population characteristics', *Archives of General Psychiatry*, 41: 934–941.

Slade, M. and Glover, G. (2000) 'The needs of people with mental disorder', in Thornicroft, G. and Szmukler, G. (eds) *Textbook of community psychiatry*, Oxford: Oxford University Press.

Slade, M. and Thornicroft, G. (1999) 'User-friendly assessment of need', *Nursing Times*, 95: 52–53.

Slade, M., Loftus, L., Phelan, M., Thornicroft, G. and Wykes, T. (1999) *The Camberwell Assessment of Need*, London: Gaskell.

Stevens, A. and Gabbay, J. (1991) 'Needs assessment needs assessment', *Health Trends*, 23 (1): 20–23.

UK700 Group (1999) 'Predictors of quality of life in people with severe mental illness. Study methodology with baseline analysis in the UK700 trial', *British Journal of Psychiatry*, 175: 426–432.

Wing, J. (1986) 'The cycle of planning and evaluation', in Wing, J. (ed.) 'Long-term community care: experience in a London borough', *Psychological Medicine Monograph Supplement* No. 2: 41–55.

# FURTHER READING

Barker, P.J. (1997) *Assessment in psychiatric and mental health nursing*, Cheltenham: Stanley Thornes.
Provides a detailed model for nursing assessments.

Newell, R. and Gournay, K. (eds) (2000) *Mental health nursing: an evidence-based approach*, Edinburgh: Churchill Livingstone.
Places needs assessment in the context of evidence-based nursing.

Slade, M., Loftus, L., Phelan, M., Thornicroft, G. and Wykes, T. (1999) *The Camberwell Assessment of Need*, London: Gaskell.
Step-by-step guide to using the CAN.

# CHAPTER 16

# RISK, DECISION-MAKING AND MENTAL HEALTH

*Andy Alaszewski*

---

## SUMMARY OF KEY POINTS

- Risk assessment and management are key components of community mental health nursing.

- Risk can be misused to disempower service users.

- Community mental health nurses should use their professional judgement to assess the risks and make the decisions which minimise harm and maximise the empowerment of users.

---

## INTRODUCTION

Risk is an extremely powerful concept and used carefully can have positive and liberating effects for support of people experiencing mental health problems. However, used without care and sensitivity risk can be repressive and disempowering. Mental health nurses are expected to assess and manage risk, and the ways in which they do this have a major impact on the users of their services. I will start my discussion of risk with a consideration of the different ways in which risk can be defined and used. I will then consider the factors which shape the day-to-day management of risk. I will end the chapter with a broader consideration of the underlying social processes that shape the definition and management of risk in contemporary society.

# DEFINING RISK

While risk appears to have entered the English language during the seventeenth century, its use and meaning have changed over time. Initially risk was associated with probability, especially with gambling and games of chance whose study created a specialist branch of mathematics, statistics (Douglas 1990). In modern society interest in risk is more generalised and links to desire to use knowledge gained from the past to predict and manage the future (Giddens 1990), and to allocate responsibility and blame when this process fails (Douglas 1986). In the twentieth century research generated new forms of technical expertise in risk, which have been applied across a bewildering range of areas of policy and practice (Lupton 1999).

For the purposes of this chapter, I define risk as:

> The possibility that a given course of action will not achieve its desired and intended outcome but instead some undesired and undesirable situation will develop.
>
>                    (adapted from Alaszewski and Manthorpe 1991, p. 277)

While it is possible to provide a broad definition of risk, it is important to recognise that such a definition may not command wide support, even within expert or professional circles. In the medical and health care literature the dominant approach is in terms of the 'risk of' specified adverse health events assessed in terms of mortality and morbidity. This involves the identification of factors associated with such events within populations – 'risk factors' or personal characteristics that make individuals 'at risk' (see, for example, the BMA's influential guide, British Medical Association 1990). However, it is also possible to identify another approach: 'risk in' health care, in which the emphasis is on the social processes which shape and influence health outcomes. These processes include 'risk communication', 'risk perception' and 'risk management', and it is these aspects of risk which form the basis of my discussion.

While some commentators have argued that such variations seriously limit the utility of risk as a concept (see, for example, Dowie 1999), an alternative approach is to acknowledge such variations and examine the range of meanings that people find in risk issues. These meanings are linked both to the symbolic associations of risk and the variety of perspectives which individuals and groups use in making sense of risk (Petts *et al.* 2001). While social scientists initially tended to uncritically accept 'common-sense' definitions of risk as anxiety-provoking danger, there is increasing awareness that risk is not only a contested concept, but in practice the experience of risk offers many attractions to individuals: it can provide opportunities for excitement, challenge and personal fulfilment (Lupton 1999).

# RISK IN COMMUNITY NURSING

In a study funded by the English National Board for Nursing Midwifery and Health Visiting (Alaszewski *et al.* 1998, 2000) we examined the ways in which community nurses supported vulnerable adults (including older people, people with mental health needs and people with learning disabilities) in the community and assessed and managed risk. We started by examining the ways in which nurses, users and carers conceptualised risk. Risk appeared to be a concept that most nurses in our study (72) took for granted rather than considered to be problematic. When asked to define risk most nurses did not have a ready response, they needed to pause to consider it and indeed some were initially reluctant to provide a definition. When they did articulate their reply, the majority (59, 82 per cent) saw risk in terms of hazard and harm, especially the negative consequences of decisions or actions. For example, a nurse managing a mental health team defined risk in the following way:

> Right, I think risk is multi-faceted . . . being a manager . . . I have to be aware of risk to clients in terms of self-harm and harm to others and that in this team doesn't focus on people who are depressed and may have suicidal tendencies or to people who are psychotic and may be at risk of self-harm . . . we also deal with people with dementia and being aware of the risks they carry . . . they may forget to eat and they are at risk of dehydration and malnutrition, loss of awareness about safety issues so that they might walk in front of a bus . . .

Nurses using this approach tended to see it as self-evident or 'common sense'. However, other nurses recognised that risk was a contested concept and that there were different ways of approaching it. For example, a lecturer on the mental health branch of a pre-registration course made the following response when asked to define risk:

> That's the 50 million dollar question. What may be a risk for me may not be for another person – it very much depends on your point of view of what risk is. The definition causes me problems. The other thing I have a problem with is who has the right to define it because that will affect what you do about it.

Some nurses (22, 31 per cent) used their awareness of the contested nature of risk to argue for a more positive approach in which risk-taking was seen as a potentially liberating experience and an essential part of human growth and development. For example, one learning disability nurse contrasted the 'official' approach to risk with a more positive approach:

> What I understand by risk and what the health authority understands is two different things. To me risk is a way of clients gaining know-ledge, being able to develop, learn new things . . . often staff as well – the staff taking risks they actually learn things by that and learn what the clients can do from risks. The health authority thinks of risk as . . . protecting their backs.

Nurses using this approach tended to emphasise both the 'normality' of risk-taking and its benefits in terms of personal learning benefits and development and as a source of pleasure. For example, a learning disability student described risk in the following way:

> [It] depends on your point of view and style of life and philosophy. I might see going to the casino and gambling as a risk but someone else might not. A result of circumstances involving an activity. There is a risk in everything and it is what is 'acceptable'. Taking a gamble – the idea of being bad being more fun than being good. It's an aspect of life which most people enjoy – a bit of fear, getting the adrenalin going can be a good thing.

'Risk as a hazard to be identified and avoided' versus 'risk-taking as an opportunity for learning and development' represent two very different and apparently irreconcilable approaches. However, we were able to identify an intermediate position in which nurses (38, 58 per cent) recognised both dangers and opportunities and saw risk management as a process of balancing the two. A nurse providing care for older people described this process in the following way:

> If you've got a patient who has been walking with guidance and that patient wants to get to be mobile again, independently, you may decide or in conjunction with the physios to let that patient take that risk – it's just weighing up whether, yes, dare I risk doing it or not really?

Within all the specialisms of community nursing included in our study, the common-sense approach of 'risk as a hazard to be identified and avoided' predominated. However, there was a difference between different groups of nurses. Mental health nurses tended to place the greatest emphasis on this approach. Learning disability nurses appeared more ready to recognise the positive aspects of risk-taking, while nurses caring for older people were the most willing to recognise the balancing approach (Table 16.1).

The mental health nurses in our study did acknowledge that their approach to risk emphasised the potentially harmful consequences of the actions of acutely ill clients. They felt that this emphasis was a product of external pressure. In particular they identified the impact of high-profile incidents in which acutely ill individuals had harmed themselves, members of the public or individuals providing them with support. Such incidents had resulted in public inquiries which

*Table 16.1* Definitions of risk

|  | Hazard | | Balance | | Opportunity | |
|---|---|---|---|---|---|---|
| Mental health n=24 | 21 | (87.5%) | 15 | (62.5%) | 5 | (21%) |
| Older people n=24 | 20 | (83%) | 16 | (67%) | 7 | (29%) |
| Learning disability n=24 | 18 | (75%) | 7 | (29%) | 10 | (42%) |
| All nurses n=72 | 59 | (82%) | 38 | (53%) | 22 | (31%) |
|  | (in some interviews more than one definition was identified) | | | | | |

Reproduced by kind permission of the English National Board for Nursing, Midwifery and Health Visiting had attracted considerable media coverage. For example, the Ritchie Inquiry (1994) highlighted the failure to effectively assess the danger posed by Christopher Clunis. It recommended that in the case of patients who had been violent, aftercare plans should include 'an assessment . . . as to whether the patient's propensity for violence presents any risk to his own health or safety or to the protection of the public' (Ritchie Inquiry 1994, para. 45.1.2). Mental health nurses in our study saw a link between high-profile media coverage and a narrow, defensive approach to risk. One group of mentors for students on a post-registration mental health course articulated this link in the following way:

*Interviewer*:    What's happening that's made people more aware [of risk]?
*Mentor A*:    It's probably because there's less hospital beds and closing down of institutions.
*Mentor B*:    High media profile.
*Mentor A*:    And ever since Ben Sillcot . . . just jumped into the lion's den it's become a very hot topic . . . So a lot of it's to do with media coverage . . . and that has made management more aware and that filters down to clinicians' level . . .

Respondents clearly felt that there was pressure from the government to prevent such incidents and to ensure that professionals identified and managed risks effectively.

## RISK AND DECISION-MAKING

Mental health nurses need to decide how they respond to these pressures to mini-mise harm and ensure safety in their everyday practice. This tension is particularly evident in the decision-making process. As Narayan and Corcoran-Perry observe, 'Decision-making tasks of interest in professional domains are characterised by complexity, ambiguity, and uncertainty' (1997, p. 354). Despite the centrality of decision-making and risk to professional practice, in our study we could find little evidence that nurses were systematically prepared for this aspect of practice (Alaszewski *et al*. 1998, pp. 58–82). Nurses had to acquire appropriate skills through trial and error in practice.

The complexity of task and skills required was evident when we analysed the decisions which nurses had to make in their everyday practice: it was clear both that they were complex and that they required developed skills. I have selected one example that illustrates this complexity. It involves an experienced community mental health nurse who decided to support his client, a single mother with young children, when she wanted to come off her medication. The nurse summarised the key components of the decision and made explicit reference to risk assessment in his justification of his decision:

I feel that I have a good knowledge of the client and a very good relationship with [her] . . . the decision really was to reduce her medication, and not to stop, and I think that if she had been irresponsible she would have said I'm not taking any again, she wasn't saying that she was saying she wanted to reduce . . . so I felt that was an appropriate risk.

In making the decision, the nurse had to identify and balance a number of factors, including the client's aims and intentions, the possible consequences, especially harm to her children, and the actions and reactions of other professionals involved with the client. While nurses and other professionals are being encouraged to ground their decisions in evidence, most of the key factors were unique to the circumstances of the decision, such as the client's intentions and the response of other professionals. Thus the nurse had to draw on his personal experience and use his professional judgement to assess the risks and make the decision. He described this process in the following way:

> I suppose the potential outcome, negative one, is that she may have another psychotic episode which she has only ever had one in her life, which is good, but we could have another one where she would have become suspicious, perhaps neglected herself, there was two young children at home who you could argue maybe were potentially at risk. I think I balanced that up because when she was mentally ill before . . . she had actually taken the children to the casualty department, wanting them to be looked at because she felt they had been poisoned . . . I felt that there was less risk this time because I was visiting in addition to social services, in addition to consultant psychiatrist's appointments, where before she has a breakdown with nobody so she could have floundered for far longer where this time there was support and screening.

The decisions we observed were often the product of negotiation – in this case negotiated with the client – but the nurse was not willing to negotiate with the other professionals involved, especially the client's consultant, as he felt that primacy should be given to the client's wishes:

> Maybe if I was honest I was a bit annoyed by the consultant's suggestion to [the client] that because she's a single mother she should stay on medication . . . it had offended the client and it had alienated the client and then really the client had made up her own mind that she was going to stop her medication.

He described the ways in which he negotiated with his client:

> We [nurse and client] drew up an agreement, contract, care plan, call it what you wish, where I would monitor her really looking for signs of illness . . . and looking at supporting her . . . she was quite willing that if she felt the illness was coming back on I would be acting as an advocate and stepping in. I did notify the GP and a copy went to the consultant.

It was evident from our study that from the earliest stages of their practice, mental health nurses were involved in complex and often challenging decisions. They placed a high priority on identifying and meeting their clients' interests and this involved making appropriate assessments of risk and balancing conflicting interests and assessments. While most practitioners felt that they had acquired the necessary skills and understanding through experience, more systematic preparation would reduce the anxieties which difficult and complex decisions often create.

## SOCIETY, RISK AND MENTAL HEALTH

In earlier sections of this chapter I have made reference to the social context within which mental health nurses practise, for example referring to the external pressures that influence practice. In this final section I shall explore the nature of this wider context and the ways in which it influences the interaction between risk and mental health. A useful starting point for such a discussion is the concept of psychological states such as fear, anxiety and worry. Extreme anxiety or emotional distress is recognised as a type of mental disorder and there is consensus amongst clinicians over the symptoms which indicate 'generalised anxiety', 'panic' and 'obsessive-compulsive disorder' (Wilkinson 2001, pp. 49–50). These types of mental disorder have a major impact on modern populations; for example, an OPCS survey identified a prevalence rate of 14 per cent amongst adults between 16 and 64, and lower socioeconomic classes have higher rates (Wilkinson 2001, p. 54).

The impact of individuals who are anxious about their health, i.e. whose personal assessments are more pessimistic than those of experts, is now well recognised. Balint (1964), in his classic study of primary care, identified a group of patients who presented repeatedly with often changing physical symptoms but whose pattern of behaviour and symptoms indicated an anxiety disorder that was undiagnosed and untreated. In the 1970s the term 'worried well' was used to describe individuals who were seen as inappropriate users of medical services. The emergence of a high-profile new disease in the 1980s, AIDS, was associated with the development of AIDS anxiety. The relationship between the worried well and individuals experiencing extreme anxiety is not clear. Bowers's (1997) review of mentally ill worried well found that these patients had significant symptoms.

Recognition of the importance of such states underpins attempts to develop 'safety cultures' in public services, which are designed not only to minimise harm but also to ensure public confidence and trust and to provide individual and collective security. However, increases in objective levels of 'safety' do not necessarily lead to increases in perception of individual well-being, as demonstrated, for example, in studies of fear of crime, which consistently show that the least 'at risk' group, namely elderly females, are the most fearful. Within the social science literature a number of commentators have identified the existence of endemic anxiety as a characteristic of the 'late modern' or 'risk' society in which we find ourselves (Bauman 1993). Taylor-Gooby, in his overview of the findings of the ESRC programme on Economic Beliefs and Behaviour, refers to 'timid prosperity', in which increased levels of collective safety and welfare are associated with increased levels of anxiety about personal security (Taylor-Gooby 2000, pp. 1–6).

Wilkinson (2001) has argued that anxiety in contemporary society is closely associated with risk and especially uncertainty. As Furedi (2002) has noted, public panics have been commonplace, with scares about issues as diverse as childhood immunisation programmes, mobile phones, global warming, foot-and-mouth disease in livestock, and the risks of long-haul flights. Following the terrorist attack on the World Trade Center on 11 September 2001, the Chief Medical Officer in the UK has accepted that measures against terrorism should form part of the government's strategy for protecting the public (Department of Health 2002). Furedi (2002) has suggested that these attacks have heightened anxiety, creating a society terrified of terror.

Many regard the mass media as playing a major role in the development of anxiety about risk. Furedi (2002), for example, argues that the media emphasise the hazards associated with new technologies, foodstuffs and dangers to children. While experts can measure risk and (attempt to) communicate their measurements to the public, this information is filtered through various media and interpreted by social groups and individuals. The mass media play an important role in shaping perceptions of risk and associated behaviour. Philo (1999), for example, provides evidence that individuals give precedence to media accounts of people with mental illness as dangerous and violent over their own contradictory experiences, even when they recognise that the media accounts may be fictional, as in soap operas.

Over twenty-five years ago, for example, Cohen (1972) showed how the emergence of 'moral panics' reflects deep-seated tensions within society which find expression through the identification of 'folk devils'. Moral panics may offer an important insight into the ways in which the risks associated with mental health are constructed. Traditional accounts of mental health policy portrayed change as being associated with progress; increased knowledge results in improved treatment technologies which in turn feed into more enlightened attitudes to mental illness (see, for example, Jones 1972). In contrast, critical commentators using a Foucauldian approach see risk in terms of discourses which are used to establish and maintain social control (Foucault 1967, Lupton 1999). For example, Foucault argued that the development of new forms of treatment for people with mental illness at the end of the eighteenth century, rather than representing progress and modernisation, marked a more sophisticated mechanism of social control. At the end of the eighteenth century governments increasingly saw their populations as a resource which needed to be managed and controlled, and the emerging professions developed forms of knowledge that facilitated this control. Thus risk was used to identify and reprogramme the deviant elements of the population in the new asylums, and to internalise responsible behaviour in the remainder of the population, who were expected to follow professional advice on safe and hygienic practices. Thus, while traditional historians would see history in terms of progress and liberation, Foucauldian commentators would see the development of services in terms of increasingly sophisticated techniques of repression centred on risk.

These two polarised accounts may each tell part of the story. Turner has suggested that there is 'a perpetual cycle of regulation and deregulation' in modern society (Turner 2001, p. 16). Disasters are followed by increases in regulation, and as costs of increased regulation grow so the pressure for liberalisation increases.

In the development of mental health services it is also possible to identify cycles: periods of optimism about the care and treatment of people with mental illness followed by periods of pessimism linked to moral panics and an emphasis on risk and dangerousness. The periods of optimism have included the early nineteenth century, the early twentieth and the mid-twentieth century. The periods of pessimism have included the late nineteenth century and the late twentieth century. The optimistic periods are linked to the development of new treatment technologies, moral treatment and asylums at the beginning of the nineteenth century, psychoanalysis at the beginning of the twentieth century and new drug therapies in the mid-twentieth century. They also follow major periods of international conflict: the Napoleonic wars, the First and Second World Wars. In the first two periods there is a clear relationship between the two developments; for example, the ideologies underpinning moral treatment can be traced to developments in revolutionary France, and the 'shell shock' victims of the First World War provided 'evidence' for the effectiveness of new approaches based on psychoanalysis. In the case of the third period there appears to be an indirect relationship. In the UK the development of a wartime consensus created an environment in which the opportunities for deinstitutionalisation created by new drug therapies were exploited. The pessimistic phases appear to be linked to the apparent failures of the new treatment technologies as well as the rise of internal tensions within society. For example, at the end of the nineteenth century the asylums had failed to achieve their therapeutic objectives and were warehousing inmates. At the same time there was an increase in social and political tensions and a moral panic over the threats posed by moral defectives and other deviant groups (Alaszewski 1988).

## CONCLUSION

Risk forms an integral part of mental health. Currently social changes are serving to highlight the negative and restrictive components of risk. The awareness that the new treatment regimes developed in the 1960s and 1970s have limitations, that individuals who refuse to comply with treatments may pose a threat to themselves and others, plus the increase in social tensions evident in the 1970s and 1980s, has underpinned the development of a more pessimistic period, with ministers declaring that community care has failed and seeking new powers to increase the surveillance and control of people with enduring mental illness in the community.

As Eldridge and Hill (1999) point out, risk does not have a fixed definition and meaning. Different definitions are accepted in different contexts. If mental health nurses do not play an active role in shaping these definitions and using approaches that empower their clients, then there is a danger that a narrow, hazard-oriented approach will predominate and the main role of community mental health nurses will be policing mental illness in the community. If, on the other hand, they seek to use a broad approach, either balancing hazard and opportunity or even empowering individuals to take risks, then they will need to use developed skills in assessment, decision-making and negotiation.

# REFERENCES

Alaszewski, A. (1988) 'From villains to victims', in Leighton, A. (ed.) *Mental handicap in the community*, London: Woodhead-Faulkner.

Alaszewski, A. and Manthorpe, J. (1991) 'Measuring and managing risk in social welfare', *British Journal of Social Work*, 21: 277–290.

Alaszewski, A., Alaszewski, H., Manthorpe, J. and Ayer, S. (1998) *Assessing and managing risk in nursing education and practice: supporting vulnerable people in the community*, Research report series no. 10, London: English National Board for Nursing, Midwifery and Health Visiting.

Alaszewski, A., Alaszewski, H., Ayer, S. and Manthorpe, J. (2000) *Managing risk in community practice*, Edinburgh: Baillière Tindall.

Balint, M. (1964) *The doctor, his patient and the illness*, London: Pitman Medical.

Bauman, Z. (1993) *Postmodern ethics*, Oxford: Blackwell.

Bowers, L. (1997) 'Community psychiatric nurse caseloads and the "worried well": misspent time or vital work?' *Journal of Advanced Nursing*, 26: 930–936.

British Medical Association (1990) *The BMA guide to living with risk*, Harmondsworth: Penguin.

Cohen, S. (1972) *Folk devils and moral panics*, London: MacGibbon and Kee.

Department of Health (2002) *Getting ahead of the curve: a strategy for combating infectious diseases (including other aspects of health protection)*, London: Department of Health.

Douglas, M. (1986) *Risk acceptability according to the social sciences*, London: Routledge and Kegan Paul.

Douglas, M. (1990) 'Risk as a forensic resource', *Daedalus, Journal of the American Academy of Arts and Sciences*, 119: 1–16.

Dowie, J. (1999) 'Communication for better decisions: not about "risk"', *Health, Risk and Society*, 1: 41–53.

Eldridge, J. and Hill, A. (1999) 'Thinking about risk: a review essay', *Health, Risk and Society*, 1: 343–350.

Foucault, M. (1967) *Madness and civilization*, London: Tavistock.

Furedi, F. (2002) *Culture of fear: risk-taking and the morality of low expectations*, 2nd edn, London: Cassell.

Giddens, A. (1990) *The consequences of modernity*, Cambridge: Polity Press.

Jones, K. (1972) *A history of the mental health services*, London: Routledge and Kegan Paul.

Lupton, D. (1999) *Risk*, London: Routledge.

Narayan, S.M. and Corcoran-Perry, S. (1997) 'Lines of reasoning as a representation of nurses' clinical decision making', *Research in Nursing and Health*, 20: 353–364.

Petts, J., Horlick-Jones, T. and Murdock, G. (2001) *Social amplification of risk: the media and the public*, Contract Research Report 329/2001, Sudbury: HSE Books.

Philo, G. (1999) 'Media and mental illness', in Philo, G. (ed.) *Message received: Glasgow Media Group research 1993–1998*, Harlow: Longman.

Ritchie Inquiry (1994) *Report of the inquiry into the care and treatment of Christopher Clunis* (Chairman J.H. Ritchie), London: HMSO.

Taylor-Gooby, P. (2000) 'Risk and welfare', in Taylor-Gooby, P. (ed.) *Risk, trust and welfare*, Basingstoke: Macmillan.

Turner, B.S. (2001) 'Risks, rights and regulation: an overview', *Health, Risk and Society*, 3: 9–18.

Wilkinson, I. (2001) *Anxiety in a risk society*, London: Routledge.

# FURTHER READING

There is a substantial body of literature developing on risk, including both specialist academic journals and books. The leading journal on risk is *Risk Analysis*, which is an official publication of the Society for Risk Analysis. However, the journal is heavily dominated by highly technical papers that generally adopt a restricted approach to risk. *Health, Risk and Society* is both more accessible and includes a wide range of papers that explore a variety of different aspects of risk. It is published by Carfax and further information, including the contents pages, can be obtained from the following website: http://www.tandf.co.uk/journals

Lupton, D. (1999) *Risk*, London: Routledge.

Deborah Lupton's short review of risk is an excellent introduction to some of the more challenging issues. While you may be put off by some of the more complex theorising, it is well worth persisting as the last chapter on risk-taking and living on the edge is fascinating.

Alaszewski, A., Harrison, L. and Manthorpe, J. (eds.) (1998) *Risk, Health and Welfare*, Buckingham: Open University Press.

Alaszewski, A., Alaszewski, H., Ayer, S. and Manthorpe, J. (2000) *Managing risk in community practice*, Edinburgh: Baillière Tindall.

My own books on risk are worth looking at. Both are grounded in research but use the research findings to explore wider issues. The first book deals with the ways in which health and welfare agencies manage risk, and identifies the tensions and problems which are often left to front-line staff to resolve. The second book focuses explicitly on nursing education and practice, and provides insight into the realities of managing risk in community practice.

Kemshall, H. and Pritchard, J. (1996 and 1997) *Good practice in risk assessment and management*, 1 and 2, London: Jessica Kingsley.

Hazel Kemshall and Jacki Pritchard have edited two collections which identify good practice in risk assessment and management. These are extremely useful texts full of practical advice and guidance.

# CHAPTER 17

# PREVENTING SUICIDE

*Steve Wood*

---

## SUMMARY OF KEY POINTS

- Prevention of suicide is a priority of mental health policy, both nationally and internationally.

- The work of community mental health nurses routinely brings them into contact with people at increased risk of suicide.

- Effective identification and management of suicide risk are complex and difficult tasks, yet crucial components of that work.

---

## INTRODUCTION

Suicide is rare. In recent times, around one in every ten thousand people in England and Wales has committed suicide each year. Moreover, the rate of suicide steadily declined during the twentieth century. The overall decline masked marked increases in suicide rates among certain groups, most notably males aged under 35 years, and static rates among others, for example males of 85 and above (Cantor 2000). There is a considerably higher rate of suicide among people with a mental disorder: the National Confidential Inquiry into Suicide and Homicide by People with Mental Illness reported that 24 per cent of suicides during a two-year period had been in contact with mental health services in the year before death (Appleby 2000).

The National Confidential Inquiry argued that mental health service action could prevent some suicides, and made thirty-one recommendations in this regard.

These have many implications for community mental health nurses (CMHNs), some of which this chapter will examine. First, risk factors for suicide and the uses and limitations of predictive scales will be discussed. Secondly, specific high-risk individuals with whom CMHNs routinely have contact will be described, and implications for practice considered. Thirdly, issues involved in the assessment of suicide risk will be examined, and an outline of good practice offered. Finally, the community management of suicide risk will be discussed.

## DEFINITIONS

Suicide has been variously defined, but any attempt at definition needs to encompass three elements: an unnatural death; the deceased being the initiator of the course of action leading to death; and the motivation of self-destruction. The term 'parasuicide' was first used by Kreitman *et al.* (1969), as an alternative to 'attempted suicide', a term criticised 'for the excellent reason that the great majority of patients so designated are not in fact attempting suicide' (p. 746). Throughout this chapter, the term is used to include all instances of deliberate, non-fatal, self-injurious behaviour.

## BACKGROUND

Reduction of suicide is an explicit aim of mental health policy. *The health of the nation* (Department of Health 1992) set targets for reducing both the overall suicide rate and the rate among seriously mentally ill people. *Our healthier nation* (Department of Health 1998) modified these targets for England, and separate targets have been set in Wales (Welsh Office 1998). Internationally, both the World Health Organization (1990) and the United Nations (1996) have recognised suicide as a public health priority and advised on national strategies for its reduction.

There is probably general agreement amongst health care professionals that suicide should be prevented whenever possible. Whilst an argument can be made for respecting the wishes of someone who has made an informed choice to commit suicide, in practice it is difficult to satisfactorily establish when this is the case. Furthermore, the frequently impulsive nature of suicidal behaviour should be borne in mind, as should the finding that only a small minority of survivors of suicide attempts regret not succeeding (e.g. Bancroft *et al.* 1977).

## SUICIDE RISK FACTORS AND THE USE OF PREDICTIVE MODELS

Suicide risk factors have been established using a mixture of population-level data, psychological autopsy studies, and studies using coroners' notes and medical records. The most in-depth information is obtained using the psychological autopsy method, which gathers information through documentary evidence and interviews with key informants. Risk factors are well known. Although the age profile of completed suicides has altered considerably in recent years, suicide is still most common in the oldest age groups. Socio-demographic risk factors include male gender, single, widowed or divorced marital status, being unemployed or retired, and living alone. In addition, younger suicides have increased likelihood of living at their current address for less than one year (Appleby *et al.* 1999). Certain occupational groups are associated with high rates: typically, these are in the agricultural and caring professions. In respect of social class, earlier studies showed skews towards the highest and lowest groups; however, a recent study of suicides by people under 25 showed an excess in social classes 3 to 5 (Hawton *et al.* 1999).

Many of the clinical risk factors reported in Barraclough *et al.*'s (1974) classic study still hold true. They include psychiatric disorder, previous deliberate self-harm, alcohol and drug dependency, history of parental separation or child-hood abuse, and family history of depressive illness and suicidal behaviour. Psychosocial risk factors include recent adverse life events, particularly loss events. In younger age groups, these tend to be interpersonal and relationship difficulties, as well as legal, financial and occupational problems (Appleby *et al.* 1999). In older age groups, they are more likely to be physical illnesses and other losses, especially bereavement (Cattell 2000).

The idea of accurately estimating suicide risk on the basis of known risk factors is an attractive one. Considerable effort has been expended on the development of predictive scales, but the results have been disappointing. Pokorny (1983) and Pallis *et al.* (1984), for example, carried out large-scale studies: both reported a high rate of false positives. Goldstein *et al.* (1991) attempted to develop a statistical model to predict suicide among 1,906 people with affective disorder admitted to hospital in Iowa, but failed to identify any subsequent suicides. More recently, Powell *et al.* (2000) attempted to construct a predictive model based on the strongest risk factors identified in 97 in-patient suicides compared to 112 living controls. They found that to predict more than 50 per cent of suicides, the false positive rate would have been greater than 99 per cent. They concluded that it is inevitable that clinicians will fail to identify a high proportion of suicides, even in this very high-risk group.

There is an intractable problem of predicting infrequent events. Demographic data identifies groups with elevated risk, but is too general to be of practical use: it identifies large numbers never, in reality, at risk. Psychiatric illness is usually present in cases of suicide, but only a small minority of those with psychiatric illness commit suicide.

Most knowledge is of long-term risk factors, and most of these are not stable characteristics. It has been suggested that long-term prediction of risk based on current characteristics is somewhat illogical (Kreitman 1982). In any event, in clinical practice, the main concern is with short-term risk.

To conclude, it is unlikely that the ability of scales to predict will ever be substantial (Goldney 2000). In recent studies, attention has begun to shift towards the interaction of different risk factors, and the pathways to suicide (e.g. Appleby *et al.* 1999, Cheng *et al.* 2000). To what use, then, can knowledge of risk factors be put? Most authors cited above concluded that predictive scales were at best an aid to clinical judgement. Pierce (1981) suggested routine use of a suicidal intent scale as a screening device in the assessment of all cases of self-injury, and Beck *et al.* (1985) recommended use of the Hopelessness Scale as an important indicator of long-term risk in depressed people. Morgan (1994) recommended that a checklist of risk factors be used, to ensure caution when risk is considered insignificant in their presence.

## HIGH-RISK INDIVIDUALS WITH WHOM CMHNs HAVE CONTACT

Suicide is strongly associated with mental disorder, and contributes to the excess mortality of mentally ill people. In a meta-analysis of 249 papers, Harris and Barraclough (1997) found that, of 44 mental disorders studied, 36 had significantly raised mortality rates for suicide. In a study of suicides by people under 35 years, nearly two-thirds had a history of psychiatric treatment (Appleby *et al.* 1999). Between 10 and 15 per cent of suicides are by people who have been discharged from psychiatric hospital within the previous four weeks (Goldacre *et al.* 1993).

Depression and anxiety are the commonest mental health problems (Singleton *et al.* 2001), and are frequent reasons for referral to community mental health teams (CMHTs). In a review of seventeen studies, Guze and Robins (1970) reported the risk of suicide in primary affective disorders to be more than thirty times that of the general population. Barraclough *et al.* (1974) reported depression, uncomplicated by other disorders, in 64 per cent of suicides, and in a further 16 per cent of cases if complicated by alcoholism or terminal physical illness. It has been reported that certain clinical features of depression are positively associated with suicide in the short term: these are anxiety, panic, insomnia, anhedonia, and poor concentration (Fawcett *et al.* 1987). Several studies have found under-treatment of depression among suicide victims a major problem (e.g. Ohberg *et al.* 1996).

People currently receiving psychiatric treatment accounted for 32 per cent of suicides by people under 35 (Appleby *et al.* 1999), and 22 per cent by people under 25 (Hawton *et al.* 1999). These figures exclude people being treated by their GP, and are, therefore, people known to mental health services. King and Barraclough (1990) estimated suicide risk for people receiving treatment as being twenty-seven times higher than that for the general population.

The increasing prioritisation of people with serious mental illness has had the consequence of increasing the proportion of CMHNs' clients with a diagnosis of schizophrenia. It has been estimated that around 10 per cent of people so diagnosed commit suicide (Miles 1977). In a study of thirty suicides by people diagnosed with schizophrenia, compared to thirty living controls, the picture was one of suicide by relatively young males with a relapsing illness, in whom depression with suicidal ideation had been noted at their last contact. They were likely to be unemployed and recently discharged from in-patient care (Roy 1982). Drake *et al.* (1984) found that suicide by people diagnosed with schizophrenia tended to happen during a relatively non-psychotic stage. Most lived alone and had previously indicated suicidal intent. They tended to have had relatively high educational attainment prior to the illness, high expectations of themselves, and good awareness of the consequences of the illness.

People recently discharged from psychiatric in-patient care are at high risk. Roy (1982) found that of suicides by people in this category, 44 per cent happened within one month of discharge, 89 per cent within one year. Goldacre *et al.* (1993) confirmed this, demonstrating a significant clustering of suicide soon after discharge. However, it is difficult to predict suicide by people in this group, despite it being known that they are at high risk. In a study of suicides over twelve months in Manchester, seventy had been discharged from psychiatric hospital within the previous five years (Dennehy *et al.* 1996). These were compared with living controls, matched for age, sex, diagnosis, and date of admission. Characteristic of both groups were many variables associated with suicide, but which did not distinguish suicides from controls.

The incidence of parasuicide has increased rapidly in the past two decades, and each year more than 140,000 people are seen in hospitals in England and Wales following instances of parasuicide. The true incidence is not known, but is higher still (Samaritans 2002). Around 19 per cent of suicide attempters make a repeat attempt within the next twelve months, and about 1 per cent actually succeed (Samaritans 2002). This is, therefore, another high-risk group.

CMHNs, therefore, routinely work with people who are at increased risk of suicide. They frequently carry out the initial assessment of people referred to CMHTs, either at the person's home or at the CMHT base. It is standard practice for this to include assessment of suicide risk, as well as risk of harm to others and risk of self-neglect. Their daily work involves repeated contact, often over a prolonged period of time, with individuals with serious mental illness. They are well placed to observe changes which may indicate heightened risk. However, there is also a danger that the routine nature of many contacts may lessen acuity of observation.

CMHNs feature prominently in the provision of post-discharge follow-up. The risks inherent during this period can be compounded if good discharge planning, with proper co-ordination between in-patient and community services, does not take place. In addition, CMHNs have become increasingly involved in assessing and managing people following parasuicide since the mid-1980s. At that time, it was recommended (Department of Health and Social Security 1984) that non-psychiatrists undertake psychosocial management of parasuicide cases.

In conclusion, CMHNs are the largest professional group working in CMHTs (Sainsbury Centre for Mental Health 1997). They often have the most direct contact with people with serious mental illness and are well placed to identify suicide risk in that group. In addition, referrals to CMHTs are often preceded by relationship breakdown, bereavement, or attempted suicide: all these are associated with increased suicide risk. A CMHN is often the first point of contact and influences the response to the referral. It is important, therefore, that they are equipped to assess suicide risk effectively.

# GOOD PRACTICE IN ASSESSING SUICIDE RISK

Several potential hazards were identified by Morgan (1994). People may be angry and challenging, rather than retarded or self-blaming; they may become alienated from helping staff, especially when there have been recurrent relapses; suicidal ideation may fluctuate; people may set out to deceive, although this is unusual; and clinical improvements, without resolution of situational factors, may mislead.

The importance of an effective therapeutic relationship, ideally with key others as well as the patient, was underlined by Morgan and Stanton (1997): estimation of suicide risk has to be guided largely by what the patient says. However, particular effort should be made to obtain verification, by an informant, of details of the client's past history, current life situation and evidence of any psychiatric illness (Kreitman 1979).

It may be useful to consider 'protectors' – factors which inhibit people from committing suicide – in the process of assessment. Linehan et al. (1983) noted that individuals who had considered, or would consider, suicide differed from those who had not, or would not, in the degree to which they attached importance to a set of life-oriented beliefs and expectations. They discovered six primary groups of 'reasons for living': survival and coping beliefs; responsibility to family; child-related concerns; fear of the act of suicide; fear of social disapproval; and moral objections. They found that people with prior suicidal behaviour volunteered fewer important reasons for living than people without such a history.

Hawton (1987) recommended that all known risk factors be assessed, particularly relationship difficulties, family problems, alcohol problems and any other psychiatric disorders. Other factors which should be assessed were: the patient's attitude to the future; whether they felt that they were likely to repeat the attempt; the degree of support available to the patient; and the degree to which they were likely to engage in follow-up.

Bowers (1995) stated that all assessments of suicide risk should include five elements: risk factors, history, ideation, plan, and intent. Assessments should always err on the side of safety. Within each element, particular features will increase the level of risk. Risk is higher where relevant aspects of history are recent, severe, or frequent; where there is a pattern which is being repeated; and where the patient's attitude to negative aspects of their history is that they are reasonable or deserved. Within ideation, a high degree of prominence and preoccupation indicates greater risk. The existence of a plan, precise knowledge of how it would be carried out, and access to the necessary means, suggest successively higher levels of risk. A statement of intent is the strongest and most powerful predictor, and should not be ignored.

The importance of understanding the psychological processes going on in suicidal individuals was emphasised by Morgan et al. (1998), who stated that the ability to evaluate suicidal ideation 'may be the paramount skill required' (p. 190). They recommended a progressive narrowing of focus from the general to the specific, in the light of client responses. For example, having elicited general pessimism about the future, one should go on to explore more definite suicidal ideas, such as 'I'd be better off dead', or 'I can't face another day'. Where these are present, one should seek to establish whether the client has actually thought about committing suicide. If so, are they currently thinking that way? Have they considered by what means? If so, are the means available? Have they actually made plans? Have they made preparations? Morgan *et al.* reported that real suicide risk is not inconsistent with a willingness to discuss suicidal ideation.

The need for professionals to be able to assess suicide risk accurately has been pointed out by many authors. For example, Morgan and Priest (1991), in a study of suicides and unexpected deaths among psychiatric in-patients and people recently discharged, reported that, in 20 cases out of 27, the seriousness of the risk was not fully recognised. They highlighted the need for better training in the assessment of suicide risk, and the National Confidential Inquiry (Appleby 2000) made recommendations as to the frequency and content of training. Similarly, Dennehy *et al.* (1996) recommended improved risk assessment of people discharged from in-patient care, particularly in the first few months. Assessment of suicide risk is difficult, uncertain and complex, but an essential part of the role of all CMHNs: as Goldstein *et al.* (1991, p. 421) put it, 'At present, the knowledge of health care professionals about their own patients remains the best tool for the prevention of suicides.'

## MANAGEMENT OF SUICIDE RISK IN THE COMMUNITY

Having reached the stage, through assessment, of believing there to be a risk of suicide, the question is how best to manage that risk. Guidance is given in *The health of the nation* (Department of Health 1992). Before outlining this, it is worth considering the evidence on which it is based. To an extent, this is general evidence as to best practice in community mental health care. However, it is largely arrived at by studying completed suicides, and identifying factors believed to have contributed which may have been modifiable. In reality, unless there is testimony from the person who committed suicide, for example through a suicide note, or verbal communication prior to death, we have to rely on inference and supposition.

What measures could be employed to assess the effectiveness of different approaches? Reductions in rates of suicide by people with mental disorder might be one possibility, but one would need to assess to which factors any such drop was attributable. Ethical considerations would make the use of any control conditions in a comparative trial exceedingly difficult.

It might be thought worthwhile to look to studies of interventions designed to reduce recurrence of instances of parasuicide. This, however, raises a number of problems. First, there is continuing debate as to whether suicide and parasuicide are separate, though overlapping, phenomena. Hawton and Catalan (1987) pointed out that the rates of each changed independently of each other between 1960 and 1990, and that parasuicides and completed suicides differed in demographic characteristics and methods used. These differences, however, have become less pronounced with the recent increase in parasuicide by young males (Hawton 2000).

Second, if one wanted to draw conclusions about interventions aimed at preventing suicide, one would wish to be informed by instances of deliberate self-harm which were genuine attempts at suicide. James and Hawton (1985) demonstrated that it can be difficult to establish this: of 34 self-poisoners, 14 claimed suicidal intent, whereas only 1 out of 34 significant others agreed that this was so.

Third, Hawton *et al.*'s (1998) systematic review of treatments aimed at preventing repetition of parasuicide reported insufficient evidence on which to base recommendations. Two interventions showed significant reductions in repetition rates, albeit with small sample sizes. Promising results were reported for two further interventions.

Decisions about whether to continue maintaining an individual in the community when there is known to be some degree of suicide risk come down to weighing up the factors which favour community management against those which suggest caution. Caution would be indicated if the person is not previously known, where there is limited documentation, and where there is lack of corroborative information. Factors to consider in the person's history would be recent deliberate self-harm, particularly if planned and severe, and any instances of impulsive behaviour. Recent alcohol or substance misuse should be considered, as should whether the person's clinical syndrome is one associated with high risk. Factors connected with the person's suicidality would include: the degree of suicidal intent; fluctuations in the degree of distress, which makes assessment of risk more difficult; denial of suicidal ideas, when there is known to have been recent, serious, suicidal behaviour; psychotic ideas which might impair insight or judgement; and morbid ideas relating to others.

Psychosocial factors favouring community management would be: a preference of the person to be treated at home; possession by them of independent living skills and adequate resources; the existence of good social supports, particularly if available on a twenty-four-hour basis; and a manageable level of stress in the home environment. The presence of unresolved, adverse outside factors, or alienation from others, would suggest caution. Factors related to working with the individual would include whether a good rapport had been established, and whether the person was able to accept and utilise offered help, possibly indicated by ability to give a commitment not to harm themselves and compliance with agreed management plans.

The resources which are available to manage the risk are also important. These include sufficient, adequately trained, confident staff, with sufficient time to provide regular and flexible contact. Support to back up the identified key-worker should be available.

In management of the risk, as with assessment of risk, it is important to establish a supportive relationship, emphasising openness, acceptance, commitment, and the concept of an alliance with the patient. Where possible, family and friends should be included in the management plan. Having agreed a plan, explanations as to how this will be implemented should be given, and the person introduced to workers who will be involved. The frequency of contacts should be set, and, where necessary, obstacles to achieving this addressed. The person should be clear as to how they can make contact with the CMHT and any other appropriate agencies.

Plans should be made for activity until the next appointment. Likely difficult times should be identified. Plans should be made for dealing with them, and other unexpected difficulties which may occur, using a problem-solving approach if appropriate. A specific strategy should be developed for dealing with suicidal urges. The person's current use of alcohol and non-prescription drugs should be examined. At a time when the person is feeling relatively better, a list of reasons for living could be compiled.

## CONCLUSION

In an evaluation of suicide prevention strategies, Lewis *et al.* (1997) reported that those aimed at high-risk groups would have only a modest effect on overall rates, even where effective interventions were developed. Their conclusion was that population strategies were more likely to be effective, and that the best of these were likely to be actions to reduce availability of the means for committing suicide, and measures to reduce unemployment. They suggested that improving services and interventions for people who deliberately self-harm was likely to be the best high-risk group strategy. Nevertheless, it is salutary for those working in mental health to remember that, by definition, their client group is at high risk of suicide. It follows that identification and management of that risk are important parts of the role of the CMHN. Carrying them out calls for specific knowledge and skills, among which the ability to form and sustain a therapeutic relationship may be paramount.

## REFERENCES

Appleby, L. (2000) 'Safer services: conclusions from the report of the National Confidential Inquiry', *Advances in Psychiatric Treatment*, 6: 5–15.

Appleby, L., Cooper, J., Amos, T. and Faragher, B. (1999) 'Psychological autopsy study of suicides by people aged under 35', *British Journal of Psychiatry*, 175: 168–174.

Bancroft, J., Skrimshire, A., Casson, J., Harvard-Watts, O. and Reynolds, F. (1977) 'People who deliberately poison or injure themselves: their problems and their contacts with helping agencies', *Psychological Medicine*, 7: 289–303.

Barraclough, B., Bunch, J., Nelson, B. and Sainsbury, P. (1974) 'A hundred cases of suicide: clinical aspects', *British Journal of Psychiatry*, 125: 355–373.

Beck, A., Steer, R., Kovacs, M. and Garrison, B. (1985) 'Hopelessness and eventual suicide: a 10-year prospective study of patients hospitalised with suicidal ideation', *American Journal of Psychiatry*, 142: 559–563.

Bowers, L. (1995) *Assessing risk: good practice guidelines*, Tameside and Glossop Mental Health Service: Psychiatric Nursing Research and Development Unit (Policy document).

Cantor, C. (2000) 'Suicide in the Western world', in Hawton, K. and van Heeringen, C. (eds) *The international handbook of suicide and attempted suicide*, Chichester: Wiley.

Cattell, H. (2000) 'Suicide in the elderly', *Advances in Psychiatric Treatment*, 6, 2: 102–108.

Cheng, A., Chen, T., Chwen-Chen, C. and Jenkins, R. (2000) 'Psychosocial and psychiatric risk factors for suicide', *British Journal of Psychiatry*, 177: 360–365.

Dennehy, J., Appleby, L., Thomas, C. and Faragher, E.B. (1996) 'Case-control study of suicide by discharged psychiatric patients', *British Medical Journal*, 312: 1580.

Department of Health (1992) *The health of the nation: a strategy for health in England*, London: HMSO.

Department of Health (1998) *Our healthier nation*, London: HMSO.

Department of Health and Social Security (1984) *The management of deliberate self-harm*, London: Department of Health and Social Security.

Drake, R., Gates, C., Cotton, P. and Whitaker, A. (1984) 'Suicide among schizophrenics: who is at risk?' *Journal of Nervous and Mental Disease*, 172: 613–617.

Fawcett, J., Scheftner, W., Clark, D., Hedeker, D., Gibbons, R. and Coryell, W. (1987) 'Clinical predictors of suicide in patients with major affective disorders: a controlled prospective study', *American Journal of Psychiatry*, 144: 35–40.

Goldacre, M., Seagroatt, V. and Hawton, K. (1993) 'Suicide after discharge from psychiatric in-patient care', *The Lancet*, 342: 283–286.

Goldney, R. (2000) 'Prediction of suicide and attempted suicide', in Hawton, K. and van Heeringen, C. (eds) *The international handbook of suicide and attempted suicide*, Chichester: Wiley.

Goldstein, R., Black, D., Nasrallah, A. and Winokur, G. (1991) 'The prediction of suicide. Sensitivity, specificity, and predictive value of a multivariate model applied to suicide among 1906 patients with affective disorders', *Archives of General Psychiatry*, 48: 418–422.

Guze, S. and Robins, E. (1970) 'Suicide and primary affective disorders', *British Journal of Psychiatry*, 117: 437–438.

Harris, C. and Barraclough, B. (1997) 'Suicide as an outcome for mental disorders', *British Journal of Psychiatry*, 170: 205–228.

Hawton, K. (1987) 'Assessment of suicide risk', *British Journal of Psychiatry*, 150: 145–153.

Hawton, K. (2000) 'Sex and suicide', *British Journal of Psychiatry*, 177: 484–485.

Hawton, K. and Catalan, J. (1987) *Attempted suicide: a practical guide to its nature and management*, Oxford: Oxford University Press.

Hawton, K., Arensman, E., Townsend, E., Bremner, S., Feldman, E., Goldney, R., Gunnell, D., Hazell, P., van Heeringen, K., House, A., Owens, D., Sakinofsky, I. and Traskman-Bendz, L. (1998) 'Deliberate self-harm: systematic review of efficacy of psychosocial and pharmacological treatments in preventing repetition', *British Medical Journal*, 317: 441–447.

Hawton, K., Houston, K. and Shepperd, R. (1999) 'Suicide in young people: a study of 174 cases, aged under 25 years based on coroners' and medical records', *British Journal of Psychiatry*, 175: 271–276.

James, D. and Hawton, K. (1985) 'Overdoses: explanations and attitudes in self-poisoners and significant others', *British Journal of Psychiatry*, 146: 481–485.

King, E. and Barraclough, B. (1990) 'Violent death and mental illness: a study of a single catchment area over 8 years', *British Journal of Psychiatry*, 156: 714–720.

Kreitman, N. (1979) 'Reflections on the management of parasuicide', *British Journal of Psychiatry*, 135: 275–277.

Kreitman, N. (1982) 'How useful is the prediction of suicide following parasuicide?' in Wilmotte, J. and Mendlewicz, J. (eds) *New trends in suicide prevention*, Basel: Karger.

Kreitman, N., Philip, A., Greer, S. and Bagley, C. (1969) 'Parasuicide', *British Journal of Psychiatry*, 115: 746–747.

Lewis, G., Hawton, K. and Jones, P. (1997) 'Strategies for preventing suicide', *British Journal of Psychiatry*, 171: 351–354.

Linehan, M., Goodstein, J., Nielsen, S. and Chiles, J. (1983) 'Reasons for staying alive when you are thinking of killing yourself: the Reasons for Living Inventory', *Journal of Consulting and Clinical Psychology*, 51, 2: 276–286.

Miles, C. (1977) 'Conditions predisposing to suicide: a review', *Journal of Nervous and Mental Disease*, 164: 231–246.

Morgan, H.G. (1994) 'Assessment of risk', in Jenkins, R., Griffiths, S., Wylie, I., Hawton, K., Morgan, G. and Tylee, A. (eds) *The prevention of suicide*, London: HMSO.

Morgan, H.G. and Priest, P. (1991) 'Suicide and sudden unexpected deaths among psychiatric in-patients', *British Journal of Psychiatry*, 158: 368–374.

Morgan, H.G. and Stanton, R. (1997) 'Suicide among psychiatric in-patients in a changing clinical scene: suicidal ideation as a paramount index of short-term risk', *British Journal of Psychiatry*, 171: 561–563.

Morgan, G., Buckley, C. and Nowers, M. (1998) 'Face to face with the suicidal', *Advances in Psychiatric Treatment*, 4: 188–196.

Ohberg, A., Vuori, E., Ojanpera, I. and Lonnqvist, J. (1996) 'Alcohol and drugs in suicides', *British Journal of Psychiatry*, 169: 75–80.

Pallis, D., Gibbons, J. and Pierce, D. (1984) 'Estimating suicide risk among attempted suicides: II Efficiency of predictive scales after the attempt', *British Journal of Psychiatry*, 144: 139–148.

Pierce, D. (1981) 'The predictive validation of a suicide intent scale: a five year follow-up', *British Journal of Psychiatry*, 139: 391–396.

Pokorny, A. (1983) 'Prediction of suicide in psychiatric patients: report of a prospective study', *Archives of General Psychiatry*, 40: 249–257.

Powell, J., Geddes, J., Deeks, J., Goldacre, M. and Hawton, K. (2000) 'Suicide in psychiatric hospital in-patients: risk factors and their predictive power', *British Journal of Psychiatry*, 176: 266–272.

Roy, A. (1982) 'Suicide in chronic schizophrenia', *British Journal of Psychiatry*, 141: 171–177.

Sainsbury Centre for Mental Health (1997) *Pulling together: the future roles and training of mental health staff*, London: Sainsbury Centre for Mental Health.

Samaritans (2002) *Suicide in the UK and Ireland*. Online. http://www.samaritans.org.uktextonly.html/txtuk.html

Singleton, N., Bumpstead, R., O'Brien, M., Lee, A. and Meltzer, A. (2001) *Psychiatric morbidity among adults living in private households, 2000*, London: The Stationery Office.

United Nations (1996) *Prevention of suicide: guidelines for the formulation and implementation of national strategies*, New York: United Nations.

Welsh Office (1998) *Better health, better Wales*, Cardiff: Welsh Office.

World Health Organization (1990) *Consultations on strategies for reducing suicidal behaviours in the European region. Summary report*, Geneva: World Health Organization.

# FURTHER READING

Appleby, L. (2000) 'Safer services: conclusions from the report of the National Confidential Inquiry', *Advances in Psychiatric Treatment*, 6: 5–15.
Good, concise summary of the National Confidential Inquiry's findings and their implications.

Department of Health (2002) *National suicide prevention strategy for England*, London: Department of Health.
This recently-launched strategy document is directed towards the target of reducing the death rate from suicide in England by at least 20 per cent by 2010.

Hawton, K. and van Heeringen, C. (eds) (2000) *The international handbook of suicide and attempted suicide*, Chichester: Wiley.
Authoritative handbook of current knowledge on suicide and attempted suicide, the processes related to suicidal behaviour, and the assessment and treatment of people who are suicidal. Also reviews interventions for prevention at local and national level.

Morgan, G., Buckley, C. and Nowers, M. (1998) 'Face to face with the suicidal', *Advances in Psychiatric Treatment*, 4: 188–196.
Discussion of practical, clinical issues related to assessment and management of suicide risk, with guidelines for practice.

# CHAPTER 18

# WORKING WITH FAMILIES I: SYSTEMIC APPROACHES

*Billy Hardy*

---

## SUMMARY OF KEY POINTS

- This chapter will highlight some of the key developments within the field of family therapy, particularly the systemic family therapy field, thus drawing on areas of practice that are relevant for mental health nurses.

- Some key skills in interviewing, team working and therapy sessions are discussed. The areas of adult and child and couple work are explored.

- There are many ideas, skills and concepts that are complementary to the practice of mental health nursing. This chapter draws attention to a few of those that can be usefully applied to current practice.

---

## SETTING THE CONTEXT

There has been a long-standing connection between mental health nursing and the field of family therapy. Changes to the way many mental health nurses approach their clinical practice have included moving to a family-focused approach, through a psychosocial intervention model or other family-based interventions. This has been particularly relevant in the Child and Adolescent Mental Health Services (CAMHS) context, which has brought family therapy approaches into a sharper focus.

MacPhail (1988) sought to bring family-based approaches to care in the community to the attention of community mental health nursing, as did Parmainteny *et al.* (1985) who focused particularly on the role of community psychiatric nurses utilising ideas from systemic family therapy. A wealth of ideas has come from US and Canadian sources. Robinson (1994) and Wegner and Alexander (1993) have particularly influenced nursing practice over the past ten years. More recently in the UK, Whyte (1997) has refocused our thinking on many spheres of nursing practice, proposing a shift towards working with families, but also providing a platform for development in systemic approaches to working with families for a whole range of problems.

Within the UK, mental health nurses are seeking out training in increasing numbers in the field of psychotherapy and counselling, and many hold dual qualifications in nursing and psychotherapy. This process, coupled with the evolving formal nature of the United Kingdom Council for Psychotherapy (UKCP), has made it necessary for many nurses to hold these formal qualifications.

Definitions in the field can be found in the 'Review of psychotherapy' (Department of Health 1996), which clearly defines the place of the psycho-therapies within many NHS service contexts. The report gives some consideration to the training, practice and supervisory arrangements for practitioners, whilst attempting to clarify the different models and schools of practice which pre-dominate in the NHS. Its conclusions in terms of clinical effectiveness suggest that 'family therapy is at least as effective as other treatments for a range of problems in a range of treatment settings' (ibid., p. 89).

Many practitioners and researchers have been advocating family approaches for many years. However, it could be argued that family-based approaches in mental health nursing have been limited to the Thorn initiative, which has its emphasis on behavioural approaches to working with families (Barrowclough and Tarrier 1992, Brooker *et al*. 1993, Gournay 2000) (see also Chapter 19). The early family work of Leff *et al*. (1982) also included a systemic family therapy approach. Over the years, this has largely been forgotten in community mental health nursing, and therefore this chapter is a timely opportunity to revisit a systemic family therapy approach which has continued to flourish throughout the UK, and may provide an additional approach for the growing expertise in the field of mental health nursing.

Confirmation of the value of a family therapy approach is highlighted in *Treatment choice in psychological therapies and counselling* (Department of Health 2001), a publication placing systemic approaches in the wider context of psychotherapeutic practice.

This chapter will familiarise the reader with the underlying concepts of a systemic family therapy approach. It will highlight the approaches, methods and techniques which may be useful to practitioners in a wide variety of contexts. Three areas of clinical practice will be highlighted: working with children and adolescents; working with those with a diagnosis of depression; and working with people who have a psychosis.

## HISTORICAL DEVELOPMENT

The interest in family patterns of communication and styles of problem solving can be traced back to the end of the Second World War and the work of the

Mental Research Institute (MRI), which was the project of Don Jackson, John Weakland, Jay Haley and Gregory Bateson. The group worked on communication patterns in porpoises, analysing paradoxes, animal learning and tribal rituals. Throughout the 1950s the group, with others, worked on the double-bind theory of schizophrenia, multi-level communication patterns and the use of general systems theory as a framework for understanding family organisation. It was Gregory Bateson's collected works on natural systems – culminating in *Steps to an ecology of mind* (1972) and *Mind and nature* (1979) – suggesting that human systems could be understood like other systems of organisation, which interested the field of psychotherapy and provided the family therapy field with a foundation which still resonates today. Carr (2000) provides an excellent overview of these influences which began to show the different strands of therapy developing from Milan systemic approaches.

Other influential ideas from constructivism included Von Foerster's (1981) work on how each individual's construction of their world is partly determined by their own sense-making capabilities. At the other end of the spectrum, and more influential today, come ideas from a social constructionist perspective. Gergen (1994) suggests that individuals or families construct their knowledge within a social context through language and a strong sense of relationships within a community of ideas and beliefs with others.

## THE MILAN TEAM

These ideas influenced the team of four psychiatrists, Gianfranco Cecchin, Mara Selvini Palazzoli, Luigi Boscolo and Giuiana Prata, known as the Milan Associates, who began to set some foundation for the practice of Milan systemic approaches. Their seminal publication, *Paradox and counterparadox* (Palazzoni *et al.*, 1978), and their later papers of 1980 and work by Cecchin (1987) began a movement within the field of psychotherapy.

Its impact on the development of the approach here in the UK grew as teams formed at the Tavistock Clinic, London, the Institute of Family Therapy, London and the Family Institute, Cardiff. Many of these early teams began to develop their practice using the techniques developed by the Milan group. Over the past three to four decades many of these centres have grown into training institutions for the teaching of systemic approaches to family therapy.

## PARALLELS IN MENTAL HEALTH NURSING

Systemic approaches can largely be described as an interpersonal therapy, not only between the client and therapist, but also in the relationships clients have with other family members, close friends and other important people in their lives. It is also interpersonal in its focus on pathology. A systemic view would see the client in relation to the pathology or problems, and vice versa. This gives the client and the therapist a greater therapeutic option for change. It is this that Dallos and

Draper (2000) have suggested is one of the major contributions that systemic thinking has brought to bear on the field of psychotherapy. In a similar vein the adaptation of general systems theory and the work of Betty Neuman and Martha Rogers place mental health nursing relationships firmly alongside those of the developing systemic field. These evolving ideas present many bridges between systemic family therapy and mental health nursing, not only in the past, but also in the present.

# CONCEPTS INFORMING PRACTICE

In many models of therapy there are some central concepts which inform practice, and this is so of the systemic approaches to working with families. Palazolli *et al.* (1980) highlighted the three key elements of practice for a Milan systemic approach: hypothesising; circularity; and neutrality. These concepts form the foundation for an approach which has developed many creative ways of working.

Hypothesising is the process of utilising the information presented to the practitioner: for example, on referral, hypotheses are generated from the information as ideas and hunches, but not truths, as to what may be happening within and around the family and the defined problems or difficulty. Carr (2000) suggests it is also a mini theory, which is checked out, to find a fit with the family, but can be modified. This is a position which gives the therapist room to explore within the family the meaning of the problems with different family members, whilst at the same time not taking or siding with one story or description over another. This gives attention to all descriptions related to the problem. By doing so, the therapist can build up a picture of how the problem is located within the family. It gives attention to the organisation of information to ensure a structure for detailed enquiry for understanding and meaning within the family.

Brown (1994) suggests that there are five benefits derived from hypothesising. It gives focus to the therapist and assists in managing the complexity of information offered by the family. It helps to organise information and enable curiosity to develop. It encourages the therapist to take a broad lens to encompass wide-ranging ideas in understanding the client's position. It also ensures that the therapist's underlying beliefs and prejudices are brought into consciousness and examined. Stratton *et al.* (1990) focus on a systemic hypothesis having a variety of components, such as: it is circular in that it connects with all family members; it focuses on relationships within the family; it is concerned with what people believe and how they behave; and it is non-pathologising.

Circularity, as Jones (1993) suggests, is the way in which the interview is conducted by the therapist whose interest is fuelled by the relationships between the family members. The Milan team first introduced the idea to the practice arena. This idea was that repetitive patterns exist in both behaviour and verbal communication styles within relational systems such as families. Fleuridas *et al.* (1986) explore further the idea of circularity in an interview context, and suggest that when investigating and exploring changes and differences in family relationships over time, having a circular approach helps to gauge the interactions and patterns. It allows the family to develop an awareness of itself, its members and relationships. Its aim is to promote significant change. Andersen *et al.* (1985) suggest that the therapist's role is to help the family move from patterns which are stuck or unhelpful to a more useful new pattern.

Neutrality can be defined to some extent as a position that a practitioner may take or hold on to. Dallos and Draper (2000), Tomm (1987) and Jones (1993) describe this as a position adopted by a therapist, in the therapeutic relationship. Tomm (1987) elaborates on this with respect to meaning and values. A position of neutrality is the closest to taking the position of remaining non-committal, but attempts to hear the views of each family member. Systemic therapy has developed ideas over time. The concept of neutrality is one that involves at a pragmatic level an openness to multiple explanations of problems experienced by a family. A more commonly used description of this process is curiosity (Cecchin 1987).

Families, like other groups, are viewed by the therapist from different perspectives influenced by different ideas. However, some key ideas remain central to practice. Family therapy is therefore seen as a relational therapy. The problem is viewed in relation to every other relationship with the client. Problem formation and resolution are determined within the pattern of behaviour and beliefs which families or groups who live together evolve and create over time. This in turn will be considered within a social context.

The wider social context is considered to be important, for example, extended family networks, other social relationships and schools, health services and other institutions which frequently relate with families who have problems. Gorrell Barnes (2001) suggests that attention is paid to all levels of interaction, giving us what we refer to as the systemic approach. It is therefore multi-layered in terms of contexts, and fluid in its utility in practice.

## CHANGE

Change is an ongoing process for families as a result of life-cycle change, i.e. loss, illness, ageing children, changing schools, leaving home, and forming relationships outside the family. Families may be re-forming or fragmenting through divorce or separation, as well as contexts where children may be in care, foster care or being adopted. All of the contexts require change and adaptation for many family members and can produce challenges for everyone. Change is therefore a contextual force, with family members permitting or adjusting to change to differing degrees.

Families can get stuck as they try to negotiate these transitions. Change is, therefore, in therapeutic terms, negotiated with the family over time, during and through the therapeutic relationship.

## IDEAS IN PRACTICE

It is always useful to consider the referrer's possible motivations and ideas about referral for family therapy and to check these out alongside those of the family.

The first stage is one of searching for a definition of relationship, between family members as well as the therapist's relationship to the family. Before therapy begins, the therapist will consider and hypothesise about the possible reasons why a referral has been made now. If it is a self-referral, the same question, amongst others, will be asked.

Organising information may be done through the use of genograms – a useful assessment process for the field of mental health nursing practice. Genograms are elaborate forms of family trees which give a visual picture of relationships over time. The use of these genograms can include other contexts such as social networks or professional systems which help to map out the clients' and the therapist's contexts and their complexities for the therapy. McGoldrick and Gerson (1985) provide a unique overview of the use of genograms as a particularly useful tool for nursing practice with potential for wider applications.

# WORKING IN TEAMS

Team working has been a prominent feature of the systemic approach. Many of the techniques, methods and theories have emerged as a result of team work in clinical practice. The Milan team presented a blueprint which other teams have replicated. This is not a team as identified in community mental health, but solely a therapeutic team. The use of a one-way screen enables the therapist to have different views in the therapy and to have feedback instantly on theory and practice, with the team on one side of the screen and the family and therapist on the other. This also gives families the opportunity to hear different views on their difficulty. Sometimes families appreciate the multiple voices from a team. It can also protect the integrity of the therapy, by way of it being a public therapy, as the therapist has an ongoing observing team whose members are detached but attached to the therapeutic process. This gives the opportunity to engage in live supervision, a key element of the systemic approach.

# THE THERAPY SESSION

Team-work will vary for different groups of practitioners and clinical contexts. There are, however, some principles which are grounded in the systemic tradition. The therapy team will meet before the session and the therapist conducting the therapy will present ideas and a hypothesis to the team. This may have been generated from a previous session or from new referral information utilising the genogram process.

The team will offer further thoughts and ideas to the therapist, but will also challenge the therapist as to their idea and perceptions of how things appear for the family. This enables the therapist to entertain other possible explanations or alternative stories about what the problem/s may be about. The therapist can then conduct the session with a range of ideas, but can be open to a more useful collaborative enquiry with the family.

Sometimes the session will be punctuated by a break. This gives the therapist an opportunity to consult with colleagues, or an invitation will be made to the team to join the family and therapist in offering reflections on the session. This is known as a Reflecting Team Process (attributed to Andersen 1987); it has been developed by some teams as a common part of practice and falls into what is commonly referred to as a post-Milan approach influenced by social constructionism (Gergen 1994).

This approach creates a transparency within the therapeutic context. Following this it is usual for the team to have a post-session discussion with the therapist. This gives the opportunity for the team to highlight significant moments in the therapy and to reflect on what changed or happened between pre-session thinking, the actual session, and the post-session position. Again this is a collaborative process within the team.

## CLINICAL AREAS AND SYSTEMIC PRACTICE

Systemic approaches are practised in many clinical areas in either in-patient settings or community settings. Working with children is one area of practice which has influenced many systemic therapists. This approach comes from a strong tradition and evidence base for practice. There is a current acceptance throughout mental health services that some therapy skills are a necessary part of a professional's skill base for working with children and young people (Appleton 2000).

Wilson (1998) gives an example of systemic approaches to working with children. A framework is offered for child-focused practice, and in this approach the concern is not with the origins of the problems defined, but with how problems get defined. The influence of language and relationships, family resources and how to gain access to these resources, either as a family or as an individual, are paramount.

Many practitioners will be familiar with attempting to engage children and young adolescents in their clinical practice. This can sometimes feel like a daunting task, especially when the practitioner is a novice and is attempting perhaps for the first time to marry theory with practice. The child's voice, as discussed by Combrinck-Graham (1991), has become paramount in the evolving field of systemic therapy. In the history of working with families much time has been lost, as therapists became engrossed in the adult voices. The emphasis is on talking with the child rather than talking about the child, a common scenario in clinical practice. Changes over the past ten years have seen a refocusing on working with children.

The role of circularity remains central when conducting interviews with families and children, as highlighted by Benson *et al*. (1991). He gives three areas of practice as potentially useful for working with children: the use of children's fantasy; using concrete materials; and the application of certain techniques in practice.

It can be intimidating for children to enter therapy with their parents or other adults. Taffel (1991) emphasises that the use of oneself is a key consideration when working with children, as too much focus on 'I being the therapist' may lead to some therapeutic paralysis. Taffel goes on to say that helping a young child tell a story is like building a house block by block, asking question by question. Adolescents may also experience the process of therapy as oppressive. Being clear about the objectives at the outset can help to diffuse tensions. Being too pushy could send the wrong message to a young person. Therefore controlling the pace and keeping close to the agenda is an essential ingredient of the therapeutic process. Being able to connect with children is important from the first moment the therapist meets them.

Therapeutic ritual is also a key element in practice. This may involve some object or symbol, perhaps a toy, a teddy bear for example – or creating one. This can be a simple or complex creation, but can make a powerful connection with the child in therapy.

Working with children is not all about taking the idea that 'actions can speak louder than words', though this rings true for systemic therapists. Combrinck-Graham (1991) suggests that children should be at home in family therapy and an over-reliance on talking can be boring and disrespectful to the child.

These principles are few, and further exploration in this field would increase the repertoire of many mental health nurses, especially when many of their clients have children.

# WORKING WITH ADULTS

Many mental health nurses will only work with adults in defined services. In this context working with the seriously mentally ill is given prominence. There are, however, still variations in which other client groups can access community mental health nursing expertise for other diagnoses and problems. It is therefore significant that depression has figured a great deal in the systemic field. As with the work of the 1970s and 1980s on schizophrenia in the London Depression Trial, Leff *et al.* (2000) have provided a sound platform for developing therapeutic strategies for working with couples who have a partner diagnosed with depression. This work was ongoing during the 1990s and has produced some encouraging outcomes for systemic couples therapy which are as important as the family work approach to schizophrenia was in the 1970s and 1980s.

For Jones and Asen (2000) the utilisation of the constraints on the therapeutic process and working with specific diagnoses can prove to be indispensable for working systemically. Leff *et al.* (2000) suggest that the approach used by the therapist may be disseminated and used in training for other professions, including mental health nursing. This would be a similar process to the ways in which nurses have been trained in schizophrenia family work through the Thorn initiative.

Couples therapy has significant differences from working with families and individuals. Jones and Asen (2000) have highlighted a variety of approaches and techniques which can be utilised. As with many of the points already covered by this chapter, hypothesising is a clear part of the process of therapy. The manualisation of this work has given clear frameworks for practice, which include: the meaning of depression and of depression in the context of the referral; social and cultural contexts and family contexts; interrupting problem cycles; shifting negative attributions; and task setting. Leff *et al.* (2000) state that the main aim of this approach is to help clients/couples to gain new perspectives on presenting problems, depressive type behaviours and attempts to find different ways for the couple to relate to each other.

Circular interviewing is a clear guideline for practice. In keeping with systemic thinking and practice, therapeutic processes are given clear attention. For example, joining or engaging with clients, as with all family approaches, is significant for a clear focus on strengths and competencies, problem solving and challenge and the use of reframing.

Having taken place over many years, this work now offers the opportunity to begin to look at depression or depressions from a different clinical research perspective. It will be of use to those mental health nurses who work in primary care, especially those working in the field of postnatal depression, where a systemic approach appears to fit both from a family and a couple relationships perspective. Systemic approaches to depression can be successfully utilised alongside many of the other interventions offered by mental health nurses.

Another area of practice in which a systemic approach can be utilised is work with people with serious mental illness. Burbach and Stanbridge (1998) have highlighted systemic approaches to working with coping with serious mental illness. This is an approach which integrates family therapy and family management approaches, and gives attention to the core principles described in this chapter, but also expands into specific skills-based practices from the family management approaches.

MacDonald (1994) demonstrated the efficacy of a brief therapy approach in an adult psychiatric context. The outcomes here showed improvements in reported symptomatology, which were seen in 70 per cent (29) of cases worked with, with no discernible costs noted for provision of such therapy by existing staff. A further follow-up study of 36 referrals by MacDonald (1997) demonstrated a good outcome for 64 per cent of clients. Outcome was reported by clients themselves and also by general practitioners, who saw the problems initially referred improved.

## CONCLUSIONS

The systemic model as an approach to working with families has a long and creative tradition in the UK. The relationships with mental health nursing and other spheres of nursing are compelling. There are many bridges between systemic family therapy and mental health nursing. The literature from the United States shows a highly developed approach to family work, and in the UK the mental health nursing profession is beginning to take notice of these developments.

This chapter has highlighted some core principles in the development of the systemic model. It has also described how the core concepts are put into practice. Hypothesising, circularity, and neutrality (curiosity) are part of the history of this approach. Many of these traditions of practice still form the practice base of many systemic family therapists, and indeed many mental health nurses.

For the novice or newly qualified practitioner these are fundamental principles in practice.

Family therapy has been ever-present in CAMH services. However, new evidence is emerging which deserves attention in the adult service context. The work on depression is one area which may compel nurses to explore this further and give it the same attention the profession paid to the early family work in schizophrenia of the 1970s and 1980s.

The work in other fields familiar to mental health nurses, such as serious mental illness, adds more opportunities for practitioners to engage in family work using a systemic model. It is now clear that systemic approaches have a place alongside other psychotherapies within the NHS.

Systemic family therapy has a valuable place in growing and expanding mental health fields. Mental health nurses will need to continue developing their clinical skills. It is hoped that many will train in the field of systemic therapy, bringing to it a rich and creative professional edge which the systemic field will value.

# REFERENCES

Andersen, T. (1987) 'The reflecting team: dialogue and meta-dialogue in clinical work', *Family Process*, 26: 415–428.

Andersen, T., Danielson, H., Sonnesyn, H. and Sonnesyn, M. (1985) 'Circular questioning and shifting relationships', *Australia and New Zealand Journal of Family Therapy*, 6 (3): 145–150.

Appleton, P. (2000) 'Tier 2 CAMHS and its interface with primary care', *Advances in Psychiatric Treatment*, 6: 388–396.

Barrowclough, C. and Tarrier, N. (1992) *Families of schizophrenic patients*, London: Chapman and Hall.

Bateson, G. (1972) *Steps to an ecology of mind*, New York: Balantine.

Bateson, G. (1979) *Mind and nature: a necessary unity*, New York: Bantam.

Benson, M., Zimmermann, T.S. and Martin, D. (1991) 'Accessing children's perceptions of their family: circular questioning revisited', *Journal of Marital and Family Therapy*, 17 (4): 363–372.

Brooker, C., Tarrier, N., Barrowclough, C., Butterworth, A. and Goldberg, D. (1993) 'Skills for CPNs working with seriously mentally ill people: the outcome of a trial of psychosocial intervention', in Brooker, C. and White, E. (eds) *Community psychiatric nursing: a research perspective*, vol. 2, London: Chapman and Hall.

Brown, J. (1994) 'Teaching hypothesising skills from a post-Milan perspective', *Australia and New Zealand Journal of Family Therapy*, 16 (3): 133–142.

Burbach, F. and Stanbridge, R. (1998) 'A family intervention in psychosis service: integrating the systemic and family management approaches', *Journal of Family Therapy*, 20 (3): 311–325.

Carr, A. (2000) *Family therapy: concepts, process and practice*, Chichester: Wiley.

Cecchin, G. (1987) 'Hypothesising, circularity and neutrality revisited: an invitation to curiosity', *Family Process*, 26 (4): 405–413.

Combrinck-Graham, L. (1991) 'On technique with children in family therapy: how calculated should it be?', *Journal of Marital and Family Therapy*, 17: 373–377.

Dallos, R. and Draper, R. (2000) *An introduction to family therapy*, Buckingham: Open University Press.

Department of Health (1996) *NHS psychotherapy services in England: review of strategic policy*, London: NHS Executive.

Department of Health (2001) *Treatment choice in psychological therapies and counselling: evidence based clinical practice guidelines*, London: Department of Health.

Fleuridas, C., Nelson, S.T. and Rosenthal, D.M. (1986) 'The evolution of circular questions: training family therapists', *Journal of Marital and Family Therapy*, 12 (2): 113–127.

Gergen, K. (1994) *Realities and relationships: soundings in social constructionism*, Cambridge, MA: Harvard University Press.

Gorrell Barnes, G. (2001) *Family therapy in changing times*, London: Routledge.

Gournay, K. (2000) 'Role of the community psychiatric nurse in the management of schizophrenia', *Advances in Psychiatric Treatment*, 6: 243–249.

Jones, E. (1993) *Family systems therapy*, Chichester: Wiley.

Jones, E. and Asen, E. (2000) *Systemic couple therapy and depression*, London: Karnac Books.

Leff, J., Kuipers, L., Berkowitz, R. and Sturgeon, D. (1982) 'A controlled trial of intervention in the families of schizophrenic families', *British Journal of Psychiatry*, 141: 121–134.

Leff, J., Vearneals, S., Wolff, G., Alexander, B., Chisholm, D., Everitt, B., Asen, E., Jones, E., Brewin, C. and Dayson, D. (2000) 'The London depression intervention trial', *British Journal of Psychiatry*, 177: 95–100.

MacDonald, A. (1994) 'Brief therapy in adult psychiatry', *Journal of Family Therapy*, 16: 415–426.

MacDonald, A. (1997) 'Brief therapy in adult psychiatry: further outcomes', *Journal of Family Therapy*, 19: 213–222.

McGoldrick, M. and Gerson, R. (1985) *Genograms in family assessment*, New York: W.W. Norton.

MacPhail, D. (1988) *Family therapy in the community*, Oxford: Heinemann.

Palazzoli, M.S., Boscolo, L., Cecchin, G. and Prata, G. (1978) *Paradox and counterparadox*, New York: Jason Aronson.

Palazzoli, M.S., Cecchin, G., Prata, G. and Boscolo, L. (1980) 'Hypothesising-circularity-neutrality: three guidelines for the conductor of the session', *Family Process*, 19: 3–12.

Parmainteny, J.P., Mangen, J., Lusted, J., Sundaram, E. and Berry, J. (1985) 'Systemic family work within a community mental health centre by a community psychiatric nursing team: by tradition?' in Campbell, D. and Draper, R. (eds) *Applications of systemic family therapy*, London: Academic Press.

Robinson, C. (1994) 'Nursing interventions with families: a demand or invitation to change?', *Journal of Advanced Nursing*, 19: 897–904.

Stratton, P., Shoot-Preston, M. and Hanks, H. (1990) *Family therapy training and practice*, Birmingham: Venture Press.

Taffel, R. (1991) 'How to talk with kids', *Networker*, July/August.

Tomm, K. (1987) 'Interventive interviewing: part 1, strategizing as a fourth guideline for the therapist', *Family Process*, 26: 3–13.

Von Foerster, H. (1981) *Observing systems*, Seaside, CA: Intersystems.

Wegner, G. and Alexander, R. (1993) *Readings in family nursing*, Philadelphia: Lippincott.

Whyte, D. (ed.) (1997) *Explorations in family nursing*, London: Routledge.

Wilson, J. (1998) *Child focused practice*, London: Karnac Books.

# FURTHER READING

Dallos, R. and Draper, R. (2000) *An introduction to family therapy*, Buckingham: Open
   University Press.
This book is a very good introduction to the field of family therapy for those who are
unfamiliar with its development. It sets out to take the reader through the various strands
of development in teaching, practice and research.

Carr, A. (2000) *Family therapy: concepts, process and practice*, Chichester: Wiley.
This book takes the development of family therapy in its widest contexts and provides
excellent foundations for all levels of readers, from novice to experienced practitioners; it
provides a valuable text for both teachers and trainee family therapists.

Jones, E. and Asen, E. (2000) *Systemic couple therapy and depression*, London: Karnac
   Books.
This book by two well-known and influential figures in the field of family therapy takes a
behind-the-scenes approach to the London depression trial. It is highly accessible in its
style and is recommended for those working with people with depression, and in particular
those working with couples.

# CHAPTER 19

# WORKING WITH FAMILIES II: PSYCHOSOCIAL INTERVENTIONS

*Geoff Brennan*

---

## SUMMARY OF KEY POINTS

- Carers of people with mental health problems are recognised as having their own needs.

- Psychosocial family interventions have been utilised to assist carers who struggle most to cope with their caring role.

- Whilst generic community workers are a key resource for all carers, there are a number of carers who would benefit from specialist intervention.

---

## INTRODUCTION

The National Service Framework for Mental Health contains a standard outlining the need to assist carers of people with mental health problems in the caring role (Department of Health 1999) (see Box 19.1). It is a major challenge of any professional working with clients in terms of their wider social networks (which is arguably all professionals) to strike a balance between the needs of the client and the needs of others, particularly carers.

In this chapter we will discuss the rise of interventions aimed at increasing the ability of carer systems to cope with the carer role. It is important to note that these interventions are aimed at improving outcomes for the client and improving health and coping within the carer system itself.

**Box 19.1    Caring about carers**

*National Service Framework for Mental Health:*
*Standard 6: Caring about carers*

All individuals who provide regular and substantial care for a person on CPA (care programme approach) should:

- have an assessment of their caring, physical and mental health needs, repeated on at least an annual basis;
- have their own written care plan which is given to them and implemented in discussion with them.

(Department of Health 1999, p. 69)

Comment

1    Carer groups such as the National Schizophrenia Fellowship (now renamed Rethink Serious Mental Illness) have expressed concern over the phrase 'regular and substantial care'. The concern is that services may interpret this in a narrow manner, such as the client and carer having to live in the same household. The issue for carer groups is the level of distress and burden (be this physical, emotional or financial) that carers face in carrying out the caring role and the recognition of this burden within the statutory services.

2    The lead organisation charged with delivery of the standard is the 'local authority', and the lead officer 'director of social services', with NHS trusts being 'key partners'. Joint service teams and new social care trusts may find it easier to collaborate on achieving this standard.

3    The major focus of the standard is around very practical types of intervention and services, such as respite care, the providing of information, and checklists for primary care service providers. The types of intervention discussed in this chapter are more inferred than explicitly called for within the standard.

# THE RISE OF PSYCHOSOCIAL INTERVENTIONS FOR CARERS

The growing body of literature regarding psychosocial interventions often gives the impression of a harmonious school of interventions with a common evidence base. In reality there are a number of types of intervention housed within psychosocial interventions. In addition, there is a tendency to draw boundaries between the psychosocial and systemic-based family interventions (see Chapter 18). These boundary demarcations are disingenuous and unhelpful (Burbach

1996). The two should rather be seen as having different approaches to common needs, which are not in competition with one another. The psychosocial interventions for psychosis, which have evolved from a behavioural approach, were preceded by systemic ideas and interventions and have been greatly influenced by them.

Having said this, there are features of the psychosocial interventions that we are examining which should be considered as differentiating them from other forms of intervention:

- The psychosocial family interventions are specifically aimed at systems that are coping with the presence of a psychosis in one of its members. In the early models, this was predominantly schizophrenia. Systemic family interventions are aimed at dealing with any possible issue located within a family which has a negative affect on the system's ability to function. As such, psychosocial interventions are purpose-built for a specific issue (psychosis), and are not generic for all possible issues.
- The main difference in delivery is that the psychosocial interventions follow a structured model with key features, which will be explored.
- Within the common aspects there is a strong emphasis on the carer system developing skills to deal with psychosis. In addition, there is an emphasis on non-sufferers of psychosis within the carer system developing interests away from that of the caring role.

## BUILDING THE MODEL

Psychosocial interventions for carers evolved logically from work on what is known as 'expressed emotion', or EE for short. Although EE is now an accepted concept, it must rank as one of the worst named ever. To the uninformed, it naturally sounds like a measure of emotion, which it is not. 'Emotion' is not measurable in any true sense. Rather, EE is a systematic means by which researchers were able to differentiate between individual carers in order to predict relapse in clients.

In EE research, carers were divided into two groups by means of a structured interview process carried out with individual carers. Those who viewed the presence of schizophrenia within a loved one as the client's or their own fault were considered to be high expressed emotion carers (high EE). These carers exhibit high levels of criticism or hostility towards the client, or overcompensate for the client's needs. Those who were able to view the condition as external to their loved one's personality, and not caused by family members, were considered to be low expressed emotion carers (low EE). These carers display a high degree of awareness as to the effects of psychosis and are able to compensate to protect both the client and themselves.

Using this demarcation, researchers have been able to demonstrate that clients who have high contact with identified high EE carers are at great risk of relapse. Those in high contact with only low EE carers have a much better chance of avoiding relapse. Whilst this explanation is simplistic for the purpose of clarity, the research underpinning the results has been reproduced within many cultural groups and found to be a robust indicator of relapse (Gamble and Brennan 1997). It follows that interventions targeted at changing high EE carers in a beneficial way would assist the client. From this premise, researchers moved into delivering and evaluating interventions designed to do this. It is important to mention that, while the evidence base for EE and its link to relapse is robust, the evidence base for the efficacy of interventions designed to change high EE carers into low EE carers is less conclusive.

Whilst the need for family interventions comes from communal EE research, the interventions designed to assist high EE carers to change their management of the caring role differed. Having said this, there was a common structure to the delivery of the interventions. In order to understand the differences it is best to consider them within this common structure. The next section will explore some of the salient features of the interventions and consider where there are differences in delivery or model.

# THE STRUCTURAL FRAMEWORK OF PSYCHOSOCIAL FAMILY INTERVENTIONS: INTERVENTIONS IN THE 'HOME'

There is a consensus within psychosocial family interventions that the professional should move towards delivering therapy in the identified 'home'. This was a move away from traditional family therapy in not having the family come to a clinic to see a therapist and the supervision team assisting the therapist. In doing this psychosocial family interventions placed a degree of burden on the professional. Dealing with family systems is emotionally and psychologically difficult, both in dealing with difficult situations and in ensuring that the professional remains as neutral as possible. The way in which this has been managed is either to have a co-working system with two family workers attending each family, or in some of the more behavioural models, to have a single worker with a very structured form of intervention backed with a robust supervision system. Whichever is used, there is evidence that lack of supervision for family workers can lead the workers to stop offering the interventions (Brennan and Gamble 1997).

# A PURPOSEFULLY POSITIVE APPROACH TO CARERS

Training courses for psychosocial family interventions emphasise that families do not *cause* psychosis. They are taught that families attempt to care as best they can, even if that caring is not what is best for the client. Hence, family members who display criticism of the client are viewed as acting out of ignorance rather than design. Psychosocial family interventions have been criticised for this carer positive stance, and in carrying out the interventions there often arises a dilemma of need, in that the carer system can have an anxiety which it perceives can only be rectified with some compromise from the client. An example would be a situation where parents believe that the person is better on medication, but the person disagrees. A positive stance with regard to carers should not be interpreted as placing their needs before client needs. In the reality of family interventions, as in family therapy, there is always a complex dynamic when it comes to the individual as opposed to the collective need. Again, supervision is essential in maintaining as neutral a stance as possible.

## EDUCATION AND INFORMATION GIVING

Psychosocial family interventions are specifically designed for carer systems dealing with psychosis. Such systems are often ill-informed about the course and treatment of psychosis, and actively look for this information (Hogman and Pearson 1995). This aspect is meant to assist with this. In addition, the information is designed to reveal any misconceptions that the family members have regarding causes of the psychosis (Fadden 1998). These can then be considered to explore issues of blame and guilt. Beyond the general belief that education and information are a necessary aspect of psychosocial interventions, there is little agreement on how to deliver them. In many models the emphasis is on formal sessions, with carers and clients guided through literature on the diagnosis. Critics of psychosocial family interventions have stated that the emphasis on the biological nature of psychosis (particularly schizophrenia) and the presentation of psychosis as an illness are questionable. In practice, this criticism has some validity. The major emphasis in education should not be on getting the carer system and the client to accept the diagnosis. Rather it should be concerned with exploring the explanatory model adopted in the absence of information, and how this model influences their attitudes towards and management of the issues arising from the presence of symptoms.

## ENHANCING COMMUNICATION

The ability to communicate effectively is a prerequisite for any system. This is as true for families and informal carers as it is for any systems. Within psychosocial interventions emphasis is placed upon controlling and improving communication patterns, although the means by which this is achieved are very different. In some models, particularly those derived from Ian Falloon's work on behavioural interventions, communication skills are identified as an explicit area to work on (Falloon 1995). Within this, role-play and rehearsal are used to allow carers and clients to communicate specific requests in a calm and clear manner. Other family workers will address communication by constructing meetings in such a manner as to change the patterns of communication within the meeting itself. In this way, the family workers will negotiate ground rules regarding: turn-taking, addressing individuals rather than 'talking about them in their presence', and sharing speaking time. In sessions the family workers are also obliged to address personal criticism. For example, if a family member were to say 'she is lazy' in a session, workers should ask what the carer sees to justify this, and reframe the personal criticism as a behavioural deficit – 'So your daughter not getting up in the morning makes you feel concerned'. Often family workers will be familiar with both types of intervention and adapt their input to suit the particular situation.

# PROBLEM SOLVING

Although there is no conclusion as to what aspect of family interventions is crucial, it is commonly held that problem solving with carers and clients is an essential aspect of the intervention. The philosophy behind problem solving is that carers and clients will benefit more from tackling real, identifiable issues produced by either the psychosis or the caring role. In this, the emphasis is on the 'here and now' in that issues chosen will be from direct feedback from both clients and carers. It is in this prioritisation of issues that conflict often arises between the needs and desires of carers and the needs and desires of clients. There is no simple solution to this conflict when it becomes apparent, and subtle negotiation is required. Often this means the family worker brokering 'deals' in an attempt to break the stand-off. A typical example from my own experience is a client wishing to socialise with friends, and carers who struggle with the anxiety this would cause them. In a situation like this, the negotiation is around what the carer would need to manage the anxiety, with a common 'deal' being that the client does socialise, but rings the family home at intervals to 'help the carer cope'.

Once an issue has been identified, a structured means of problem solving is used to come to a consensus on how to move forward. This is the six-step problem-solving method described in Box 19.2. Six-step problem solving can be overtly introduced with the worker helping the family move from one stage to the next, or covertly used with the worker guiding the meeting through targeted questions. Within all models the setting of homework tasks to carry out the identified problem solution is seen as essential, and workers are charged with assisting the client and carers to identify changes to their behaviour which will assist in dealing with the issue.

---

**Box 19.2    A six-step problem-solving strategy**

Step 1: What exactly is the problem or goal?

Step 2: List all possible solutions

Step 3: Highlight the possible advantages and disadvantages

Step 4: Choose the best solution

Step 5: Plan how exactly to carry out the solution

Step 6: Carry out a review of the solution

(Falloon and Graham-Hole 1994)

# COGNITIVE RESTRUCTURING

Behaviour patterns within caring systems are attempts to deal with the problems that the psychosis can create. This can result in carers and clients acting in seemingly punitive, intrusive or uncaring ways towards each other. Although mostly a covert outcome of family interventions, the thinking behind these behaviours is challenged and alternatives sought when problem solving. Often this requires some part of the system to take a risk in order to change the pattern, and the resultant anxiety has to be acknowledged and managed. In this way, all members of the family are asked to review how they view their attitudes and beliefs regarding the management of the psychosis. It is this long-term change in attitude and belief that family interventions are ultimately interested in. It should be remembered that the low EE carers referred to earlier are able to maintain their effective caring role, due to not losing sight of the individual within the psychosis and having the ability to look after themselves whilst carrying out the caring role.

# TIME SPAN AND RESOLUTION

Family interventions take time, effort and a deep commitment. In addition, the interventions are resource-intensive and therefore should be targeted to those carers who struggle most with the psychosis. Once the carer and client have completed the interventions, workers should always leave the option of contacting services rather than formally discharging them (Kuipers *et al.* 1992). In practical experience, family workers can work with an individual family for up to two years under strict administration of the model, with nine months usually considered the minimal length of time. Research has shown that short-duration interventions do not compare favourably against the longer-term interventions described above, as initial positive gains are not maintained on follow-up. In Box 19.3, a case study illustrates the use of the model.

# THE EVIDENCE BASE

The effectiveness of psychosocial family interventions has been the subject of extensive research. The most comprehensive review of the entire school of interventions comes from a meta-analysis conducted for the Cochrane Schizophrenia Group (Pharoah *et al.* 2002). This analysis concluded that the interventions may decrease the frequency of relapse, decrease hospitalisation and encourage compliance with medication. One criticism of the Cochrane analysis was that it considered outcomes for all carer systems, regardless of whether or not they had completed the full package of identified interventions (Fadden 1998). In a previous meta-analysis, results had shown that there was significant difference with regard to delaying relapse if the carer system was able to receive the whole package of interventions (De Jesus Mari and Streiner 1994).

**Box 19.3   Case study**

The following case study highlights the family intervention model in action.

The Bernstein family

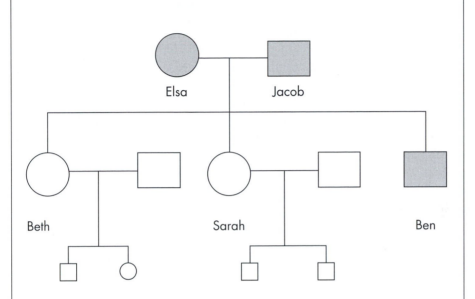

The Bernstein family consist of three generations living within close proximity. Although the shaded family members all live in a single household, there is a culture of regular contact and sharing of caring with regard to the youngest members of the family. The family has a strong and rich Jewish cultural identity and is closely integrated into their local community.

Elsa and Jacob were born in Spain but immigrated to England after their marriage. The adult children, Beth, Sarah and Ben, were all born in England, as were their children.

The index client is Elsa, the matriarchal head of the family, who has a diagnosis of late onset schizophrenia, having first become ill in her late thirties. Elsa had been known to services for fifteen years prior to interventions. Since her first episode of psychosis, Elsa has had an average of one admission to hospital every eighteen months.

An initial referral for family work was received from the family's general practitioner who identified that 'Elsa has experienced regular relapses of symptoms over the last few years, in spite of Jacob giving up work to care for her'. At the time of family interventions beginning, Jacob was also receiving treatment for high blood pressure and Sarah was reported as being burdened with assisting in caring for the household.

The process of family interventions had to give way to the immediate problem of Elsa's relapse. The symptoms described by Elsa were primarily auditory hallucinations, paranoia and suicidal thoughts. In previous years, Elsa would have been admitted. The family agreed to interventions in the home as an alternative, provided the assistance of the workers was regular and that admission could be initiated if the situation did not rectify itself.

The family workers engaged and worked with the family system for a period of eighteen months. Initially visits were twice weekly with additional telephone contact, moving to weekly once the initial crisis was resolved. After twelve months, the meetings were changed to monthly.

### Home visits

All work was carried out within the family home. Although all the adult family members had an open invitation to attend, Elsa, Jacob and Sarah were the most regular attendees, with Ben sometimes being absent due to his work which took him abroad for long periods. Beth attends least often, living furthest away and having less direct input into her mother's care.

### Education and information giving

The family had no experience of psychosis prior to Elsa's first episode. At that time, they thought it was a combination of hormonal problems and concern for Ben, who happened to be abroad. Elsa's first admission was described by the family as 'a major shock' and they were increasingly alarmed by her continuing symptoms. Although the family had picked up information regarding the diagnosis, they were confused by a majority of the literature, which they felt focused on psychosis in younger people with limited social networks. The family also divulged that they had taken over household tasks previously carried out by Elsa as a way of 'taking the pressure off . . .'. In this discussion Elsa expressed anger at being seen as 'incompetent', and a desire to reclaim her role as a mother and grandmother. The family had specific questions regarding Elsa's medication, given she was on a combination of drugs. This led to a formal session to give an explanation of medication and side effects.

### Enhancing communication

Whilst the family were polite and respectful, it was clear that Elsa was used to Jacob talking on her behalf. This was challenged by both asking Jacob to verify with Elsa that she agreed with what he was reporting and asking Elsa to talk for herself. When Elsa did speak it was often in contradiction to what Jacob reported. It was evident that Elsa's paranoid thinking revolved around Jacob. Eventually Elsa admitted that her auditory hallucinations included Jacob's voice telling her she was going to be poisoned and that he hated her. This had become worse since Jacob had given up work to care for Elsa.

### Problem solving

Throughout the interventions, several issues were 'problem solved':

#### 1 Elsa increasing medication and using relaxation tapes when suffering an exacerbation of symptoms

This was felt to be the best solution to the immediate crisis facing the family. The normal pattern of management would have been for Jacob to assume responsibility for medication and Elsa to have become more paranoid. It was agreed that Ben could prompt Elsa and that Elsa could contact the family workers if needed.

#### 2 Jacob having a 'holiday from care'

Sarah and Ben's concern for Jacob's health led to several weekends where he would spend time at Sarah's house, while Ben and Elsa stayed at the family home. Following these 'holidays', Elsa became more able to recognise the hallucinations that adopted Jacob's voice. Sarah also found these weekends beneficial as she was spending more time in her own family home, and Jacob assisted with her own children.

#### 3 Elsa cooking the Sabbath meal

As Elsa stabilised she expressed frustration at the loss of her own role of caring for her family. The Sabbath meal assumed a major importance for her and several weeks were devoted to re-skilling Elsa to be able to shop for and prepare this meal.

#### 4 Elsa and Jacob being 'normal grandparents'

As Elsa stabilised, both she and Jacob reflected on their losses as a result of Elsa's psychosis. The biggest loss was the stopping of weekend visits from the grandchildren as Sarah and Beth viewed this as too much of a burden for them. This belief was challenged. Elsa had always managed to control her psychosis in the presence of her grandchildren and their visits were viewed as valuable to both Elsa and Jacob. A period of trial visits was arranged, beginning with Jacob's birthday and increasing to a regular event.

### Early warning signs and early family management

Towards the end of the eighteen months, Elsa and her family were concerned that she was 'due for another relapse'. An early warning signs interview was conducted, and the family was then asked to rehearse what they would do in the event of these signs emerging.

### Resolution

At the end of the eighteen months, Elsa had stabilised to the extent that she was able to control her symptoms. Both she and her family were very anxious not to lose contact with the family workers. It was agreed that the interventions would stop for six months and be reviewed. In addition, the family workers would ring Elsa on a monthly basis to 'check in' regarding her early warning signs. This was done and Elsa did report one occasion when she felt vulnerable, but managed this with a temporary increase in medication.

### Conclusion

It would be wrong to give the impression of a smooth process through the steps outlined above. Both workers and the family allowed themselves to take calculated risks in order to change the pattern of Elsa's psychosis and treatment. At times throughout the interventions it seemed that these risks had not resulted in positive outcomes, such as Jacob's anxiety when asked to allow Elsa to shop without him, and Elsa's subsequent panic when faced with the reality of shopping alone for the first time in five years. In these situations it became necessary to slow the process of change and reduce the anxiety elicited by change. Elsa did have a short readmission twelve months after the completion of interventions. This admission was not under the Mental Health Act, as previously, nor was it preceded by violence towards Jacob, as had also been a previous pattern. The family did evaluate the interventions as very helpful, with positive health gains for family members other than Elsa, and particularly in relation to Jacob's identified health needs.

Within all meta-analyses of family interventions, assumptions are often made regarding comparability which are, in my opinion, questionable. Early research following from EE concerned itself with specific models of intervention, with the differences outlined above, but recent meta-analysis has tended to amalgamate these subtly different interventions together. Many studies have also been rejected due to methodological issues. This has been a common feature in meta-analysis and leads to the worry that a great deal of the research is scientifically weak. As a consequence, whilst we are right to be cautious regarding the evidence base of psychosocial family interventions, this should be seen as sometimes telling us more about the research than the intervention.

## IMPLICATIONS FOR CPNs

Many CPNs (community psychiatric nurses) support carers with skill and dedication. The issue for services with regard to widening the support for carers, as indicated in the National Service Framework, is whether we should be offering psychosocial (or indeed systemic) family intervention within generic teams or have specialist services dedicated to their delivery. The simple answer to this seems to be that we should have some form of identified specialism, as the model outlined above goes beyond that of generic working with carers. This specialist service could be provided either by a team of family workers or by individual community workers with dedicated time allocated for the interventions. Both these models exist. Avon and Wiltshire Mental Health Trust operates a Family Work for Schizophrenia Service for the whole trust, co-ordinated by Nurse Consultant Gina Smith (Department of Health 2000). Other areas have community mental health workers who have time allocated to providing family interventions whilst also working in a generic manner with other clients. Within both these service types, however, there is a realisation that the personnel need specialist training in family interventions in order to provide the services.

Providing the level of support needed for carers who are having major problems dealing with the presence of psychosis should not, therefore, be seen as a generic activity in the same way that providing open and accessible services to all carers should be. If we are to assist the population of carers who we know struggle, separate provision must be made within services to support CPN work. Many CPNs have the skill and ability to provide this service with the relevant training and support.

## CONCLUSION

In this chapter we have explored the common aspects of psychosocial family interventions. Community psychiatric nurses are key in assisting carers to support service users, and often work within their generic services to good effect. There are a number of carers who will struggle with the caring role and who will need further assistance. For this population of carers, specialist services should be provided, as they have specific needs. Psychosocial family interventions seem to be effective in assisting these carers, and community psychiatric nurses are well placed, given the proper training and service structure, to provide this support.

## REFERENCES

Brennan, G. and Gamble, C. (1997) 'Schizophrenia family work and clinical practice', *Mental Health Nursing*, 17 (4): 12–15.

Burbach, F.R. (1996) 'Family based interventions in psychosis: an overview of and comparison between family therapy and family management approaches', *Journal of Mental Health*, 5 (2): 111–134.

De Jesus Mari, J. and Streiner, D. (1994) 'An overview of family interventions and relapse on schizophrenia: meta-analysis of research findings', *Psychological Medicine*, 24: 565–578.

Department of Health (1999) *National service framework for mental health: modern standards and service models*, London: Department of Health.

Department of Health (2000) *NHS Beacon learning handbook: spreading good practice across the NHS*, London: Department of Health.

Fadden, G. (1998) 'Family interventions', in Brooker, C. and Repper, J. (eds) *Serious mental health problems in the community: policy, practice and research*, London: Baillière Tindall.

Falloon, I.R.H. (1995) *Family management of schizophrenia*, Baltimore: Johns Hopkins University Press.

Falloon, I.R.H. and Graham-Hole, V. (1994) *Comprehensive management of mental disorders*, Buckingham: Buckingham Mental Health Services.

Gamble, C. and Brennan, G. (1997) 'Working with informal carers and families of schizophrenia sufferers', in Thomas, B., Hardy, S. and Cutting, P. (eds) *Stuart and Sundeen's mental health nursing: principles and practice*, London: Mosby.

Hogman, G . and Pearson, G. (1995) *The silent partners: the needs and experiences of people who care for people with a severe mental illness*, London: National Schizophrenia Fellowship.

Kuipers, L., Leff, J. and Lam, D. (1992) *Family work for schizophrenia: a practical guide*, London: Gaskell.

Pharoah, F.M., Mari, J.J. and Streiner, D. (2002) *Family interventions for schizophrenia* (Cochrane review), in The Cochrane Library, Issue 1, Oxford: Update Software.

# FURTHER READING

Burbach, F.R. (1996) 'Family based interventions in psychosis: an overview of and comparison between family therapy and family management approaches', *Journal of Mental Health*, 5 (2): 111–134.
This article gives a comprehensive comparison of systemic and family work with regard to history, research and possible collaboration to further improve understanding.

Fadden, G. (1998) 'Family interventions', in Brooker, C. and Repper, J. (eds) *Serious mental health problems in the community: policy, practice and research*, London: Baillière Tindall.
This chapter gives a good insight into the research base and provides an in-depth analysis of the provision of family work in clinical practice.

Gamble, C. and Brennan, G. (1997) 'Working with informal carers and families of schizophrenia sufferers', in Thomas, B., Hardy, S. and Cutting, P. (eds) *Stuart and Sundeen's mental health nursing: principles and practice*, London: Mosby.
T his chapter gives a major overview of EE and family work, including an in-depth analysis of early research.

# CHAPTER 20

# COGNITIVE BEHAVIOUR THERAPY FOR PSYCHOSIS

*Norman Young*

---

## SUMMARY OF KEY POINTS

- Cognitive behaviour therapy is gaining increasing support for its use in the routine care of psychosis.

- CBT is best implemented pragmatically, and offered alongside a comprehensive range of evidence-based psychosocial interventions.

- CMHNs have an important role in helping people adjust to and recover from psychosis.

---

## INTRODUCTION

The last ten years have seen a rapid rise of interest in the cognitive psychology of psychosis and consequently the application of cognitive behaviour therapy (CBT) in its treatment. The evidence supporting the use of this psychological therapy over others is growing. However, its application and effectiveness in routine care remain uncertain.

There is a long history to the development of cognitive and behavioural therapies. A landmark publication was Aaron T. Beck's *Cognitive therapy for depression* and subsequent treatment manual for anxiety disorders and phobias (Beck *et al.* 1979, Beck and Emery 1985). Now CBT for the treatment of anxiety disorders and depression has become firmly established. What has been responsible for the success and appeal of this psychological approach has been the allied rapid growth of cognitive psychology (Eysenck and Keene 2000), the openness of

CBT's theoretical basis to empirical testing, and exposure of the therapy to randomised controlled trials.

There are now a number of excellent CBT training manuals for psychosis and these should be referred to for a comprehensive account of the application of the therapy (see 'Further reading' at the end of this chapter). This chapter will provide an overview of CBT for psychosis, one that provides a quick reference guide and addresses some of the difficulties and dilemmas particular to community mental health nurses (CMHNs).

## CONCEPTUALISING PSYCHOSIS

In order to understand why the techniques used in CBT work, it is necessary to touch on the foundations of cognitive psychology, in particular the important interdependent roles that attention and emotion play.

Our appreciation of the mind is highly dependent on the comparisons made with the way that computers work (although such an analogy is more contentious when applied to emotions). People draw together and process various types of information in order to construct a personal understanding of the world. Because the world conforms to fairly constant physical and social rules we are able to construct schemas; these are ways of processing information bound to a fixed set of conventions. This allows many everyday tasks to be anticipated and therefore processed automatically, with little attention. This is a very useful skill and ultimately enables complex tasks to be carried out simultaneously – for example, driving a car while listening to the radio or functioning in social situations.

Schema theory has been used to account for emotional states, in particular anxiety and depression. It is proposed that dysfunctional schemas are formed during our development and lie dormant until activated by a significant life event (Beck and Clark 1988). Once activated they produce biases in the way that the person views the world (a cognitive bias).

In cognitive therapy the term 'schema' is used interchangeably with the notion of a 'core belief' people have about themselves, for example 'I'm worthless'. Such core beliefs are not freely available to the person's consciousness and must be 'uncovered'. This is achieved through a process of guided discovery where the therapist helps the person become aware of their automatic thoughts and assumptions, which arise from their core belief. Williams *et al.* (1997), whilst recognising the role of schemas in processing information, have found attention biases in people who are anxious and depressed. Depressed people process information with a tendency to interpret events negatively and recall more negative past events. People who are anxious not only possess a bias to interpret ambiguous events as threatening but also have an attention bias to threatening stimuli. This remains an interesting area of research, which clinically means that CBT may benefit by focusing on the client's skills in processing information rather than solely on the beliefs they hold.

The same research approach has been adopted for those with psychosis, and a number of cognitive differences have been found to exist between those who have been diagnosed with schizophrenia and those who have not (Garety and

Freeman 1999). These differences can be separated into two groups: cognitive deficits and cognitive biases (Box 20.1). Cognitive deficits are more closely linked to physiological changes associated with negative symptoms and may benefit from cognitive remediation therapy (Wykes and Van der Gaag 2001). Cognitive biases can be transitory and more closely linked to a person's degree of distress and stress.

As yet there appears to be no clear psychological explanation for these observations. However, Garety and Freeman (1999) direct therapy to focus first on halting the client's tendency to jump to conclusions, and then on developing skills in generating alternative explanations for other people's actions or events. Beck's cognitive therapy utilises such an approach in developing and maintaining functional schemas.

Cognitive behaviour therapy encourages clients to process material that is not consistent with their automatic thoughts and mood. As a result, mood changes and greater flexibility in the interpretation of events are achieved. Additionally it forces clients to practise attention-focusing skills. When applied to psychosis the therapy has proven itself effective in reducing symptomatology and relapse; it can help improve social functioning, insight and medication adherence (National Institute for Clinical Excellence (NICE) 2002).

Despite modest but encouraging results there remains a need for longer prospective studies alongside trials that examine the effectiveness of the therapy in routine care. Additionally the finding that CBT is particularly useful in patients with treatment-resistant symptoms will encourage research into the synergistic effects of cognitive remediation therapy and CBT (research into this area is currently being conducted by Til Wykes's team at the Institute of Psychiatry, King's College London).

---

**Box 20.1   Changes in cognition in psychosis**

Cognitive deficits

*   People diagnosed with schizophrenia have difficulty in maintaining and directing their attention.
*   Some of those diagnosed with schizophrenia find it difficult to understand how other people view the world.

Cognitive biases

*   People who are defined as paranoid tend to see negative events as being caused by other people.
*   People who are classified as deluded are often more likely to jump to conclusions.
*   Some people who hear voices are more likely to attribute inner speech to another person.

The following sections will provide an overview of the key elements of CBT for psychosis, starting with the need to adopt a bio-psychosocial model explaining the development and maintenance of psychosis.

## STRESS AND VULNERABILITY

The stress vulnerability model has been one of the most important developments in our understanding of mental ill-health. Zubin and Spring's (1977) seminal paper, and its later development by Neuchterlein and Subotnik (1998), gives us a framework with which to develop a formulation of the causes and maintenance of a person's mental illness.

The model simply proposes that the development of psychosis is derived from an interaction between our genetic inheritance and our environmental experiences. Our genetics determine many characteristics, for which our ability to discriminate and process information is important for psychosis. Environmentally, having experiences that allow us to construct a good sense of self-identity, efficacy and worth is important in maintaining good mental well-being. By the time we reach adolescence we have matured to a point where we will have developed a personal vulnerability to psychosis, one which has a threshold, which once passed gives rise to psychosis.

What causes this threshold to be crossed is usually a critical event such as personal injury, a period of substance use, or physical illness, but typically a stressful life incident. Because we all come to an individual threshold, no one incident will affect two people in the same way. Figure 20.1 illustrates this concept for two people, Mark and Phillip. Each possesses an individual vulnerability curve; for each there is a threshold, which, once passed, dramatically increases the risk of developing psychosis.

Looking at the graph we can see that at stress level A Mark is at significant risk of developing psychosis compared to Phillip's small risk. Although there is still a slim chance that Phillip will develop psychosis, this is far more likely at stress level B.

Once psychosis has developed it can follow a variety of courses, including remission, a relapsing course or continuance of psychosis. The course a person follows will be predicted by the interaction between the degree of recovery from the first episode and the stressful psychosocial factors that surround them. Overall the experience of psychosis can be considered toxic, and in effect shifts the person's curve to the left, making them more susceptible to life's stresses and future relapses.

## THE CONTEXT OF THERAPY

Typically, CMHNs work with people who have seemingly intractable problems which result from the interaction between a multitude of difficulties, which may include poverty, social isolation, disability, victimisation, substance use, and poor mental and physical health (see Keene 2001 for an overview of clients with complex needs).

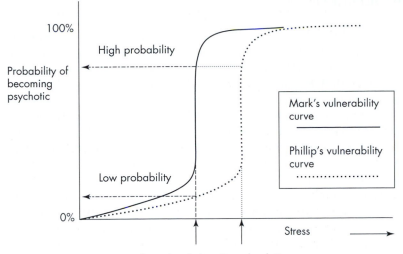

*Figure 20.1*  Stress vulnerability

In order to work effectively with clients, CMHNs need to adopt a holistic and pragmatic approach that is sensitive to their clients' fluctuating and interacting needs. They must be able to frequently re-evaluate the work they are engaging in with their clients, and be prepared to suspend one area of work to focus on another. Such pragmatism is also required in the application of cognitive behavioural therapy (see Box 20.2 for an overview), where it may be necessary to dip into and out of therapy according to the priority of the client's concerns.

This is the real world of routine care, one in which CMHNs not only need to be skilled in CBT but need to have expertise in integrating and applying therapy across a wide range of settings and against competing demands. This expertise differentiates the community mental health nurse from the cognitive behavioural therapist.

---

**Box 20.2   Overview of CBT for psychosis**

- Engagement
- Cognitive behavioural assessment
- Socialisation into therapy and the development of a shared understanding of psychosis
- Strengthening existing positive coping strategies and reducing social stigma
- Anticipating the impact of developing alternative explanations of psychotic experiences
- Detailing the evidence that supports the person's beliefs
- Developing alternative explanations, historically and in the present
- Creating new experiences that strengthen new beliefs and self-esteem
- Promoting recovery and relapse minimisation

# ENGAGEMENT

Engagement is gaining a client's involvement in a collaborative relationship with the aim of perusing the client's goals. Like all working relationships this is built on trust and purpose. CMHNs can facilitate the process of gaining trust by using the interpersonal skills of openness, a non-judgemental approach, self-disclosure and active listening. Important to this whole process is the use of a common language with an agreed way of describing and framing problems and experiences. Identifying and focusing on the client's key concerns, a willingness to offer practical help, and explaining your role can all complement the process of engagement.

This latter point raises the issue of the purpose of the relationship. Not everyone wants someone to call on them week after week without it making sense to them. This is the key to engagement and is discovered by identifying the client's goals and even aspirations. However, one must be mindful that at times clients' goals might be viewed as unrealistic, or against the morals of society. It is essential that the CMHN understands their own motives and goals for engaging with clients, and is prepared to adapt their approach along a continuum of styles which range from coercion through persuasion to collaboration.

The priorities for clients in the community often start at the level of social functioning with the improvement of their social network, finances and housing. As progress is being made on this it will be possible to introduce other areas of work, in particular, goals that relate to the person's voices or unusual beliefs. For the client these typically take the form of reducing distress, trying to act on the belief or instructions, encouraging the experience, or finding meaning in the experience.

CMHNs will be comfortable with the reduction of distress and the search for meaning; however, it is more difficult to help reconcile grandiose aims such as flying out to the United States of America to fight Mike Tyson because the client believes that they are the best boxer in the world. At these times it is necessary to demonstrate a willingness to discuss the person's aspirations in order later to develop a deeper understanding of the meaning attached to this goal. However, one cannot work outside one's public responsibilities. Therefore, managing the tension between the suspension of one's own beliefs and the sharing of them with the client is a major skill. One's honesty in the relationship will work as a currency in obtaining trust over the long term. It will also set clear boundaries, promote consistency, help identify areas on which to agree to disagree, and promote the opportunity to offer cognitive behavioural therapy.

# ASSESSMENT

The purpose of assessment is to enable a formulation. A formulation is a conceptualisation of a client's situation; it is a way of drawing links between the factors in the client's past and present, and ultimately will help map out the maintaining factors for particular problems. Working together on a formulation is a good way of coming to a shared understanding of the person's psychotic experience, and this will be dealt with shortly; in order to do this the CMHN needs to ask questions that elicit specific information about the client.

Assessment is not a static process, and whilst a great deal of information may be acquired from the initial assessment, the questioning style will need to be re-employed throughout one's work with the client. Initially a comprehensive account of the person's circumstances will be sought through interview and recourse to their personal history, from which one will identify factors that led to them developing a psychotic illness.

Cognitive behavioural assessments ask questions that inform the ABC approach to functional analysis (Richards and McDonald 1990, Fox and Conroy 2000). From the start the interviewer is interested in taking a problem, one identified by the client, and focusing in on it. Functional analysis takes a view that behaviour cannot be seen in isolation but is triggered and maintained by other events. So following the question 'What is the main problem?' we are interested in what makes the problem worse or better. The problem can be further examined by using the other four Ws of questioning; after this the impact of the problem can be assessed (an overview and prompt card for this are given in Box 20.3).

Next the problem needs to be narrowed from the broad to the specific. This can be achieved by highlighting an incident that has occurred in the past week or month. Ask your client to detail what was going through their mind, how they felt, and how they behaved before, during and after the event. This questioning will elicit triggers for the experience, the person's strengths, and what the person finds supportive.

---

**Box 20.3   Overview of problem assessment**

*Problem*

What is the main problem? What makes it worse? What makes it better?

Where is the problem worse? Where is the problem better?

When is the problem worse? Better?

With whom is the problem worse? Better?

Why do you think you have this problem?

*Impact*

Avoidance: What do you find yourself doing less of because of this problem?

Behavioural increasers: What do you find yourself doing more of because of this problem?

Frequency: How often have you experienced this over the last month, week, day?

Intensity: On a zero to eight scale, where eight is the most intense it has been, where would you say this feeling lies?

Duration: How long is it before the problem goes away?

Occurrence: Are there particular instances when it occurs?

*Explore a specific event*

Looking at a time over the last month/week, I'd like to look at an incident in more detail.

A. Activating event: Tell me what was going on before you had the problem?
   a. Affect:        How did you feel, what sensations did you experience?
   b. Behaviour:     What were you doing or did you do?
   c. Cognitive:     Thoughts/images/voices

B. Behaviour:        Tell me what happened next?
   a. Affect:        How did you feel, what sensations did you experience?
   b. Behaviour:     What were you doing or did you do?
   c. Cognitive:     Thoughts/images/voices

C. Consequences:     Tell me what happened next?
   a. Affect:        How did you feel, what sensations did you experience?
   b. Behaviour:     What were you doing or did you do?
   c. Cognitive:     Thoughts/images/voices

*Course*

Over the time that you have had this problem has it got any worse? Has it been better? Is there anything you have found that leaves you feeling better?

The application of functional analysis to the assessment of voices and beliefs is one that can be quite demanding for clients and will place significant strain on the rapport one has developed and the sensible pacing of sessions. Chadwick *et al.* (1996) provide a detailed account of the process, and usefully include a functional assessment interview for voices alongside their 'Beliefs about Voices' questionnaire, which has now been revised (Chadwick *et al.* 2000).

As with all CBT work, the process of ongoing assessment is vital. The rationale for further assessment needs to be valued by the client and serves to deepen the understanding of their situation. Self-monitoring is an important process here and can be achieved through various strategies (see Box 20.4). The client can provide an account of the frequency and nature of their voices or preoccupation with a particular line of thinking. The ABC model can be applied to diaries as an invaluable way for the clinician to gain further information about symptoms, and furthermore socialise the client into the CBT process by framing their experiences within the stress vulnerability model of psychosis.

Box 20.4  Ongoing monitoring

This can be achieved through diaries, taping, or the use of pictures. Monitoring usefully starts when the person notices that they become emotionally uncomfortable (anxiety, low mood or anger), or encounter a distinct event, e.g. hear a voice.

Focus on capturing:

- events (triggers) that precipitated the voice or discomfort
- the person's interpretation of triggers
- the identity of the voice
- the power of the voice over them
- the strength of conviction in a belief
- frequency of the voice or discomfort
- what occurred after the voice or discomfort
- what the person does to encourage or reduce the voice or discomfort

## DEVELOPING A SHARED FORMULATION OF THE PSYCHOTIC EXPERIENCE

As clinicians we use information gleaned from our assessments to develop a formulation of a client's situation; from this we hypothesise links and consider areas to focus on. In routine care the pace of work often sacrifices any depth to this process. However, the stress vulnerability model provides a template on which to hang our assessment.

Continuing with the example of Mark (Box 20.5), who believed that he was being followed and would ultimately be attacked, using the key factors of precipitating, maintaining, vulnerability and protective factors it is possible to draw a Mind Map® (Figure 20.2) which produces an overview or formulation of Mark's main problem. From this we can draw links between factors and suggest areas to work on. (Mind Maps® are a visual thinking tool created by Tony Buzan (2000.)

It is invaluable, although not always possible, to work on a formulation with the client, and for them to have to keep the copy. Initially it is useful to adopt a naïve approach to their problem and look at their view of it. Through careful exploration it will be possible to map out a functional model of their distress and from this an opportunity may appear. This could prove to be an area where the client expresses a degree of uncertainty or where they are keen to reduce the impact of the problem. At this point it will be possible to extend their construction of the problem by introducing concepts of stress, vulnerability and mental ill health. This will need to be done tentatively and with attention to the possible impact of such a reformulation.

## Box 20.5   Vulnerability

Growing up, Mark had a normal development with no major illnesses. He enjoyed school and made friends; however, home life was difficult because of unemployment and hardship. His mother and father both have depression and his grandmother has been diagnosed with schizophrenia. He is one of three boys and two girls all living in the same four-bedroomed house in a socially deprived ex-mining village.

### Stress A

Mark was 18 years old when he was caught for a second time driving without insurance and tax. He was sentenced to three months' community service, fined £200 and banned from driving for a year. Mark had been saving for his own car and much of his social life revolves around driving.

### Manifestation

Following the conviction Mark began to withdraw and over the next six months increasingly became suspicious about people he passed on the street. He noticed that people looked at him when he passed them and on one occasion he felt sure that someone said 'that's him'. Mark's parents became increasingly worried and asked the GP to see Mark; the GP referred him on to the community mental health team.

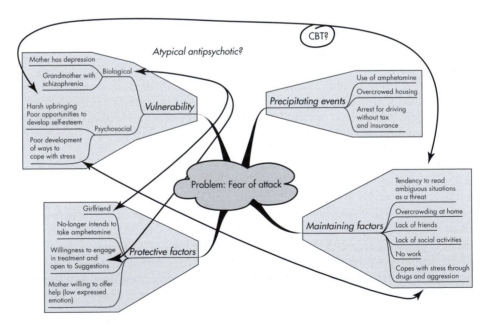

*Figure 20.2* The development of an ongoing formulation using Mind Maps ®

## SOCIALISING THE CLIENT TO THE COGNITIVE BEHAVIOURAL MODEL OF PSYCHOSIS

One problem faced by clinicians working with people who are psychotic is in explaining what CBT entails and why they should engage in its demands. Clients value the interest and opportunity in telling someone about their predicament, but when this is moved on to looking at alternatives to explain events this may be seen as argument or rejection. First and foremost one must come to a common understanding that one's role is to reduce distress and social exclusion. Focusing in on the formulation and drawing connections between events can highlight these areas.

Psycho-education forms a vital part of the initial phases of CBT. This is not a lecturing process, and does not mean telling the person that they have schizophrenia. Psycho-education is achieved through the use of metaphor and analogy in the integration of cognitive behavioural theory into the initial formulation. Early on it is useful to ask the client to explain what they would feel, think and do if they heard the sound of glass smashing outside their window late at night. The scenario can be developed through the use of guided discovery (asking questions that lead the person to certain foreseen conclusions). In this example one would ask questions that elicit various explanations for the noise. These could then be developed to define different consequences in affect and action. The conclusion we are after is that thinking something does not necessarily mean that it is true, and what we base truth on is evidence, of which there are many kinds. The success of CBT is dependent on the client buying into this and demonstrating flexibility in their interpretation of events.

## PROMOTING THE PERSON'S STRENGTHS, ASPIRATIONS AND CURRENT WAYS OF COPING

Clients possess strengths, which can often be applied to overcome their problems. For Mark it was his interest and motivation to drive again; he could use this interest as a goal, which would not only serve as an aspiration but be a source of distraction from his preoccupation with people outside his home. People with psychosis often employ a number of ways of coping with voices or distress. It is helpful to ask about these and look to whether they can be applied to other problems (one client informed me that he coped with voices by hoovering with a loud vacuum cleaner, which also helped reduce the number of critical comments from his family). This way of working shares much with the strengths approach to case management (Kanter 1989), and not only facilitates the process of engagement but also helps discover functional aspects of the person rather than focusing on problems.

Because some clients cannot entertain contradictions to their experiences it may be possible to work on the level that says you are there to help them manage the distress caused by their persecution. This will focus on practical ways of coping (see Box 20.6) which the client can assimilate into their existing beliefs. In using this approach the person can still be socialised into the CBT model of managing distress, and strategies can be employed that tackle the person's attention and interpretations whilst side-stepping the causes of their distress. Of course, if successful, it may provide an opportunity at a later time to discuss why it should have worked.

---

**Box 20.6   Coping strategies for voices or paranoia**

- Earplug in one or both ears
- Speaking over the voices
- Focusing on the sound of the voice rather than the content
- Telling the voices to go away
- Scheduling the voices
- Distraction (walkman)
- Exercise
- Relaxation or scheduling enjoyable events
- Asking for other people's views on situations
- Using flash cards with positive statements

---

# EXPLORING DIFFERING VIEWPOINTS ON EVENTS

If the client displays a readiness to see that how they interpret events is important to how they feel and act, then therapy can move on. It is now useful to engender self-awareness in the client. We know from experimental work that they will experience cognitive biases and deficits. Through our knowledge of the client, and the use of guided discovery, clients can be offered the hypothesis that they are more likely to jump to conclusions or have certain styles of thinking which lead to or support the beliefs they hold. Following such an awareness, clients can be asked if they would wish to work with you on making better judgements in order to manage their distress, improve their self-esteem or come to a deeper understanding of their situation.

Returning to the example of Mark. His feelings of anxiety left him hypervigilant, which, through guided discovery, he understood as a factor that led to him jumping to conclusions more readily. Mark was prepared to test his hypervigilance out through homework. It is desirable to engender a strong rationale and motivation for homework with the client, and this can be helped by constantly reformulating the person's main concern by using a Mind Map®. Through a thought diary Mark was able to identify an assumption he held, 'if someone stares at me then they're in on it'. This assumption was put into the developing formulation and linked to the headings of thoughts, feelings and actions, under the subheading assumptions.

Once a degree of awareness of styles of thinking, and attention to events that confirm this style, has been attained, then it may be possible to train the person to adopt a more objective stance to events. The person is encouraged to generate alternative explanations for events, and by doing so will halt their automatic processes, and distance themselves from their automatic thoughts. This standing back from thoughts reduces the emotional salience attached to them; the person can then move their attention to other explanations for events and weigh up or even test the evidence associated with each explanation. Finally a compromise between the explanations can be made. The continuance of this work outside of therapy sessions will lead to the person turning their mind to an alternative understanding of their experiences.

One concern raised about challenging a person's beliefs is that they in some way serve to protect their self-esteem. The evidence for this is not conclusive but for some individuals this may be true. However, it is always sensible to work out the possible implications of therapy through one's formulation and by asking hypothetical questions in advance.

When increasing flexibility in thinking through generating alternatives, each alternative will have a deeper meaning. So if Mark adopts the view that someone staring at him may mean they think he looks attractive, this will reduce his conviction in the belief that he is being persecuted. Before we develop alternatives we will have checked out what were his reasons for his persecution, for they may be because he sees himself as special and is therefore compensating for a (hypothesised) low self-esteem. If this were the case, therapy would look to addressing self-esteem early on and move tentatively forward.

## SUMMARY

Individual cognitive behavioural therapy for psychosis is at an early stage of development, but is now mature enough for CMHNs to consider learning and applying the techniques. Integrating psychological therapies for people with psychosis is difficult because of the complex and interacting needs that they have. CMHNs therefore need to appreciate and develop skills in case management, social care, family interventions, and psychopharmacology, which will enable them to remain engaged with the clients as the focus of work changes (as discussed in other chapters in this book).

The integration of cognitive behavioural therapy into routine care is a key area of research. An important question is whether CBT in routine care can adhere to the formats found in experimental research and so improve quality of life and demonstrate itself a worthy addition to routine care. In addressing this and similar questions, nursing can draw on its strong qualitative tradition to investigate what part CBT plays in people's recovery from psychosis. For many, recovery is not a road to the abolishment of symptoms but adjustment to them.

# REFERENCES

Beck, A.T. and Clark, D.A. (1988) 'Anxiety and depression: an information processing approach', *Anxiety Research*, 1: 23–36.

Beck, A.T. and Emery, G. (1985) *Anxiety disorders and phobias*, New York: Basic Books.

Beck, A.T., Rush, A.T., Shaw, B.F. and Emery, G. (1979) *Cognitive therapy for depression*, New York: Guilford Press.

Buzan, T. (2000) *Use your head*, London: BBC Consumer Publishing.

Chadwick, P., Birchwood, M. and Trower, P. (1996) *Cognitive therapy for hallucinations, delusions and paranoia*, Chichester: Wiley.

Chadwick, P., Lees, S. and Birchwood, M. (2000) 'The revised Beliefs About Voices Questionnaire (BAVQ-R)', *British Journal of Psychiatry*, 177: 229–232.

Eysenck, M.W. and Keene, M.T. (2000) *Cognitive psychology: a student's handbook*, 4th edn, Hove, Sussex: Psychology Press.

Fox, J. and Conroy, P. (2000) 'Assessing clients' needs: the semi-structured interview', in Gamble, C. and Brennan, G. (eds) *Working with serious mental illness: a manual for clinical practice*, London: Baillière Tindall.

Garety, P. and Freeman, D. (1999) 'Cognitive approaches to delusions: a critical review of theories and evidence', *British Journal of Clinical Psychology*, 38: 113–154.

Kanter, J. (1989) 'Clinical case management: definition, principles, components', *Hospital and Community Psychiatry*, 40 (4): 361–368.

Keene, J. (2001) *Clients with complex needs: interprofessional practice*, Oxford: Blackwell Science.

National Institute for Clinical Excellence (NICE) (2002) *Schizophrenia: core interventions in the treatment and management of schizophrenia in primary and secondary care, National Clinical Practice Guideline Number 1, Second consultation*, London: NICE/National Collaborating Centre for Mental Health.

Neuchterlein, K.H. and Subotnik, K.L. (1998) 'The cognitive origins of schizophrenia and prospects for intervention', in Wykes, T., Tarrier, N. and Lewis, S. (eds) *Outcome and innovation in psychological treatment of schizophrenia*, Chichester: Wiley.

Richards, D. and McDonald, B. (1990) *Behavioural psychotherapy: a pocket book for nurses*, Oxford: Heinemann.

Williams, J.M.G., Watts, F.N., Macleod, C.M. and Mathews, A. (1997) *Cognitive psychology and emotional disorders*, Chichester: Wiley.

Wykes, T., and Van der Gaag, M. (2001) 'Is it time to develop a new cognitive therapy for psychosis – cognitive remediation therapy (CRT)?' *Clinical Psychology Review*, 21 (8): 1227–1256.

Zubin, J. and Spring, B. (1977) 'Vulnerability – a new view of schizophrenia', *Journal of Abnormal Psychology*, 86: 103–126.

# FURTHER READING

British Psychological Society (2000) *Recent advances in understanding mental illness and psychotic experiences*, Leicester: British Psychological Society.
This publication draws together many of the leading psychologists in this field to produce a balanced overview of the present knowledge base for psychosis. This is a very good introduction to psychosis. Also available at the BPS website: http://www.bps.org.uk

Fowler, P., Garety, P. and Kuipers, L. (1995) *Cognitive behaviour therapy for psychosis, a clinical handbook*, Chichester: Wiley.
This book is part of an excellent series published by Wiley throughout the 1990s. It guides the practitioner through a logical progression of steps and hence provides one of the clearest 'manual' approaches.

Gamble, C. and Brennan, G. (eds) (2000) *Working with serious mental illness: a manual for clinical practice*, London: Baillière Tindall.
A comprehensive resource for practitioners in mental health, which contains an excellent chapter on CBT for psychosis by Jem Mills.

# CHAPTER 21

# RELAPSE PREVENTION IN PSYCHOSIS

*Michael Coffey*

---

## SUMMARY OF KEY POINTS

- Mental health service users frequently self-manage their own illnesses to prevent relapse.

- There is sufficient research to support CMHNs engaging in relapse planning with service users to promote greater self-efficacy and control.

- Relapse planning should form one element of personal recovery from mental illness and CMHNs can help facilitate this.

---

## INTRODUCTION

Relapse in psychosis is not inevitable. Relapse prevention is not only possible, it is a daily fact of life for many service users engaged in recovery from mental illness. Relapse prevention embodies a number of overlapping concepts such as symptom self-management, crisis plans/cards, self-advocacy and living wills. From a professional standpoint it is informed by research evidence on early signs and relapse triggers, and it is more than anything testimony to the emergence of the service user voice in securing interventions which are individual, contextual and extend beyond prescription of antipsychotic medication. Community mental health nurses (CMHNs) have an opportunity in relapse planning with service users to positively influence the lives of those they work with, by reducing lengthy hospitalisation and limiting the devastating social consequences of relapse.

Planning for relapse is facilitated by CMHNs giving due credence to interpersonal relationships and is founded upon trust, negotiation and collaboration. It is something that service users do which CMHNs can assist them with.

To a certain extent the concept of relapse prevention as applied to serious mental illnesses such as psychosis is a misnomer. The term is evident within the addictions literature (Annis 1986) and is used widely in a number of health-related arenas as well as in forensic work with offenders (Laws 1989). It may even be criticised for perpetuating a belief that relapse is completely avoidable, and as such can engender feelings of frustration and exasperation among both service users and those working with them. It may be wise, then, to reconsider the use of the term and adopt the more accurate title of relapse planning. This itself may be criticised for implying that relapse is inevitable, and no such implication is intended. As such the term may be viewed negatively by some service users, and terms such as symptom management and self-care agency have been used (Cutler 2001) and may be more acceptable. Whatever the phrase used, the process is essentially psycho-educational and provides an opportunity for CMHNs to provide tangible benefit to service users.

Service users are keen to know more about their illness and to have a greater say in how they are treated when ill (Garcia Maza 1996). Relapse planning has its roots in service user groups developing self-management techniques. This has been the case for a number of years and community mental health nurses have been slow to recognise its potential. According to Sutherby and Szmukler (1998) the International Self Advocacy Alliance and Survivors Speak Out launched the first crisis card in the UK in the 1980s, and this has been followed up by other organisations such as the Manic Depression Fellowship.

In constituting what this intervention might be, I am proposing that relapse is viewed as a learning opportunity and that plans for relapse are informed by lessons from previous experiences so that relapses are recognised by both service users and CMHNs and efforts are made to limit the destructive quality of them. The main aim of relapse planning is to prepare for future possibilities of relapse. This is not a new construct. Service users, as indicated, have been concerned with recognition of and planning for relapse for some time. Mental health nurses are also being drawn to considering the area; for example, Watkins (2001) conceptualises this area of work within a humanistic framework that will appeal to many in the profession.

It has been suggested that mental health nurses make efforts to align themselves with service users in offering interventions that are informed by the experience of mental illness (Department of Health 1994). Although government policy has tended to view the benefits of such efforts solely from the perspective of risk management, as evidenced in the National Service Framework (Department of Health 1999), more tangible therapeutic outcomes are clearly possible. Indeed I have been personally guilty of this emphasis on risk (Coffey and Bishop 2000). In this chapter, however, I want to avoid this obsession with risk that so undermines therapeutic intervention and instead explore the components of relapse planning, its role in recovery from psychosis and the potential role of the community mental health nurse.

# RELAPSE IN PSYCHOSIS

Relapse for the purposes of this chapter is defined as a deterioration in a person's condition which may place them in need of added support and requires steps to be taken to prevent or treat further deterioration. Theoretically relapse planning is based upon the work of Caplan (1970). The focus is on crisis resolution and the aim is to resolve current problems and help the service user to develop their coping abilities to better deal with future problems.

Relapse in psychosis appears to be preceded by subtle changes in mental functioning up to four weeks before the event (Malla and Norman 1994) and is perceived as a loss of well-being by the person. Relapse planning does not necessarily require professional involvement; indeed in the absence of professional attention service users initiate symptom monitoring and a range of responses to this monitoring (McCandless-Glincher *et al.* 1986). Service users therefore are attempting to gain control and recognise symptoms of their illness (Eckman *et al.* 1992, Meuser *et al.* 1992). So why get involved at all, you might ask. It seems that while some service users engage in symptom monitoring, many who could benefit from such techniques do not, and some of those who do may be helped to refine their coping strategies to facilitate better personal control. It should be acknowledged, however, that some service users may have no interest whatsoever in nurses interfering in their illness. Relapse prevention is no panacea nor is it a template for all interactions with all service users.

As a first step, CMHNs could start by disinvesting themselves of the gloom and pessimism that often accompanies work with people with psychosis. Watkins (2001) suggests that the missing ingredient in much mental health work is hope, and a belief in the ability of people to change and grow. Having low expectations of what service users can achieve limits the choices open to them within services. Deegan (1993) suggests that the existential challenges faced by people with mental illness who have held expectations for their lives, only to see them come to nothing, require that those who work with them should offer hope. There is now evidence that mental illnesses such as schizophrenia may not have the chronic unremitting course previously believed, and as such there are real grounds for hope (Kruger 2000). Appleby (1992), in a review of suicide and self-harm studies, found that an absence of hope or hopelessness was the most significant indicator for completed suicide. Clearly, then, hope can play an important role in the experience of mental illness and in recovery (Nunn 1996). Kirkpatrick *et al.* (2001) argue that hope is an essential turning point in recovery from mental illness but accept that little is known about how mental health professionals can instil hope. Service users' experiences of hope, what for them constitutes hope and how they value and use it may help us understand the role it plays in recovery. More importantly it may also help mental health professionals to facilitate the development of hope.

We should incorporate into our practice an awareness that the experience of living with mental illness can contribute meaningfully to the management of that illness. CMHNs should recognise that many service users with whom they work are interested in actively self-managing their condition and will want to combine this self-management with standard interventions. In this regard, then, service users should be seen as experts by experience, and CMHNs can aspire to being experts by profession (Romme and Escher 2000).

# STRESS VULNERABILITY AND EXPRESSED EMOTION

The role of stressful life events as potential triggers for relapse in psychosis is a constant feature of the literature. Zubin and Spring (1977), for example, propose a stress-vulnerability hypothesis in which individuals when encountering circumstances they find stressful may be vulnerable to relapse of their illness. The proposition is that being aware of the role of stress vulnerability in the onset of relapse can provide a means to avoid becoming ill. Expressed emotion (EE) is one source of environmental stress for people with schizophrenia within families, which appears to be amenable to intervention (Kavanagh 1992). Therapeutic efforts that address EE in families (Smith 1992) and in hostel staff (Ball *et al.* 1992) have been demonstrated to reduce relapse and need for hospital admission. It is perhaps a reflection of the complexity of working with serious mental illness that, on the one hand, social supports may buffer against certain life stresses, while, on the other, they may exacerbate them. While the concept of EE is not new, its utility in practice remains problematic. It is doubtful whether many CMHNs actually use it as a measure within practice, and where specific training has been given, mental health professionals have found difficulty incorporating into practice many of the interventions which potentially could deliver a reduction in relapse rates (Fadden 1997). EE is therefore a concept with some utility (although it is questionable whether this actually extends beyond research studies) and may be usefully considered as a factor when relapse planning. CMHNs, however, must be aware of family sensitivities when considering its use, so that the family is not blamed for the presence of the illness (Johnstone 1993). Perhaps Brennan's (see Chapter 19) emphasis on helping carers to cope with the effects of mental illness within the family may offer a route to avoiding blame.

Johnstone (1993), despite strong rebuttals (Leff and Vaughn 1994), has highlighted a number of valid concerns about assertions made in regard to relapse prevention in schizophrenia family work. These largely centre upon the supposed prophylactic properties of antipsychotic medication. Antipsychotic medication has demonstrated its value in the treatment of acute schizophrenic episodes and the prevention of relapse (Wyatt 1991, Kane 1996). Although neuroleptics control symptoms in up to 80 per cent of cases, the nature of the improvement varies considerably between individuals and in some cases the benefits are outweighed by the unpleasant and disabling side effects (Kane 1996). The prophylactic effect of medication can be limited. Relapse rates of 30 to 40 per cent within the first one to two years of treatment have been reported (Leff and Wing 1971, Johnson 1979), and later studies continued to support these findings (Schooler *et al.* 1980, Hogarty 1984). Overall there will be some 20 to 30 per cent of people who will not respond to antipsychotic medication (Anon. 1995). A considerable number of people continue to experience hallucinations and delusions with no improvement of the symptoms despite taking antipsychotics (Curson 1985). It is apparently generally accepted, following the work of Hogarty and Ulrich (1977), that medication will not prevent relapse but will instead lengthen the period between relapses. So it appears that medication has a role in relapse prevention, but this is often highly individual and may vary depending on a number of contextual factors, such as stressful life events, coping abilities and previous experiences.

The inclusion of early signs monitoring data (Birchwood *et al.* 1989) in plans aimed at managing crisis and relapse may prove useful. Essentially this involves working with the person and their family to elucidate and record the range of experiences that the individual recognises prior to relapse. In many cases these will include seemingly unrelated events – for example, disturbed sleep or recurrent arguments with others – and assistance may be required so that these are recognised as meaningful. Hamera *et al.* (1992) suggest that early identification of symptoms has the potential to avoid disease exacerbation and relapse. They propose an intervention wherein the individual is helped to recognise the symptoms they experience before onset of illness and then take action to alter these symptoms in an attempt to regulate their illness. Hamera *et al.* (1992) sought to describe the factors which individuals with schizophrenia (n=51) identified, and then sought to evaluate the stability of these factors at one-year follow-up. They found that the most frequent indicators were auditory hallucinations (n=11) and anxiety symptoms (n=9). Forty-one per cent (n=21) of the primary indicators were coded as anxiety-based, 28 per cent (n=14) as depressive and 31 per cent (n=16) as psychotic. Confidence in the indicators was high, with 73 per cent reporting that their primary indicator always occurred with relapse (sensitivity), and 60 per cent saying they did not experience relapse unless the primary indicator was present (specificity). A significant relationship existed where the individual who identified a psychotic primary indicator also tended to be more confident that the indicator occurred when getting ill. After one year, 28 of the original subjects were interviewed and 24 of these again identified a primary indicator, and of these 10 identified the same indicator again. Two further respondents gave a primary indicator in the same category. Although this suggests that the indicators do not on the whole remain stable, it may also be taken to mean that if subjects had further input and indicated more than one primary indicator, the intervention may prove clinically useful.

Relapses can be highly idiosyncratic and CMHNs should be wary of a 'one size fits all' approach to developing relapse plans. Even if this were not the case, many individuals will vary in their commitment and motivation over time, in much the same way as we all do when, for example, making new resolutions. As early signs of relapse or prodromes vary from person to person, the service user should only be measured against their own baseline (Subotnik and Neuchterlein 1988). This distinctive and individual assessment has been termed 'relapse signatures' and can be elucidated by interview to identify the changes in behaviour or thinking leading up to an episode of illness (Birchwood *et al.* 1998).

Birchwood *et al.* (1989) have developed measurement scales for recording prodromal changes. These include involving a chosen observer such as a carer who may note behavioural changes where the person loses insight or under-reports prodromal changes. It is important to note that this is not meant to imply that the service user is somehow devious in ignoring or failing to report signs of relapse, but rather an acknowledgement that relapse can be a frightening experience which may in some cases prompt denial in an individual. Service users may have unhappy experiences of previous relapse and hospitalisation, and the prospect of this recurring may motivate them to under-report concerns they have about their mental health. CMHNs should recognise this and reassure service users about the range of options available, of which hospitalisation will only be one – for example, increased formal and informal support, changes to routine to improve sleeping pattern, community respite facilities or a review of medication could all be appropriate options.

Identifying and monitoring for signs of relapse should be a shared responsibility between the CMHN, the service user and the carer. In one study where the responsibility was not shared, drop-out rates were as high as 50 per cent (Carpenter *et al.* 1990). This of course means spending real time working on relationships with service users and their support networks. Frank and Gunderson (1990) have shown that in themselves therapeutic alliances with service users have real and measurable benefit, and this should not be ignored.

---

**Box 21.1    Five fundamental principles of relapse prevention**

1    It should be based upon the individual service user's experience.
2    It should facilitate skill development and mastery.
3    It should be negotiated and collaborative.
4    It should be informed but not restricted by empirical findings.
5    It should facilitate personal control over the illness.

---

# RELAPSE PREVENTION AND THE CONCEPT OF RECOVERY

The concept of recovery within mental health is one that is only beginning to emerge in the literature within the UK (Chadwick 1997), although it has a longer tradition within the US (Deegan 1988, Anthony 1993). It is largely service user-defined and is concerned with reclaiming a sense of personhood that transcends thinking of oneself as just being mentally ill. Anthony (1993) argues that the seeds of the recovery movement were sown in the failure of mental health services to address anything other than the symptomatology needs of those with mental health problems. The multiple and often complex needs of those with serious mental illness require professionals to take account of much more than attempts at addressing symptoms. From a professional standpoint it seems that recovery has been conceptualised within a rehabilitation framework – for example, addressing the needs people have to regain and maintain a sense of independence. Rehabilitative services have tended towards a broader view of mental health, and to this end focus upon the consequences of the illness as well as treatment of it. Service users, while recognising these elements as fundamental, tend towards a more existential construct, that is, wanting to regain a sense of oneself as a valued person (Deegan 1988). Warner (1994) argues that mental health service users need to be helped to develop mastery over their condition. This means achieving personal control over one's life and personal control over one's illness as a feature of one's life. Relapse prevention can be seen as forming just one part of the person's recovery, offering this sense of control and facilitating the development of significant new skills. It is focused upon facilitating movement in how the person deals with these relapse episodes.

Recovery is also about developing new meaning and purpose; in a sense it is an epiphany in which the person starts to make sense of their experience and from it begins to build a new life for themselves. In doing so they must overcome and accommodate not just the limitations of their condition but also the consequences and strengths of that condition. Anthony (1993) is at pains to point out that recovery is not about cure or removal of symptoms, but rather that exacerbations of the person's condition may still occur. Illness forms only part of the person and is not the only way in which the person is conceived. Recovery can occur without professional help and some service users may choose such a route.

## WHAT CAN CMHNS ACTIVELY DO TO ASSIST AND SUPPORT THIS?

CMHNs need to be aware that the mental health system itself acts in ways that restrict opportunities for recovery. It does this by use of disempowering treatment practices, removing choice and exerting indiscriminate coercion. Mental health services are now so obsessed with the supposed risk posed by the mentally ill that treatment options of CMHNs are likely to narrow rather than expand (Rose 1998). Despite this, however, useful constructions of relapse within a recovery model of mental health nursing are emerging (Watkins 2001). Repper (2000), for example, suggests a clear role for the profession in facilitating recovery. Mental health nursing should, I believe, be about improving the lot of those with mental health problems and ultimately should be judged by what service users say they find helpful. Relapse planning may be that rare opportunity to offer interventions that service users want, which are evidenced-based and which are uniquely provided by CMHNs.

Mental health nurses can help service users to learn about their condition and the difficulties this presents while fostering a sense of hope that a measure of personal control is possible. It will also be necessary to assist service users to overcome the social consequences of the mental illness. In planning for potential relapses CMHNs can help service users achieve these aims. It means facilitating access to those aspects of life we might take for granted but from which the mentally ill have been excluded by virtue of their diagnosis. This will mean seeing relapse planning as one element of the person's overall recovery and offering assistance to enable the person to access suitable housing, income, education, employment and relationships. In Box 21.1, I have suggested what I see as five fundamental principles of relapse prevention in community mental health nursing, and these essentially summarise the discussion offered.

It is important to introduce an air of realism here. People can become frustrated and depressed by constant failure to prevent relapse, and it is important that the ebb and flow inherent in a recovery model is communicated at the outset. Personal accounts of recovery from mental health service users indicate that recovery is not linear and setbacks will occur. It is also clear from these accounts that service users value having someone who believes in them, who is consistent and who is gently encouraging (Deegan 1988). This may be a difficult role for CMHNs to fulfil, and the value of good-quality clinical supervision should not be underestimated, as we too can become frustrated, defensive in our therapeutic responses and unwittingly limiting in our treatment options. Repper (2000) outlines a reasonably straightforward and logical strategy for helping service users work towards gaining the wished-for control over their symptoms (Box 21.2). This should be viewed as a starting point and not an end in itself. It is an ongoing process and should be reviewed at intervals and especially after a relapse or a life event which threatens a relapse.

---

**Box 21.2   Strategies for helping manage illness**

1   Recognise the triggers of relapse.
2   Recognise the warning signs of relapse.
3   Construct an action plan to avert relapse.
4   Develop coping strategies.
5   Compile an advance directive.

(Repper 2000, p. 583)

---

# CONCLUSION

The focus on relapse, as evidenced in government mental health policy, may be on risk prevention not relapse prevention. Mental health services may see the primary rationale as being one of admission prevention. While it would be foolish to suggest that CMHNs ignore such concerns, neither emphasis should dominate the work of assisting service users with recovery. Helping service users to develop their own recoveries may ultimately lead to better risk management and prevent long admissions to hospital, but this is not the primary goal and we should try to avoid being distracted by emotive calls for safety at all costs. To do this we should develop our understanding of, and knowledge base on, relapse and its role in recovery. We need to determine what it is that helps and hinders this process and in what contexts we should seek to intervene. CMHNs may also feel they need educational preparation for such an undertaking and many courses already provide this. Transferring these approaches from education into practice may also prove to be problematic and as such we will have to strive to overcome barriers to meet the needs of service users.

# REFERENCES

Annis, H.M. (1986) 'A relapse prevention model for the treatment of alcoholics', in Miller, W.R. and Heather, N. (eds) *Treating addictive behaviours: processes of change*, New York: Plenum.

Anon. (1995) 'The drug treatment of patients with schizophrenia', *Drug and Therapeutic Bulletin*, 33: 81–86.

Anthony, W.A. (1993) 'Recovery from mental illness: the guiding vision of the mental health service system in the 1990s', *Psychosocial Rehabilitation Journal*, 16 (4): 11–23.

Appleby, L. (1992) 'Suicide in psychiatric patients: risk and prevention', *British Journal of Psychiatry*, 161: 749–758.

Ball, R.A., Moore, E. and Kuipers, L. (1992) 'Expressed emotion in community care staff. A comparison of patient outcome in a nine month follow-up of two hostels', *Social Psychiatry and Psychiatric Epidemiology*, 27 (1): 35–39.

Birchwood, M., Smith, J., MacMillan, F., Hogg, B., Prasad, R., Harvey, C. and Bering, S. (1989) 'Predicting relapse in schizophrenia: the development and implementation of an early signs monitoring system using patients and families as observers, a preliminary investigation', *Psychological Medicine*, 19: 649–656.

Birchwood, M., Smith, J., MacMillan, F. and McGovern, D. (1998) 'Early intervention in psychotic relapse', in Brooker, C. and Repper, J. (eds) *Serious mental health problems in the community: policy, practice and research*, London: Baillière Tindall.

Caplan, G. (1970) *The theory and practice of mental health consultation*, London: Tavistock.

Carpenter, W.T., Hanlon, T.E., Summerfelt, A.T., Kirkpatrick, B.M., Levine, J. and Buchanan, R.W. (1990) 'Continuous versus targeted medication in schizophrenic patients', *American Journal of Psychiatry*, 147: 1138–1148.

Chadwick, P.K. (1997) 'Recovery from psychosis: learning more from patients', *Journal of Mental Health*, 6 (6): 577–588.

Coffey, M. and Bishop, N. (2000) 'Crisis plans in forensic mental health nursing', *Mental Health Practice*, 4 (4): 22–25.

Curson, D. (1985) 'Long term depot maintenance of chronic schizophrenia outpatients', *British Journal of Psychiatry*, 146: 464–480.

Cutler, C.G. (2001) 'Self-care agency and symptom management in patients treated for mood disorder', *Archives of Psychiatric Nursing*, XV (1): 24–31.

Deegan, P. (1988) 'Recovery: the lived experience of rehabilitation', *Psychosocial Rehabilitation Journal*, 11 (4): 12–19.

Deegan, P. (1993) 'Recovering our sense of value after being labelled', *Journal of Psychosocial Nursing*, 31: 7–11.

Department of Health (1994) *Working in partnership: a collaborative approach to care. Report of the Mental Health Nursing Review Team*, London: HMSO.

Department of Health (1999) *National service framework for mental health: modern standards and service models*, London: Department of Health.

Eckman, T.A., Wirshing, W.C., Marder, S.R., Leiberman, R.P., Johnston-Cronk, K., Zimmerman, K. and Mintz, J. (1992) 'Technique for training patients in illness self-management: a controlled trial', *American Journal of Psychiatry*, 149: 1549–1555.

Fadden, G. (1997) 'Implementation of family interventions in routine clinical practice following staff training programs: a major cause for concern', *Journal of Mental Health*, 6 (6): 599–612.

Frank, A.F. and Gunderson, J.G. (1990) 'The role of the therapeutic alliance in the treatment of schizophrenia: relationship to course and outcome', *Archives of General Psychiatry*, 47: 228–236.

Garcia Maza, G. (1996) 'Structuring effective user involvement', in Heller, T., Reynolds, J., Gomm, R., Muston, R. and Pattison, S. (eds) *Mental health matters: a reader*, Basingstoke: Macmillan.

Hamera, E.K., Peterson, K.A., Young, L.M. and McNary Schaumloffel, M. (1992) 'Symptom monitoring in schizophrenia: potential for enhancing self-care', *Archives of Psychiatric Nursing*, 6 (6): 324–330.

Hogarty, G.E. (1984) 'Depot neuroleptics: the relevance of psycho-social factors', *Journal of Clinical Psychiatry*, 45: 36–42.

Hogarty, G.E. and Ulrich, R.F. (1977) 'Temporal effects of drug and placebo in delaying relapse in schizophrenic outpatients', *Archives of General Psychiatry*, 34: 297–301.

Johnson, D.A.W. (1979) 'Further observations on the duration of depot neuroleptic maintenance therapy in schizophrenia', *British Journal of Psychiatry*, 135: 524–530.

Johnstone, L. (1993) 'Family management in "schizophrenia": its assumptions and contradictions', *Journal of Mental Health*, 2: 255–269.

Kane, J.M. (1996) 'Schizophrenia', *New England Journal of Medicine*, 334: 34–41.

Kavanagh, D.J. (1992) 'Recent developments in expressed emotion and schizophrenia', *British Journal of Psychiatry*, 160: 601–620.

Kirkpatrick, H., Landeen, J., Woodside, H. and Byrne, C. (2001) 'How people with schizophrenia build their hope', *Journal of Psychosocial Nursing*, 39 (1): 46–53.

Kruger, A. (2000) 'Schizophrenia: recovery and hope', *Psychiatric Rehabilitation Journal*, 24 (1): 29–37.

Laws, R.D. (ed.) (1989) *Relapse prevention with sex offenders*, New York: Guilford Press.

Leff, J. and Vaughn, C. (1994) 'Critics of family management in schizophrenia: their assumptions and contradictions', *Journal of Mental Health*, 3 (1): 115–116.

Leff, J. and Wing, J.K. (1971) 'Trial of maintenance therapy in schizophrenia', *British Medical Journal*, 3 (755): 599–604.

McCandless-Glincher, L., McKnight, S., Hamera, E., Smith, B.L., Peterson, K. and Plumlee, A.A. (1986) 'Use of symptoms by schizophrenics to monitor and regulate their illness', *Hospital and Community Psychiatry*, 37: 929–933.

Malla, A.K. and Norman, R. (1994) 'Prodromal symptoms in schizophrenia', *British Journal of Psychiatry*, 164: 487–493.

Meuser, K., Bellack, A., Wade, J., Sayers, S. and Rosenthal, K. (1992) 'An assessment of the educational needs of chronic psychiatric patients and their relatives', *British Journal of Psychiatry*, 160: 668–673.

Nunn, K.P. (1996) 'Personal hopefulness: a conceptual review of the relevance of the perceived future to psychiatry', *British Journal of Medical Psychology*, 69: 227–245.

Repper, J. (2000) 'Adjusting the focus of mental health nursing: incorporating service users' experiences of recovery', *Journal of Mental Health*, 9 (6): 575–587.

Romme, M. and Escher, S. (2000) *Making sense of voices*, London: MIND.

Rose, N. (1998) 'Living dangerously: risk thinking and risk management', *Mental Health Care*, 1 (8): 263–266.

Schooler, N.R., Levine, J., Severe, J.B., Brauzer, B., DiMascio, A., Klerman, G.L. and Tuason, V.B. (1980) 'Prevention of relapse in schizophrenia: an evaluation of fluphenazine decanoate', *Archives of General Psychiatry*, 37: 16–24.

Smith, J. (1992) 'Family interventions: service implications', in Birchwood, M. and Tarrier, N. (eds) *Innovations in the psychological management of schizophrenia*, Chichester: Wiley.

Subotnik, K.L. and Neuchterlein, K.H. (1988) 'Prodromal signs and symptoms of schizophrenic relapse', *Journal of Abnormal Psychology*, 97: 405–412.

Sutherby, K. and Szmukler, G. (1998) 'Crisis plans and self-help crisis initiatives', *Psychiatric Bulletin*, 22: 4–7.

Warner, R. (1994) *Recovery from schizophrenia: psychiatry and political economy*, London: Routledge.

Watkins, P. (2001) *Mental health nursing: the art of compassionate care*, Oxford: Butterworth Heinemann.

Wyatt, R.J. (1991) 'Neuroleptics and the natural causes of schizophrenia', *Schizophrenia Bulletin*, 17 (2): 325–351.

Zubin, J. and Spring, B. (1977) 'Vulnerability: a new view of schizophrenia', *Journal of Abnormal Psychology*, 86: 103–126.

# FURTHER READING

Initiative to Reduce the Impact of Schizophrenia (IRIS): http://www.iris-initiative.org.uk
This website resource is the work of Max Birchwood and colleagues and offers accessible information on early intervention and relapse prevention. More specifically it offers what it refers to as a Tool Kit for clinical practice to assist in relapse planning.

Perkins, R. and Repper, J. (1998) *Dilemmas in community mental health practice: choice or control*, Oxford: Radcliffe.
This is an erudite, comprehensive and critical treatise on the tensions in modern community mental health care.

Read, J. and Reynolds, J. (1996) *Speaking our minds: an anthology*, Basingstoke: Macmillan.
An excellent source book of first-person accounts of experiences of living with mental health problems.

# CHAPTER 22

# CASE MANAGEMENT AND ASSERTIVE OUTREACH

*Steve Morgan*

---

## SUMMARY OF KEY POINTS

- Case management and assertive outreach originated in the USA in the 1970s.

- Case management provides a framework for the identification of needs, the provision of interventions, and the evaluation of effectiveness.

- The 'team approach' is a key component for effective implementation of assertive outreach.

---

## INTRODUCTION

What is in a name? Case management (intensive, brokerage, clinical, rehabilitation, strengths), assertive community treatment, intensive community treatment teams, care management, assertive outreach – the names are numerous, and the confusion is rife. Defining models of clinical practice should provide a degree of simplicity for practitioners in a complex world. In reality, academic research may be offering nothing more than greater complexity in an already confusing workplace.

Broadly speaking, the task for most mental health practitioners should be a simple one to describe. However, any such simplicity is hidden by an extremely complex range of variables and functions, which need careful co-ordination if they are to be targeted and delivered effectively.

# HISTORICAL DEVELOPMENTS

The origins of most of the ideas can be traced back to a single source – the programme of 'Training in Community Living', initiated in 1970 as an ambitious twenty-year evaluated programme of alternatives to hospital treatment by Stein and Test (1980). 'Case management' became more widely recognised as a concept in American psychiatric services through federal legislation in 1976 and 1978. Increasing interest through the 1980s in the delivery of care gave rise to a number of models of case management (Intagliata 1982, Bachrach 1989), most notably the 'strengths' (Rapp 1988) and 'clinical' (Kanter 1989) models.

In the UK, 'intensive case management' (Ryan *et al.* 1991), applied to the adult mental health population, denoted a development focused more on direct care and support, as opposed to the co-ordination function of brokerage. The NHS and Community Care Act 1990 (House of Commons 1990) established responsibility on social services departments nationwide to adopt a brokerage model known as 'care management'. To add to the subsequent confusion in the UK, some of the intensive models adopted the same title, responding to real or perceived criticisms of inferring that people are 'cases to be managed'. The whole shift was one of highlighting the emphasis on managing the process and delivery of care, not managing people.

'Assertive outreach' is believed to specifically originate from the Thresholds Bridge programme in Chicago (Witheridge and Dincin 1985); and subsequently through the principles of the strengths model (Rapp 1988). The first references in UK literature appear in the early 1990s (Onyett 1992, Morgan 1993), and it gained prominence through the publication of *Keys to engagement* (Sainsbury Centre for Mental Health 1998). Its influence on government policy for mental health services is evident since assertive outreach teams have become one of the cornerstones of comprehensive and integrated systems of community care (Department of Health 1999, 2000).

# RESEARCH DEVELOPMENTS

Models of case management and assertive outreach are some of the most widely researched elements of mental health services. They have been demonstrated to be effective and efficient responses to meeting the needs of people most disabled by their mental distress, needing long-term intensive community support (Mueser *et al.* 1998).

Robust evidence demonstrates the effectiveness of assertive outreach in:

- engaging and retaining service users in treatment and care;
- reducing hospitalisation;
- improving housing stability;
- improving user satisfaction.

The results are mixed in relation to:

- symptom reduction;

- improvements in social functioning;
- improvements in quality of life.

The literature specifies the concept of 'fidelity to the model' (Teague *et al.* 1998), whereby effectiveness is clearly linked to the application of the identified core components of the model. Yet, in the UK, less enthusiastic results have been published, particularly where the core components have not been so closely adhered to (PRiSM Psychosis Study 1998, UK700 Group 1999). These specific critical reports have themselves been challenged (Marshall *et al.* 1999, Sashidharan *et al.* 1999) for the flawed research methodology in relation to the negative conclusions they are reporting.

# CONTEMPORARY 'CASE MANAGEMENT'

With all the attention paid to it, case management could easily be confused as being a method of treatment. However, it is not an 'intervention'; case management is a 'framework' within which treatment, care and support can take place. It is the framework for co-ordinating the identification of needs, decisions about the nature and delivery of appropriate interventions, and the evaluation of their effectiveness.

Broadly, the functions of case management are:

- comprehensive assessment of needs;
- direct casework, including elements of outreach work;
- co-ordination of service delivery;
- advocacy for services to meet user needs, and to respond to the identified unmet needs;
- monitoring and review;
- working with caseloads of approximately fifteen upwards.

Case management has come to shape all aspects of mental health service delivery for the group of people experiencing severe and enduring mental health problems. What started three decades ago as a radical way of working has arguably become the routine work of community mental health teams across the UK, subconsciously at least. 'Standard case management' is seen as the term for the functions of such teams (PRiSM Psychosis Study 1998), and is largely indistinguishable from the mechanisms of the care programme approach.

Assertive outreach has come to take on the mantle of intensive work with smaller caseloads, in UK services. However, nothing is that simple; it is still possible to define the complexity of service needs across a system as including 'intensive case management' and assertive outreach. The functions of the two will be largely blurred, with the main distinction being the definition of client group. Intensive case management will involve working with people experiencing very complex needs, requiring skilled co-ordination, but who do engage with services.

# ASSERTIVE OUTREACH

## Definition

> Assertive (Active) Outreach is a flexible and creative team-based approach to working with the complex needs and wishes of a clearly defined group of people. This group is frequently referred to as experiencing severe and enduring mental health problems, and as being hard-to-engage or resistant to services. They have generally been inadequately served in the mainstream development of community and inpatient mental health services.
>
> (Graley-Wetherell and Morgan 2001, p. 5)

## Functions

Essentially the function of assertive outreach is to work with service users who, whilst not engaging readily with services, nevertheless experience a complex range of needs leading them to utilise disproportionately high levels of service contact in a largely involuntary and unco-ordinated fashion.

The primary function is to engage in a mutually trusting working relationship, through providing a flexible and creative approach to client-centred care. It is about taking the service to the person, where they feel most comfortable, rather than expecting their attendance at service-based appointments. Engagement is a distinct and separate function working towards a shared purpose, frequently based on unstructured, informal and conversational styles. It is about sharing common ideas and interests, in order to establish a basis for future practical and evidence-based clinical functions (Morgan 1996).

Assertive outreach services are open to wide-ranging interpretations, particularly with the differences of terminology used, e.g. assertive community treatment. This latter term holds connotations of 'control'. Assertive is not 'aggressive' outreach, i.e. it is not narrowly restricting risks through enforcing medication compliance. The concern for risk and medication compliance is important, but needs to be seen within a broader context of service user needs and service delivery. The term 'assertive' should be applied more to the service provider than to the service user. It is a requirement for services to take a more active role in adjusting to meet the needs of the individual person, rather than vice versa.

Whilst recognising the rare occasions where public safety is an issue, assertive outreach approaches recognise the complexity of service users' lives, and the need to work with reasonable and practical priorities within a complex picture. It is not about reducing the complex social, cultural and environmental factors down to a narrow identification of symptoms, risk factors and strategies for restrictive management (Morgan 2000).

# Critical success factors

Responsiveness to local area needs, and resource constraints, cannot be ignored when attempting to initiate new assertive outreach services. The Sainsbury Centre for Mental Health (1998) outlines the rationale for stand-alone teams in the more densely populated urban areas, and for seeing assertive outreach as a function of the community mental health team in the less populated semi-rural area services. This latter possibility may be open to question, because of the very different ways of working of assertive outreach and community mental health teams (Morgan and Juriansz 2002).

Whatever service configuration is adopted, straying from the critical components identified in the research and literature is likely to reduce their successful implementation and effectiveness. The key is to demonstrate how the following core components are delivered in any locally identified model of practice:

- clearly targeted client group;
- one point of access to the service;
- engagement as a primary function;
- flexible, creative and persistent approaches;
- working on the client's own territory;
- manageable caseloads (approximately 1: 10);
- team approach, with keyworker co-ordination functions;
- range of practical tasks, and evidence-based interventions;
- 'no close' policy;
- adequate staff skill mix (personal and professional);
- individual, team and peer supervision;
- integration into a comprehensive area mental health service.

# Implementation issues

## 1  Targeting

Within a broad description of severe and enduring mental illness assertive outreach services will work with the 'most complex' and 'hard-to-engage' individuals. Many of these people will already be known to existing services, across all sectors, but some needy populations may be less well known. A study of the local demographics of the population will need to be sensitive to the needs of frequently excluded or isolated populations, particularly the issues of social exclusion experienced by black and other ethnic minority communities. For many, the issues of isolation stem from a lack of cultural sensitivity to the different needs of their groups.

Inclusion and exclusion criteria for assertive outreach should be clearly communicated to all potential referrers, in order for it to find its niche within a comprehensive and integrated area mental health service. The known populations may be generally described as people exhibiting many of the following characteristics (not an exhaustive list):

- not always responsive to conventional treatment options;
- poor general health status;
- lower life expectancy;
- long periods of unemployment;
- low income;
- risk of homelessness;
- poor social networks;
- frequent contact with criminal justice agencies;
- dual diagnosis (mental health and substance misuse);
- requiring assistance with practical tasks of routine functioning.

Locally developed operational policies will need to clearly reflect the definition of the client group that assertive outreach services are being set up to work with. Shifting goalposts and expectations only serve to undermine their effectiveness.

## 2 Staffing

The debate about statutory versus voluntary sector suitability for effectively providing assertive outreach services is sterile and unhelpful. The challenge is one of identifying the service components and qualities that underpin effective service delivery, and creating an environment that supports their implementation. As a specialised and demanding area of work, we need to ensure, as far as possible, that we are attracting staff with the attitudes and qualities that equip them to work in different and challenging circumstances. Simply appointing existing staff within the service to a new area of work is no guarantee that they can achieve the change of values and attitudes required to deliver a different service.

Staff must adopt a positive and persistent approach to seemingly intransigent circumstances. They need to feel comfortable working outside of the traditional expectations of their role. They must work across artificial boundaries – e.g. primary–secondary care, and health–social care – in order to create appropriate solutions. They need to network and co-ordinate diverse provider agency contributions – e.g. statutory and voluntary mental health services, housing, social security, criminal justice system.

The optimal size of team would be six to eight staff, from a diverse range of backgrounds, enabling the tapping of a pool of personal and professional expertise. Larger numbers only make it more difficult to co-ordinate the team, and to achieve the benefits of a team approach to knowing all the clients accepted into the service.

## 3 Management

Assertive outreach is a specialised area of mental health service delivery, requiring appropriate clinical and managerial leadership. The team manager may come from any professional background, but their leadership role in relation to the responsible medical officer will need to be clearly articulated and supported. Protocols will need to reflect and support managerial and supervisory responsibilities across professional boundaries, whilst also supporting the need for individual clinicians to seek appropriate external professional supervision, as necessary.

## 4  Style of working

A flexible and creative client-centred approach to complex needs requires a service that differs from the conventional community mental health team in a number of ways:

- flexible hours, working beyond the 9.00 a.m. to 5.00 p.m. tradition;
- primary emphasis on establishing and maintaining trusting working relationships with service users who otherwise do not want to know;
- active responses to service user-stated wishes and aspirations, not just professionally assessed problems;
- persistence in the face of adversity;
- a mobile response, largely working outside of traditional service settings;
- a time-unlimited focus, rather than discharge-oriented; taking a long-term perspective, whilst being aware of the potential for less intensive service options with time;
- offering practical help with daily activities of functioning, including recreational activity;
- implementing evidence-based clinical interventions in non-clinical settings;
- responding to crises experienced by people on the team caseload.

## 5  Location

If the assertive outreach function is to live up to its claim of being a different experience for the service users, it must be largely performed outside of traditional mental health service settings to be most effective, e.g. in people's homes, in parks, cafés, streets, police stations, housing departments, social security offices. Ideally the service would also be based outside of the traditional clinical settings, e.g. in a converted house, shop or office, in a location not identified as a usual clinical service.

## 6  Integration within a comprehensive service system

Assertive outreach should not be considered as a 'bolt-on' service, where people considered too resistant and complex can be dumped by other components of the area service. The complex needs of the target client group mean that a range of agencies and service providers may have to be involved in a co-ordinated network of care and support. No single agency will hold the key to all the needs.

An example of close integration is offered by crisis responses. Assertive outreach teams will be expected to respond to crises presented by users of their services, but will call on the back-up of dedicated crisis response services when a greater short-term intensity of contact is required. Integration with generic community mental health teams will be essential for enabling appropriate transfer of people when they reach a point of requiring lower intensity of input than is normally envisaged through assertive outreach. The assertive outreach function will also require workers to follow the service user through pathways in the system occasionally involving admission to in-patient care. A pronounced hospital–community divide is prejudicial to the continuity of care for many service users. 'Inreach' describes the regular visiting of a service user by the community service while they are an in-patient, and should greatly contribute to diminishing this divide.

## 7  Local service management responsibilities

The essential first step is a thorough assessment of local needs and resources. The aims should be: to identify the client populations for whom assertive outreach would be the most effective method of service delivery; and to identify the organisational and clinical expertise to develop, support and sustain a specialised service function.

Identifying target populations requires:

- defining local interpretations of 'complex needs' and 'hard-to-engage';
- identification of current 'heavy' users of services in a properly co-ordinated manner;
- identifying gaps in services that may be contributing to frequent relapses for these individuals;
- connecting with local voluntary sector and community resources, which may identify potential unknown needy populations;
- acknowledging real and potential causes for exclusion from services.

A service-based assessment of local expertise needs to identify the best partnerships for developing effective assertive outreach services across statutory and voluntary sector agencies. Responsive and relevant services may be determined by:

- an ability to offer real or perceived accessibility, rather than a sense of alienation, to the prospective service users;
- a readiness to adopt the necessary cultural change of service delivery, i.e. being able to step outside of the more traditional methods;
- the robustness of their service delivery structures;
- the ability to sustain delivery of the core components of assertive outreach in the longer term;
- their readiness to reach out to particularly disadvantaged groups, e.g. homeless populations, black and other ethnic minority communities.

The subsequent emerging assertive outreach services will have a number of requirements in relation to the senior management of the local area services:

- clarity of expectations regarding priorities and purpose;
- consistency of expectations and purpose;

- realistic expectations in relation to risk management, i.e. risk minimisation not risk elimination;
- clearly articulated statements of accountability and responsibility, integrated between the individual, team and organisational levels;
- clearly expressed and supported relationship to the other components of a comprehensive area mental health service;
- inter-agency understanding and agreement between health, social services and voluntary sector agencies about the purpose and function of assertive outreach;
- long-term funding, to sustain the reality of the work with people described as hard-to-engage.

# A 'TEAM APPROACH'

This is one of the most significant components contributing to the effectiveness of an assertive outreach method of working. All the team are encouraged to know and work with all the clients accepted by the team, supporting continuity of the service for each service user through the team, rather than through an individual keyworker in isolation. It is based on the premise that continuity of service is best offered through shifting the fostering of dependency of the service user, from the individual worker, to the team as a whole.

All the staff will perform core tasks of the service, and will be expected to get to know the team caseload, not just an individual caseload. Specialised skills may be held by individuals, but are seen as a team resource to be shared or supervised within the team. Not all service users will wish to relate to all staff members, so the team approach will offer degrees of flexibility in its approach to engagement.

This approach needs a managerial overview that does not lose sight of the external service connections within a broader network of care, treatment and support, as well as a strong ethos of support and supervision. Keyworker coordination roles are essential to ensure that the broader range of identified needs is being met by the team and wider service system. The role of the keyworker is not to do all but to ensure that all is done.

However, an assertive outreach team should not be seen to develop as a collection of individuals working solely with their own individual keyworker caseload. Similarly, appointing an individual assertive outreach worker attached to a team presents greater potential for staff member isolation and burnout. Adhering to critical components becomes more difficult when in an isolated position. The result is dilution of the assertive outreach function, as the worker seeks closer identification with the rest of the team, or becomes pulled by conflicting priorities to cover other team functions.

# A CASE STUDY IN TEAM-WORKING

The 'team approach' is a controversial issue. Adopting the title 'team', or working within a team, does not necessarily correspond with working as a team. Many teams function as a collection of individuals, team in name only. Function-led community service developments do not necessarily guarantee the best examples of team-working. Maybe an outcome-led approach is needed. If we wish for service users to experience a 'team approach' rather than an individual keyworker system, because of the inherent benefits it may offer, we may need to design a service with this outcome specified from the outset.

The assertive outreach team in Kettering (Northamptonshire) began as a function within a community mental health team, and will be used here as an illustration of some of the controversies of assertive outreach and effective team-working. The first issue is whether they should be stand-alone teams or a function within the community mental health team. Morgan and Juriansz (2002) outline the rationale for a countywide assertive outreach service, enabling it to function alongside rather than within the community mental health teams. The two parts of the system work with distinctly different client groups, in distinctly different ways, attracting practitioners with very different outlooks and attitudes. Placing assertive outreach within a community mental health team only sets the conditions for conflicting priorities when the total team workload is pressured.

The current literature indicates a multidisciplinary team encapsulating the broad range of professional expertise in one stand-alone team. Whilst this is justified in an urban context, it is believed that the number of clients and corresponding practitioners is too small in semi-rural areas (Sainsbury Centre for Mental Health 1998). The size of urban-based teams may generally be ten to twelve people, in the suggested configuration. Optimum functioning of a 'team approach' may only be possible with six to eight staff. It becomes more difficult to co-ordinate the workloads, and to hold sufficiently detailed information about the increasing number of service users taken on by larger teams. Ten to twelve may well be a highly functioning community mental health team, not necessarily an assertive outreach team.

Arguably, we need to be prioritising personal qualities and experience, above the mix of all professions. In the event of not having a particular profession represented, the team need to be more creative in how they access the necessary expertise. The 'can do' attitude, thinking the unthinkable and then doing it, is a vitally important ingredient which is more valuable than having people who know their professional boundaries and how to stay within them.

The Kettering team has five core members (three nurses, one health-based support worker, and one social services-based support worker). The broader range of professional expertise can be accessed through other parts of the local service, and through developing strong identity through links across a countywide assertive outreach service.

The highly effective 'team approach' requires careful co-ordination through daily information sharing with all members of the team. The white board becomes the focal point of daily handover meetings in the team base. All service users are listed, and daily work planning can be addressed, and made easily accessible to those who need to know. With a team caseload of up to thirty-five people, the Kettering team is able to hold a morning handover every day, with all staff being up-to-date with the daily progression of needs and planning of interventions for all service users. This one-hour meeting is the focal point for all the work, with detailed service user reviews being managed in other forums. The team are able to flexibly respond to individual needs, including taking account of fluctuating engagement issues, if a service user does not wish to be seen by all team members.

## CONCLUSIONS

Case management has become integrated into the ways of thinking and working across UK community mental health service delivery, even if it is not the term widely adopted by managers and practitioners to describe what it is they actually do. Arguably, case management and the care programme approach have become indivisible in terms of how treatment, care and support are currently delivered. Assertive outreach has more recently become synonymous with a specialised type of service to meet the complex needs of people for whom traditional approaches have been less successful.

Intensive case management and assertive outreach are widely researched and evaluated elements of international mental health services. 'Fidelity to the model' has come to sound like an inflexible mantra. The reality of clinical situations should be focusing our attention on how we can best implement the core components, not how we implement the research project in all its exact details, many of which may not be possible within local service structures and resources (Morgan and Juriansz 2002).

A new way of looking at team-working and individual worker contributions has emerged. Staff with more open attitudes and ethical appreciation of their practice appear better equipped to deliver the necessary flexible and creative approaches to engagement, persistence and effective service delivery.

Graley-Wetherell and Morgan (2001) argue that the importance currently placed on the research and theory agenda negates the vitally important messages that come from the service users, carers and practitioners about what really works, and how. This is not an argument against the value of the research, but one for a more balanced appreciation of how we measure potential successes.

Finally, Morgan (2000) argues against the implied agenda of using assertive outreach services, and case management systems, as the new face of the mental health risk business. Linking assertive outreach to a restrictive policy of tracking resistant people, and enforcing medication compliance through coercive means, is not a guarantee of reducing risks posed by people experiencing mental health problems. This approach offers additional disincentives for people to engage with services, potentially increasing risks to all by driving service users further away from services which may be of some help to them.

Conversely, positive risk-taking can have very beneficial effects. Understanding the consequences of different courses of action, supporting people to make decisions based on choice, backed up by adequate and accurate information, may be an essential key to engaging the trust of many service users.

# REFERENCES

Bachrach, L.L. (1989) 'Case management: toward a shared definition', *Hospital and Community Psychiatry*, 40 (9): 883–884.

Department of Health (1999) *National service framework for mental health: modern standards and service models*, London: Department of Health.

Department of Health (2000) *The NHS Plan: a plan for investment, a plan for reform*, London: The Stationery Office.

Graley-Wetherell, R. and Morgan, S. (2001) *Active outreach: an independent service user evaluation of a model of assertive outreach practice*, London: Sainsbury Centre for Mental Health.

House of Commons (1990) National Health Service and Community Care Act, London: HMSO.

Intagliata, J. (1982) 'Improving the quality of care for the chronically mentally disabled: the role of case management', *Schizophrenia Bulletin*, 8 (4): 655–673.

Kanter, J. (1989) 'Clinical case management: definition, principles, components', *Hospital and Community Psychiatry*, 40 (4): 361–368.

Marshall, M., Bond, G.R., Stein, L.I., Shepherd, G., McGrew, J., Hoult, J., Rosen, A., Huxley, P., Diamond, R.J., Warner, R., Olsen, M., Latimer, E., Goering, P., Craig, T.K., Meisler, N. and Test, M.A. (1999) 'Prism psychosis study – design limitations, questionable conclusions', *British Journal of Psychiatry*, 175: 501–503.

Morgan, S. (1993) *Community mental health: practical approaches to long-term problems*, Cheltenham: Nelson Thornes.

Morgan, S. (1996) *Helping relationships in mental health*, Cheltenham: Nelson Thornes.

Morgan, S. (2000) 'Assertive outreach: risk-making or risk-taking?' *Openmind*, 101: 16–17.

Morgan, S. and Juriansz, D. (2002) 'Practice-based evidence', *Openmind*, 114: 12–13.

Mueser, K.T., Bond, G.R., Drake, R.E. and Resnick, S.G. (1998) 'Models of community care for severe mental illness: a review of research on case management', *Schizophrenia Bulletin*, 24 (1): 37–73.

Onyett, S. (1992) *Case management in mental health*, Cheltenham: Nelson Thornes.

PRiSM Psychosis Study (1998) Papers 1–10, *British Journal of Psychiatry*, 173: 359–427.

Rapp, C.A. (1988) *The strengths perspective of case management with persons suffering from severe mental illness*, Lawrence, KS: NIMH, University of Kansas.

Ryan, P., Ford, R. and Clifford, P. (1991) *Case management and community care*, London: Research and Development for Psychiatry.

Sainsbury Centre for Mental Health (1998) *Keys to engagement: review of care for people with severe mental illness who are hard to engage with services*, London: Sainsbury Centre for Mental Health.

Sashidharan, S.P., Smyth, M. and Owen, A. (1999) 'PRiSM psychosis study – thro' a glass darkly: a distorted appraisal of community care', *British Journal of Psychiatry*, 175: 504–507.

Stein, L.I. and Test, M.A. (1980) 'Alternatives to mental hospital treatment', *Archives of General Psychiatry*, 37: 392–397.

Teague, G.B., Bond, G.R. and Drake, R.E. (1998) 'Program fidelity in assertive community treatment: development and use of a measure', *American Journal of Orthopsychiatry*, 68 (2): 216–232.

UK700 Group (1999) 'Intensive case management for severe psychotic illness: a randomised trial', *The Lancet*, 353: 2185–2189.

Witheridge, T.F. and Dincin, J. (1985) 'The Bridge: an assertive outreach team in an urban setting', *New Directions for Mental Health Services*, 26: 65–76.

# FURTHER READING

Burns, T. and Perkins, R. (2000) 'The future of case management', *International Review of Psychiatry*, 12: 212–218.
Charting the historical development and functions of case management and assertive outreach, nationally and internationally, this paper explores the fundamental need to engage the relationship within which evidence-based practice can be implemented effectively. In looking at the future of case management and assertive outreach, it argues that they provide a bridge between what psychiatry offers and the holistic needs that service users express.

Dodd, T. (2001) 'Clues about evidence for mental health care in community settings – assertive outreach', *Mental Health Practice*, 4 (7): 10–14.
This paper argues that the process of implementing evidence-based practice is extremely complex, and requires a realistic long-term view of effective outcomes. In relation to assertive outreach, we need clarity about what the critical elements are, and which elements can withstand adaptation to local circumstances without having a negative impact on outcomes. Integration of a whole systems approach is made more vital with a health and social services division of responsibilities.

Galvin, S. (2000) 'Justifying the use of a model of assertive community treatment: a critical appraisal of the effectiveness literature', unpublished working paper, Ipswich: Local Health Partnerships NHS Trust (copies available from Ipswich Outreach Team, 72 Foundation Street, Ipswich, Suffolk, IP4 1BN).
A succinct summary and analysis of the national and international research into case management and assertive outreach. The paper summarises the main points from the effectiveness literature, as well as examining the bases for conflicting outcomes in the UK research.

# CHAPTER 23

# PSYCHOPHARMACOLOGY AND MEDICATION MANAGEMENT

*Richard Gray, Elizabeth Brewin and Daniel Bressington*

---

## SUMMARY OF KEY POINTS

- Pharmacological treatments have revolutionised the treatment of mental health problems.

- Novel antipsychotics and antidepressants are better tolerated and may offer efficacy advantages over older treatments.

- Many service users are concerned about psychiatric medicines and often stop taking them, causing unnecessary morbidity.

---

## INTRODUCTION

The introduction of psychopharmacological treatments since the late 1940s has undoubtedly revolutionised the treatment of psychosis, affective disorders and other mental health problems. However, as in many other areas of health care, pharmacotherapy often requires long-term maintenance treatment to maintain health and prevent relapse. This can be problematic because service users are often uncertain about taking medication, especially long term. Mental health nurses have always had an important role to play in medication management, working with service users to help them manage their treatment so that it fits in with their lifestyle and maximises their health. This chapter will discuss pharmacological treatments for psychosis, affective disorder and other mental health problems, and also address how mental health nurses can work with service users to explore their uncertainty about taking medication and raise awareness about the importance of pharmacotherapy to maintain health.

# PSYCHOPHARMACOLOGY

Nerve cells communicate with each other by electrical impulses. An impulse travels along the nerve axon and stimulates the release of chemical messengers known as neurotransmitters. They are released from storage vesicles in the presynaptic nerve and released into the synapse. The synapse is the gap between the pre-synaptic cell and the postsynaptic cell at a transmission site (Figure 23.1). The neurotransmitter travels across the synapse and binds with the appropriate receptor on the postsynaptic cell membrane. Receptors are selective cellular recognition sites for neurotransmitters, hormones and many drugs. This usually sets up an electrical impulse (an excitatory effect) in the postsynaptic nerve cell and so the message is passed on. Sometimes neurotransmitters have an inhibitory effect and stop further transmission of the message. After transmission, the neurotransmitter usually leaves the receptor and is taken back up into the pre-synaptic cell (reuptake) or destroyed by enzymes such as monoamine oxidase (MAO) in the synapse. Some of the most important neurotransmitters in mental disorders are dopamine, serotonin (5-hydroxytryptamine or 5-HT), noradrenaline and gamma-aminobutyric acid (GABA).

It has been hypothesised that over- or under-response within neuro-transmission may be linked with some mental health problems. For example, psychosis may involve excessive dopamine neurotransmission, whilst depression and mania may involve disruption in the normal patterns of neurotransmission of noradrenaline and serotonin. This thinking about neurotransmission has led to the development of a range of pharmacological strategies to try to treat mental health problems. For example, antipsychotic drugs stop the neurotransmitter from binding to the postsynaptic receptor site by blocking those receptors. This reduces the transmission of the message and activity of the nerves in that structure of the brain.

Antidepressants stop the reuptake of noradrenaline and serotonin and regulate areas of the brain that make them. Monoamine oxidase inhibitors (MAOIs) prevent enzymatic metabolism of noradrenaline and serotonin. Both these actions result in increasing levels available at the synapse, thus increasing the activity between nerve cells. The clinical effects of medicines used in psychiatry do not, however, confine themselves to the specific areas of the brain associated with mental health problems. Medicines will often interact with many other receptors, causing unwanted symptoms or side effects and potential drug inter-actions during concomitant drug therapy.

# ANTIPSYCHOTICS

Antipsychotic medication has been the mainstay of treatment for schizophrenia since the 1950s when it was discovered that the dopamine antagonists, haloperidol and chlorpromazine, exert antipsychotic effects.

Dopamine is a neurotransmitter mainly associated with reward and control of movement. A deficit of dopamine (as a result of the degeneration of the substantia nigra in the mid-brain) results in Parkinsonism. This is characterised

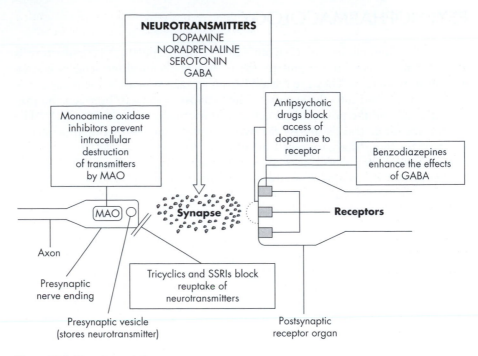

*Figure 23.1* Neurotransmission
Source: adapted from Taylor and Thomas 1997

clinically by movement disorders, including tremor, shuffling gait, stiffness and bradykinesia (slowed movement). Excessive dopamine results in symptoms of psychosis such as delusional beliefs and hallucinations. This can be demonstrated by administration of L-dopa (the precursor of dopamine) or amphetamines (dopamine agonists) in healthy subjects.

The dopamine hypothesis of schizophrenia proposes that excessive dopamine activity, or hyperdopaminergia, is associated with the pathophysiology of schizophrenia. Therefore, reducing this activity should reduce symptoms. Drugs that are known to block these receptors are advocated as treatment for psychotic symptoms. This is supported by reports that the clinical potency of antipsychotics is proportional to the extent to which they block dopamine receptors.

Some reports suggest that a high affinity for $D_2$ receptors may not be the only basis for efficacy in antipsychotic agents. Although these drugs typically occupy these receptors within a few hours of administration, there is often a one- to three-week delay before therapeutic benefits are reported. This suggests that these drugs act via a series of secondary, and as yet unknown, processes that evolve over days to weeks. There are suggestions that a number of other neuroreceptors, peptides, and amino acid systems may be involved. This is further supported by the fact that changes in systems other than the dopamine system have been implicated in the aetiology of schizophrenia.

Chlorpromazine, the first effective pharmacological treatment for the symptoms of schizophrenia, was introduced during the 1950s. Since then, a variety of antipsychotic agents have been developed (for example, haloperidol, trifluoperazine and sulpiride), some of which are available in a long-acting depot formulation (for example, flupenthixol and zuclopenthixol). Controlled clinical trials have repeatedly shown that these drugs are generally efficacious for the positive symptoms of schizophrenia. However, tolerability problems – especially acute extrapyramidal symptoms (EPS; dystonias, akathisia and Parkinsonism), raised prolactin levels (for example, sexual dysfunction and amenorrhoea), anticholinergic symptoms (dry mouth, blurred vision, sedation and constipation), cardiac problems (including QTc prolongation) and the potential to cause tardive dyskinesia – encountered with these so-called conventional agents have prompted further research into the development of improved novel and atypical agents such as clozapine, risperidone, olanzapine and quetiapine.

By definition atypical antipsychotics cause fewer EPS, in fact they are no more likely than a placebo drug to do so. However, that is not to say that they are side effect-free. One of the atypical antipsychotics, sertindole, was voluntarily withdrawn by its manufacturers in 1998 because of fears over cardiac safety (Gray 2001a). The side effects of clozapine, specifically the risk of neutropenia, are potentially so serious that it is only licensed for use in patients who are treatment-resistant, where the benefits of treatment are thought to outweigh the risks. In contrast, clinical experience with risperidone, olanzapine and quetiapine over a number of years has shown them to be exceptionally well tolerated (Gray 1999). Problems caused by raised prolactin, such as sexual dysfunction and period problems in women, are rare, although these symptoms have been seen in some patients taking risperidone (Gray 1999). Clozapine and risperidone can both cause postural hypotension, especially during the early part of treatment. Clozapine, olanzapine and quetiapine are clearly sedative, and anticholinergic effects such as dry mouth and blurred vision are fairly common in patients taking clozapine and are occasionally seen in patients taking olanzapine (Gray 2001b). Importantly risperidone, olanzapine and quetiapine do not have the cardiac side effects reported with sertindole, thioradazine or droperidol (Gray 2001a). Finally, in the long term, atypical antipsychotics seem to cause much less tardive dyskinesia than traditional antipsychotics (Gray 2001b).

A dramatic reduction in side effects is not the only difference between conventional and atypical antipsychotics. When the data from a large number of clinical trials are pooled together it is clear that risperidone, olanzapine and quetiapine (Gray 2001b) are effective treatments for schizophrenia, producing clinically meaningful improvements in symptoms and preventing relapse. However, they are no more effective at doing this than conventional antipsychotics such as chlorpromazine or haloperidol. Clozapine shows that uniquely it is more effective than typical antipsychotics but cannot be widely used because of its side-effect profile. There is emerging evidence that atypical antipsychotics may also be effective in treating negative symptoms such as social isolation and withdrawal. There is also interesting preliminary work suggesting that atypicals may be useful in treating cognitive symptoms, reducing violence and aggression, suicidality, craving for illicit substances and alcohol and, perhaps most importantly, improving patients' health-related quality of life (Gray 2001b). Based on this compelling evidence the most recent edition of the South London and Maudsley NHS Trust prescribing guidelines (Taylor et al. 2001) recommends that atypical antipsychotics should be the treatment of choice for people with schizophrenia.

## Implications for clinical practice

- Antipsychotics are effective in reducing psychotic symptoms for the majority of service users.
- Atypical antipsychotics cause fewer side effects than conventional treatments.
- Atypical antipsychotics may offer additional therapeutic benefits over traditional treatments.

# ANTIDEPRESSANTS

It has been proposed that depression is caused by a reduction in either serotonin or noradrenaline, and mania by an excess of noradrenaline. MAOIs (monoamine oxidase inhibitors) effectively inhibit the metabolism of these neurotransmitters (Figure 23.1), whilst tricyclic antidepressants and SSRIs (selective serotonin reuptake inhibitors) prevent their reuptake at the presynaptic neurone (Figure 23.1). Both these mechanisms increase the amount of neurotransmitter at the synapse. Although this theory is widely taught to mental health nurses, there are a number of substantial problems with it. Perhaps most important is the observation that 20 to 30 per cent of depressed service users do not derive any benefit from the medicines. Although mainly used in the treatment of depression and related mental health problems, there is evidence that they may also be useful in the treatment of other illnesses such as obsessive–compulsive disorder. It is important to remember that all antidepressant medicines may take four to six weeks to begin to work and service users cannot expect to realise a quick response to treatment.

Tricyclic antidepressants (TCAs) have been the mainstay for the treatment of depression for many years. Although clearly very effective in the treatment of depression, it has long been known that they are poorly tolerated (common side effects include sedation, weight gain and anticholinergic symptoms) and, because of cardio-toxicity, are potentially fatal in overdose. Perhaps because of tolerability problems psychiatrists and general practitioners have tended to prescribe doses of TCAs that are known to be sub-therapeutic. Over the past decade their use in both primary and secondary care settings has reduced dramatically.

TCAs have now been largely replaced by SSRIs (such as citalopram, fluoxetine and sertraline), a group of drugs that inhibit the reuptake of serotonin at the presynaptic membrane, promoting the neurotransmission of serotonin in the brain. Because they have specific affinity for serotonin receptors they have little effect at the transmission sites for other receptors and consequently are as effective as TCAs but have fewer side effects. Venlafaxine is another newer antidepressant and is an SNRI (selective noradrenaline reuptake inhibitor). It increases levels of both serotonin and noradrenaline. Although claims of increased efficacy have been made for this medicine, in practice it appears to be equally as effective as SSRIs and TCAs. SSRIs do not cause many of the side effects associated with traditional TCAs and they are much safer in overdose. The main side effects associated with SSRIs are nausea and agitation; they have also been associated with sexual dysfunction in both men and women and less commonly with dry mouth and sedation.

The final group of antidepressant drugs to consider are monoamine oxidase inhibitors (MAOIs; for example, phenelzine and tranylcypromine). Although available for many years, and generally well tolerated, they have not been widely prescribed because clinicians are worried about the hypertensive crisis when tyramine-containing foods and some other medicines are taken with these drugs. More recently, moclobemide, a new MAOI, has been marketed. Unlike previous MAOIs it only temporarily inhibits monoamine oxidase and consequently the tyramine reaction is substantially reduced and there are no dietary restrictions.

## Implications for clinical practice

- Antidepressants are effective in the treatment of depression.
- SSRIs are safer and better tolerated than TCAs.
- It takes several weeks for antidepressants to begin to ameliorate depressive symptoms.

# MOOD STABILISERS

Mood stabilisers are the most widely used drugs to treat bipolar affective disorder and other related conditions such as unipolar depression and schizoaffective disorder. There is also evidence that lithium is effective in treating some non-affective mental health problems such as borderline personality disorder. Lithium has been the front-line drug for bipolar disorder for many years, although increasingly carbamazepine and sodium valproate are becoming more popular. There is also emerging evidence that some other drugs – most notably the atypical antipsychotics clozapine, olanzapine and risperidone – may be effective in the treatment of bipolar disorder.

Lithium has been used as a mood stabiliser since the late 1940s when it was first recognised to have antimanic properties. However, the exact mechanism of action is poorly understood. It has been proposed that lithium corrects ion exchange abnormality, alters sodium transport in nerves and muscle cells, normalises synaptic neurotransmission of noradrenaline and changes receptor sensitivity. Lithium can be a complex drug to use. At high doses it can cause renal damage and reduce renal function. Hypothyroidism is also seen in service users taking lithium, even at therapeutic doses. The maintenance dose for lithium must be individually tailored and carefully monitored and adjusted over time. Lithium is associated with a range of acute (such as tremor and fatigue) and long-term (such as thyroid dysfunction) side effects as well as the potential for toxicity (a clinical emergency).

Typically lithium is first-line treatment; however, two anticonvulsants, carbamazepine and sodium valproate, have been shown to be effective mood stabilisers. Typically these drugs are only used if service users have not responded to lithium therapy or if it is contraindicated.

## Implications for clinical practice

- Lithium is an effective mood stabiliser but requires close monitoring.
- Lithium toxicity is an emergency situation.
- Carbamazepine and sodium valproate are also well tolerated and effective mood stabilisers.

# ANTI-ANXIETY AND SEDATIVE-HYPNOTIC DRUGS

Benzodiazepines are the most widely prescribed group of drugs in the world, although in recent years their popularity has waned because of their potential to cause tolerance and dependence. Benzodiazepines have a wide range of uses including for anxiety, anxiety-related phobias, alcohol withdrawal, and sleep disorders. They are also widely used in the treatment of acute agitation and aggression in service users with psychosis.

Benzodiazapines (for example, diazepam, lorazepam and temazepam) reduce anxiety by potentiating the inhibitory neurotransmitter GABA. There are few clinical differences between the different types of benzodiazepines except for different half-lives (the time for the plasma level of drug to reduce to half of peak level). Overdoses of benzodiazepines are almost never fatal (unless taken in conjunction with other central nervous system depressants such as alcohol and opiates), and the effect can be reversed by the specific antagonist flumazenil. Side effects are rare and tend to be dose-related. When used regularly tolerance increases, therefore people need higher doses to obtain the same level of symptomatic relief. Prolonged use can result in physical dependency. Withdrawal symptoms range from insomnia and anxiety, to extreme agitation and convulsions. It may be fatal if not treated appropriately. However, if prescribed over a short term (around two weeks), dependence should not be an issue, especially if treatment is stopped gradually. It is also useful to advise service users to use benzodiazepines intermittently rather than regularly to reduce the risk of tolerance and dependence.

The use of barbiturates has largely been replaced by benzodiazepines as anti-anxiety and sedative-hypnotic drugs because of tolerability and safety issues (the range between therapeutic and toxic dose, leading to coma and respiratory arrest, is very narrow). Two drugs not structurally related to benzodiazepines which are licensed for the treatment of insomnia are zopiclone and zolpidem. Other drugs that may be useful anti-anxiety and sedative-hypnotic drugs include some antihistamines, propranolol and buspirone.

# MEDICATION MANAGEMENT

There is compelling evidence that psychiatric medicines are effective in treating a range of mental health problems including affective disorders and psychosis. More modern treatments offer the potential for effective treatment with few side effects.

Generally psychiatric medicines need to be taken continuously over a sustained period of time if patients are to derive maximum benefit from treatment. However, studies consistently seem to suggest that many service users stop taking medication of their own accord. It is generally agreed that around half of all patients will stop antidepressant medication within six months of treatment being started, and the same is true of service users with psychosis. Stopping medication in people with psychosis is associated with a substantial increase in relapse rates, more frequent hospitalisations and a generally poorer outcome (Helgason 1990). Stopping medication is typically referred to as non-compliance or non-adherence. Definitions of non-compliance vary from complete cessation or verbal refusal, to any significant deviation from prescription, including dosage errors or failure to attend appointments. Given these definitions it is perhaps not surprising that for many service users the words compliance and adherence have many negative connotations, inferring a power imbalance where service users are not free to make choices themselves.

A number of factors have been identified that seem to affect whether or not service users take medication. Factors that have a negative impact on taking medication include:

- negative beliefs about medication;
- lack of awareness and understanding of the problem (or insight);
- unwanted side effects from medication;
- non-prescribed substance use (e.g. cannabis or alcohol);
- complexity of the treatment regimen.

Factors that seem to make people more likely to take medication include:

- a good relationship with clinicians;
- family and carer involvement in treatment;
- effective treatment;
- awareness of the positive effects of medication;
- awareness of the indirect benefits of medication.

Based on these factors a number of different types of pragmatic intervention have been tested to try to help service users to be better at taking their medication. Much of this work has focused on service users with psychosis. A detailed systematic review of the literature on interventions to improve the taking of pre-scribed medication can be found in the Cochrane Library (Haynes *et al.* 2002). Interventions can broadly be divided into three categories: educational, behavioural, and cognitive–behavioural.

Educational interventions aim to provide information to service users about both their illness and their medication, with the goal of increasing understanding and promoting compliance. Group and individual service user education has been evaluated using a variety of methodologies including a number of randomised controlled trials (Macpherson *et al.* 1996, Gray 2000). Results of these studies have consistently shown that just giving information will improve service users' understanding of their illness and medication but will not reduce the number who stop taking medication.

Behavioural interventions aim to simplify treatment regimens and minimise side effects to help service users tailor their treatment to suit their daily routine. For example, encouraging service users to take medication last thing at night before they go to bed to minimise the sedative effects of medication, or linking taking medication with a routine behaviour (such as making a cup of tea first thing in the morning). There is some evidence that this approach can be useful (Boczkowski *et al.* 1985).

In recent years research into improving the taking of medication has focused on cognitive behavioural approaches. These interventions focus on working collaboratively with service users to explore their beliefs about illness and treatment. Lecompte and Pelc (1996) tested a cognitive–behavioural programme based around five therapeutic strategies: engagement; psycho-education; identifying prodromal symptoms and developing coping strategies; behavioural strategies for reinforcing compliant behaviour; and correcting false beliefs about medication. In a randomised controlled trial service users who received the cognitive–behavioural intervention spent significantly less time in hospital than those in the control group, suggesting that this approach has promise.

Along similar lines Kemp *et al.* (1997, 1998) devised compliance therapy based on motivational interviewing and cognitive–behavioural techniques. Key principles include working collaboratively, emphasising personal choice and responsibility, and focusing on service users' concerns about treatment. The intervention is divided into three phases, which acknowledges that readiness to change is on a continuum. Phase 1 deals with patients' experiences of treatment by helping them to review their illness history. In phase 2 the common concerns about treatment are discussed and the good and bad things about treatment are explored. Phase 3 deals with long-term prevention and strategies for avoiding relapse. Compliance therapy was evaluated in a randomised controlled trial (Kemp *et al.* 1998). Seventy-four psychotic in-patients were randomly assigned to receive either compliance therapy or non-specific counselling. Patients received four to six sessions with a research psychiatrist lasting, on average, forty minutes. Treatment adherence was significantly better in the compliance therapy group, resulting in enhanced community tenure, with patients in the compliance therapy group taking longer to relapse than those who received non-specific counselling.

## Implications for clinical practice

Based on the available evidence, medication management should aim to help maximise the clinical potential of medication. It is not about improving compliance but collaboratively working with service users to help them make choices that are right for them. When clinicians work in this way service users are less likely to stop taking medication. This process can be considered as building concordance. Gray (2002) has described the components of good medication management:

- a collaborative approach to working with service users;
- a careful assessment of the service user's views about treatment, response to medication and side effects;

- medication review;
- giving tailored information about the illness and treatment;
- working with the service user to tailor their medication to suit their individual circumstances;
- use of motivational interviewing and cognitive–behavioural strategies.

Mental health nurses in both community and in-patient settings spend a considerable amount of time addressing and discussing medication issues with service users and the rest of the multidisciplinary team. Developing and enhancing the medication management skills that nurses already have may lead to improved clinical outcome for users of mental health services. Box 23.1 summarises some useful assessment measures and therapeutic approaches.

---

**Box 23.1   Medication management**

*Useful assessment measures*

Psychopathology

- KGV-M (Krawiecka, Goldberg and Vaughn-Modified) (Krawiecka *et al*. 1977)

Side effects (general)

- Liverpool University Neuroleptic Side Effects Rating Scale (LUNSERS) (Day *et al*. 1995)

Side effects (EPS-specific)

- Simpson Angus (Simpson and Angus 1970)

- Barnes Akathisia (Barnes 1989)

Side effects (TD (Tardive dyskinesia)-specific)

- AIMS (Abnormal Involuntary Movement Scale) (Guy 1976)

Beliefs about treatment and insight

- Drug Attitude Inventory (DAI-30, Hogan *et al*. 1983)

- Insight and Treatment Attitude Questionnaire (ITAQ, McEvoy *et al*. 1989)

*Example therapeutic techniques*

*Addressing practical issues*

Sorting out practical issues should be a priority. For example, is the service user able to get hold of medication? Do they remember to take it? Can they dispense their medication accurately?

---

*Medication review*

Regularly reviewing and evaluating the service user's medication with the multidisciplinary team is important to ensure that they are on the minimum effective dose and are not prescribed any unnecessary medicine. It can often be useful to compare a service user's drug chart with local or national guidelines (such as the South London and Maudsley NHS Trust guidelines, Taylor *et al.* 2001).

*Illness timeline*

Exploring previous experiences of treatment may teach service users what treatment strategies have been helpful in the past. The service user should identify when they or others first recognised that they had mental health problems and plot the course of those problems over time.

*Exploring ambivalence*

Most service users are uncertain about the importance of taking medication. It may be helpful to explore the not-so-good and the good things about medication and the good and not-so-good things about stopping medication. The aim is to help the service user explore their personal reasons for taking or not taking medication.

*Long-term prevention*

In order to help develop an understanding of the long-term need for medication, service users should be asked to set themselves a goal or target that they want to achieve (for example, returning to work). A problem-solving approach can then be used to identify broad and specific tasks that need to be undertaken, and any potential barriers that might be in the way and need to be addressed to help them achieve this goal.

## Implications for education and research

A survey of medication management practice (Gray *et al.* 2001) has shown that the majority of community mental health nurses do not report using measures of antipsychotic side effects in their day-to-day practice. These findings should not be interpreted as critical of nurses but rather as an observation of the challenge of getting new health technology into day-to-day clinical practice. There may well be a need for education providers to be more responsive to emerging clinical interventions and to provide appropriate courses to develop mental health nurses' skills, enabling them to make use of this technology for the benefit of the service users they are working with. However, it is all too easy to assume that training will be effective in developing clinical skills, but this is not always the case (Gournay and Brooking 1994). Trials of the effectiveness of training packages in producing improved clinical outcomes need to be conducted. If the results of such trials are positive, then training can be rolled out nationally.

## SUMMARY

Modern medicines offer safe and effective treatment for service users suffering from a range of mental health problems. However, these medicines are only effective if service users continue to take them. Many are ambivalent about the benefits of long-term treatment. Mental health nurses have a vital role to play in working collaboratively with service users to consider experiences of treatment and explore their ambivalence about medication.

## REFERENCES

Barnes, T.R.E. (1989) 'A rating scale for drug induced akathisia', *British Journal of Psychiatry*, 154: 672–676.

Boczkowski, J.A., Zeichner, A. and De Santo, N. (1985) 'Neuroleptic compliance among chronic schizophrenic outpatients: an intervention outcome report', *Journal of Consulting and Clinical Psychology*, 53: 666–671.

Day, J.C., Wood, G., Dewey, M. and Bentall, R.P. (1995) 'A self-rating scale for measuring neuroleptic side-effects. Validation in a group of schizophrenic patients', *British Journal of Psychiatry*, 166: 650–653.

Gournay, K. and Brooking, J. (1994) 'Community psychiatric nurses in primary health care', *British Journal of Psychiatry*, 165: 231–238.

Gray, R. (1999) 'Antipsychotics, side effects and effective management', *Mental Health Practice*, 2 (7): 14–20.

Gray, R. (2000) 'Does patient education enhance compliance with clozapine? A preliminary investigation', *Journal of Psychiatric and Mental Health Nursing*, 7: 285–286.

Gray, R. (2001a) 'Medication related cardiac risks and sudden deaths among people receiving antipsychotics for schizophrenia', *Mental Health Care*, 4 (9): 302–304.

Gray, R. (2001b) 'Medication for schizophrenia', *Nursing Times*, 97 (31): 38–39.

Gray, R., on behalf of the medication management dissemination project group (2002) 'Sweetening the pills', *Mental Health Today*, February, pp. 22–23.

Gray, R., Wykes, T., Parr, A.M., Hails, E. and Gournay, K. (2001) 'The use of outcome measures to evaluate the efficacy and tolerability of antipsychotic medication: a comparison of Thorn graduate and CPN practice', *Journal of Psychiatric and Mental Health Nursing*, 8: 191–196.

Guy, W. (1976) *Assessment manual for psychopharmacology*, Washington, DC: Department of Education and Welfare.

Haynes, R.B., Montague, P. and Oliver, T. (2002) *Interventions for helping patients follow prescription for medications* (Cochrane review), in The Cochrane Library, Issue 6, Oxford: Update Software.

Helgason, L. (1990) 'Twenty year follow-up of first psychiatric presentation for schizophrenia: what could have been prevented?' *Acta Psychiatrica Scandinavica*, 81: 231–235.

Hogan, T.P., Awad, A.G. and Eastwood, R. (1983) 'A self-report scale predictive of drug compliance in schizophrenics: reliability and discriminative validity', *Psychological Medicine*, 13: 177–183.

Kemp, R., Hayward, P. and David, A. (1997) *Compliance therapy manual*, London: Maudsley Publications

Kemp, R., Kirov, G., Everitt, B., Hayward, P. and David, A. (1998) 'Randomised controlled trial of compliance therapy. 18-month follow-up', *British Journal of Psychiatry*, 172: 413–419.

Krawiecka, M., Goldberg, D. and Vaughn, M. (1977) 'A standardised psychiatric assessment scale for rating chronic psychotic patients', *Acta Psychiatrica Scandinavica*, 55: 299–308.

Lecompte, D. and Pelc, I. (1996) 'A cognitive-behavioural programme to improve compliance with medication in patients with schizophrenia', *International Journal of Mental Health*, 25: 51–56.

McEvoy, A.P., Apperson, L.J., Applebaum, P.S., Ortlip, P., Brecosky, J., Hammill, K., Geller, J.L. and Roth, L. (1989) 'Insight in schizophrenia: its relationship to acute psychopathology', *Journal of Nervous and Mental Disorders*, 177: 43–47.

Macpherson, R., Jerrom, B. and Hughes, A. (1996) 'A controlled study of education about drug treatment in schizophrenia', *British Journal of Psychiatry*, 168: 709–717.

Simpson, G.M. and Angus, J.W.S. (1970) 'Drug-induced extrapyramidal disorders', *Acta Psychiatrica Scandinavica*, 45 (supplement 212): 11–19.

Taylor, D. and Thomas, B. (1997) 'Psychopharmacology', in Thomas, B., Hardy, S. and Cutting, P. (eds) *Stuart and Sundeen's mental health nursing: principles and practice*, London: Mosby.

Taylor, D., McConnell, D., McConnell, H. and Kerwin, R. (2001) *The South London and Maudsley NHS Trust 2001 Prescribing Guidelines*, London: Martin Dunitz.

# FURTHER READING

Haynes, R.B., Montague, P. and Oliver, T. (2002) *Interventions for helping patients follow prescription for medications* (Cochrane review), in The Cochrane Library, Issue 6, Oxford: Update Software.

A detailed review of interventions to enhance compliance. Essential reading if you are interested in the quality of research in this area.

Kemp, R., Hayward, P. and David, A. (1997) *Compliance therapy manual*, London: Maudsley Publications

A useful, straightforward manual that will enable clinicians to deliver compliance therapy.

Taylor, D., McConnell, D., McConnell, H. and Kerwin, R. (2001) *The South London and Maudsley NHS Trust 2001 Prescribing Guidelines*, London: Martin Dunitz.

The most widely used prescribing guidelines in the UK. Offers useful practical advice to clinicians.

# CHAPTER 24

# CREATIVITY AND THE THERAPEUTIC USE OF THE CREATIVE ARTS

*Tony Gillam*

---

## SUMMARY OF KEY POINTS

- Community mental health nursing can be considered a creative activity.

- Community mental health nurses need to have an understanding of how the creative arts and creative arts therapies can help people with mental health problems.

- There are opportunities for community mental health nurses to become actively involved in using the creative arts in their own practice.

---

## INTRODUCTION

### The relevance of the creative arts to community mental health nursing

This chapter will consider how the creative arts are relevant to community mental health nursing. There are three elements to the discussion. The most obvious of these is the creative arts therapies (such as art therapy and music therapy), with which many nurses will have some familiarity as potential interventions for their patients. Less obvious are the ways in which nurses might become involved in the creative arts themselves (be this through using them as part of an intervention with patients, or for their own personal or professional development). Less obvious still are the ways in which nurses can become more aware of creativity and its benefits in their own everyday practice. First, then, I will explore creativity itself.

# CREATIVITY

Creativity is such a broad-ranging concept that it can be difficult to define. A quick search of the Amazon books website, for example, using 'creativity' as the keyword, will bring up a long list of books on subjects as diverse as cookery, gardening and creative writing, as well as a host of self-help, popular psychology, and 'new age' approaches to personal development and management. Creativity is clearly not something that applies solely to traditionally artistic activities such as drama or painting; it can be applied to almost any aspect of life – including community mental health nursing. Cropley (2001) has usefully identified three key aspects of creativity: novelty, effectiveness and ethicality.

## Novelty, effectiveness and ethicality

First, whether we are considering a creative product, a course of action or an idea, Cropley suggests that that which is creative is inherently *novel*, i.e. it necessarily departs from the familiar. Second, it must be *effective* (i.e. it must work, in the sense that it achieves some end). The effectiveness may be aesthetic, artistic or spiritual, but it may also be material, such as winning or making a profit. Third, it must be *ethical* (the term 'creative' is not usually used to describe selfish or destructive behaviour) (Cropley 2001).

## Exceptional and everyday creativity

Cropley's recent work is concerned not so much with creativity as the production of 'acclaimed work' as with 'the psychological factors within the individual that give the person in question the potential to behave creatively' and 'the aspects of the environment that promote turning potential into creative behaviour' (Cropley 2001, p. 27). It follows from this that creativity can be exceptional and acclaimed (as in the case of great literature, music, inventions or discoveries), but it can equally be an everyday phenomenon in any walk of life. Barker (1995) describes how, when people are asked what the word 'creativity' suggests, their initial answers imply that it is thought of as something exceptional (e.g. 'being a genius', 'producing a work of art'). In other words, 'creativity is often seen as rare: some magical power that only a few possess' (Barker 1995, p. 4). When, at the end of a course on creative thinking, people were invited to review their definitions of creativity, their answers suggested a much wider, more achievable range of connections with everyday experience (e.g. 'being daring', 'unlearning', 'challenging assumptions', 'making novel associations', etc.).

# COMMUNITY MENTAL HEALTH NURSING AS A CREATIVE ACTIVITY

If creativity can be an everyday behaviour, and one not necessarily related to artistic activity, then there is no reason why community mental health nursing cannot be creative. There may be obstacles, but creative thinking itself may offer ways around these. For example, 'being daring' may be interpreted as 'risk-taking'. Flexibility or willingness to take risks was identified by Sternberg (1988) as one of the 'facets' of creativity. Sternberg saw willingness to take risks as a facilitatory aspect of personality. I have argued, elsewhere, that while risk assessment and risk management have become a preoccupation for community mental health nursing, the positive aspects of risk-*taking* – for patients and for nurses – have been marginalised (Gillam 2002). Reasserting the importance of taking risks could be seen as one aspect of promoting more creative community mental health nursing.

Other aspects of 'everyday creativity', such as 'unlearning', 'challenging assumptions' and 'making novel associations', might be viewed as quintessential to the concept of the 'reflective practitioner'. Again, the ability to unlearn, challenge assumptions and make novel associations need not be related to any particular artistic activity, but I will go on to discuss how, for instance, creative writing or storytelling might be deployed to promote reflective practice.

# CREATIVE ARTS THERAPIES

Practically any art form can be – and has been – used as a therapy. Drama and theatre arts have given rise to dramatherapy and psychodrama. The visual arts have spawned art therapy (which may include not only painting and drawing, but sculpture and pottery). Music has produced music therapy, while movement and dance have led to dance therapy. Storytelling and creative writing are used as therapeutic activities. Other art forms which combine elements of more than one (such as puppetry) and creative work in media such as film, video and digital technology have all been used to achieve therapeutic ends. Some of the creative therapies have developed into professions in their own right (notably art therapy, music therapy and dramatherapy) with their own training courses, recognised qualifications and professional bodies. Others have remained more peripheral and have become the domain of artists-in-residence, community arts workers, interested professionals from other disciplines (occupational therapy, nursing, medicine, psychology), or of patients themselves in a form of self-help.

# THE ART AND THE THERAPIST

Thomson observed that:

> when Adrian Hill first coined the term 'art therapy' in 1938, he meant simply that art does the therapeutic work. . . . By the time I first heard

of this term it had found a companion: 'art therapist'. This personage complicates matters, for is it now the art or the therapist that initiates the healing process?

(Thomson 1989, p. 3)

The use of the terms 'therapy' and 'therapist' is problematic in discussing creative arts therapies. Warren believes that much of the problem has been caused:

> by attempting to define what individual creative therapies are, rather than looking at what they do. As a result a great deal of time has been spent attempting to answer the question 'what is Art Therapy, Music Therapy, etc.?' Moreover, rather than establishing the benefits to health and well-being of artistic activity itself, the 'therapeutic legitimacy' of artistic activity has been established, defined and calibrated in terms of other bodies of knowledge, most notably psychotherapy, medicine and psychology.

(Warren 1993, p. 5)

## CREATIVE ARTS THERAPIES AND NURSING

There are parallels between the creative arts therapies and nursing. Community mental health nursing has had similar problems in trying to define itself in terms of those other bodies of knowledge ('most notably psychotherapy, medicine and psychology') mentioned by Warren, and in trying to create an underpinning scientific body of theory. Clarke has argued that community mental health nurses have tried to validate what they do by mimicking psychologists and psychiatrists. This trend has been exacerbated, he believes, by the increasing focus on severe and enduring mental illness, as a result of which he fears:

> interventions are either going to be cognitive-behaviourist in nature, thus edging nursing towards a psychological mode of practice, or they are going to be of a nature which will return nurses to the role of interminable second-fiddle to a medical speciality which enduringly controls diagnosis and prescription.

(Clarke 1999, p. 5)

Could engagement in creative arts provide community mental health nurses with a way of avoiding the 'role of interminable second-fiddle' to other, arguably higher-status, mental health disciplines? Warren identified a similar tendency among creative arts therapists, complaining that 'many creative specialists have tried to demonstrate just how much they are like psychotherapists and psychoanalysts. However, few creative specialists accentuate their greatest strength, the thing that makes them different, their expertise in their art form' (Warren 1993, p. 5). It might be argued that what makes community mental health nurses different is their expertise in *their* art form – the art form being community mental health nursing. This requires us to view nursing not as an activity with a scientific basis, like medicine, but as a creative art.

## SCIENCE, ART, SPIRITUALITY, CREATIVITY . . .

It would be easy, at this point, to sink into the rather tired debate of whether community mental health nursing is an art or a science. Clarke has written of the 'delusion of scientific respectability' under which nursing labours, balanced against all the 'dubious talk of spirituality' and holism (Clarke 1999, p. 9). He suggests that a theory of nursing might become:

> a resigned acceptance of essentially unique encounters between nurses and patients, individual renditions of problems and ills against a background of the basic humanities which define our culture. Certainly, it has not been possible to concoct a definition to which a majority (of nurses) could subscribe and the endless models and frameworks proposed, entertained and then abandoned are testimony to the mystery which lies at the heart of nursing.
>
> (Clarke 1999, pp. 8–9)

I would not wish to add to the 'endless models and frameworks', but simply to concur with Clarke that we work 'against a background of the basic humanities which define our culture' and that, because there is a 'mystery at the heart of nursing', it is fitting that we be creative, and that our work be considered as akin to the arts and humanities. Moreover, if the creative arts can help us in the task (whether we deploy them directly in patient care or use them as a tool for our own professional development), then so much the better.

Not wishing to prolong discussion about theories of nursing, let us move on to focus on two of the creative art forms in detail and how these might inform community mental health nursing. The first of these is music, the second creative writing and storytelling.

## THE ROLE OF MUSIC AND MUSIC THERAPY IN MENTAL HEALTH

Bunt explains how music 'has been used extensively throughout history as a healing force to alleviate illness and distress' (Bunt 1994, p. 3). It is only in recent times, however, that music therapy as a specific discipline has evolved. In the early twentieth century music was used in hospitals 'mainly to boost morale, as a general aid to convalescence and as an entertaining diversion' (ibid.). Bunt goes on to describe how:

> physicians invited musicians to play to large groups of patients on the vague assumption that it might activate metabolic functions and relieve mental stress. Listening to music could provide an aesthetic experience of quality and was regarded by many as a very humane way of occupying patients' time. Anecdotal accounts of music's inherent worth abound in the early literature on music in medicine.

> There seems to be a general consensus that exposure to music could
> do nothing but good.
>
> (Bunt 1994, pp. 3–4)

The 1940s saw the development in the USA of music therapy as an emerging profession, with its own training courses for musicians wanting to become music therapists; and by the 1950s there were professional associations of music therapy in both the USA and the UK. By the 1960s the UK also had professional training courses in music therapy. It was only really in the last decades of the twentieth century, however, that Bunt and others argued for the need for a strong research base in music therapy.

## EVIDENCE-BASED PRACTICE, VALUE FOR MONEY AND THE ARTS

As discussed above, there are parallels with other professions involved in health and social care, which are increasingly feeling the need for an 'evidence base' to underpin practice. Evidence-based practice is also about practitioners being seen to provide 'value for money'. There would seem to be a paradox, though, in seeking hard, scientific evidence to support the value of arts and arts therapies. Artists are, perhaps, by nature more likely to rely on intuition and impression. If a session of music-making – or a painting or a poem – evokes a powerful emotional response, this may be indication enough that it has 'inherent worth', though this so-called 'wow factor' is hard to quantify. Ansdell and Pavlicevic write:

> as funders generally become more insistent on 'evidence' that what
> we do makes a difference, and that it makes economic sense to support
> our work, it is no longer enough for us just to be practising and
> presenting our work. The 'Wow!' is over.
>
> (Ansdell and Pavlicevic 2001, p. 243)

## THE MUSIC WORKSHOP PROJECT

My own project, the Music Workshop Project, thrived for five years on what Ansdell and Pavlicevic might have described as 'pure wow!' Essentially, the project encourages people with mental health problems to make their own music. Co-ordinated by a service user and me, it has two main aims – first, to help people with mental health problems by involving them in musical activities, and second, to present a more positive image of mental health to the public, in order to reduce fear and stigma. The backbone of the project has always been a monthly improvisational group session, but out of this grew the ambition to produce and release CD albums. To coincide with the release of its first album, *Organised Chaos*, the project also launched its own website. Interestingly, the cover design was a piece of computer-generated art produced by a project member, while the text on the website was also the work of a project member. Thus, although primarily a music project, it has also inspired both writing and visual art.

The Music Workshop Project provides regular opportunities for people with a range of mental health problems to express themselves through music. Along with the therapeutic effects of being creative, it aims to encourage people to develop interpersonal skills through improvisational group-work. From the start, the project was not intended for competent musicians. It did not set out to teach people to be proficient musicians, but to promote an interest in making music and exploring its potential for personal expression and interpersonal communication. Moreover, the group was expressly not for passively listening to music but for actively creating it. It sought to enhance active listening skills through playing in a group, being sensitive to the emotional, psychological and creative needs of other members of the group.

The Music Workshop Project has received considerable coverage in the nursing and mental health press since its inception in 1995 (Mason 1999, Everett 2000, Gillam 2002). In 1997, we received a national award from the MIND Millennium Fund, and in 1998, we achieved international acclaim as the only UK winner of the Lilly Schizophrenia Reintegration Award. The subsequent local, national and international media interest in the project has helped to present a positive image of mental illness, and has acted as a catalyst, encouraging greater user involvement and participation in the planning and expansion of the project.

Awards and recognition for artistic achievements certainly boost the 'wow factor'. It is often within the simple context of the monthly improvisational work-shops, though, that moments of 'pure wow' occur; when a small group of people with mental health problems who do not normally consider themselves musicians come together to produce moments of breathtaking, inspired creativity.

For all its sheer delight in pure and simple music-making, even the Music Workshop Project began to succumb to the pressure for a modest 'evidence base', as if to agree with Ansdell and Pavlicevic that it might no longer be enough simply to be practising and presenting our work. Accordingly, in 2000 we carried out a small piece of research, which surveyed the views of project members, service users who were not yet using the project and mental health workers. Results from this research were of immediate practical help in illuminating how best to use resources to meet the needs and wishes of service users. The findings of the survey suggested that there was a real appetite for further recordings, hence work began on a second CD, *Late in the Morning*. This turned out to be very different from *Organised Chaos* in that it focused on developing the skills of certain members of the project in songwriting, performing and recording.

More recently, in response to the many requests for support and advice from others wanting to start similar projects, a one-day conference was held – *Using music in mental health* – which discussed the development of the project as well as covering the aspects of group facilitation and the practicalities of recording. It was through organising the conference that I became more fully aware of the vibrant community music movement which has grown up in recent years alongside professional music therapy.

# THE EMERGING COMMUNITY MUSIC MOVEMENT

While music therapy and other arts therapies have become more and more professionalised (with increasingly advanced training courses, professional bodies, journals and bodies of research), there has arisen a parallel movement of community arts. This movement is less about using art forms to *treat* mental health problems and more about user involvement and empowerment. It involves artists and sometimes mental health workers who are not professional creative arts therapists, and it also involves service users themselves.

The community music movement upholds the belief that everyone should have the opportunity to make music and explore their musical potential. It is concerned with the value of music and the arts, not just to individuals, but to communities. Rather than using music *therapists*, in community music professional musicians such as drummers, singers, songwriters, composers and music technicians are often employed. These musicians then work with people with any level of musical experience (or none at all) to create and sometimes to perform or record music, in a wide range of settings, including schools, youth clubs and day centres as well as more traditional performance venues. Community music organisations act as initiating and developing agencies for innovative participatory music and work towards improving access to music-making. Often they work in partnership with both arts organisations and disability organisations.

There are a number of key features in the philosophy of the community music movement. These include a belief in providing opportunities for individuals and communities, inclusiveness, forging links with community settings, promoting innovation and participation, facilitating access to creativity for people with disabilities, and possibly providing the means for the resulting music to reach a wider audience. Some of these aims are common to music therapy approaches, and the Music Workshop Project is one example of an initiative which has, almost organically, grown away from a 'therapy' model and towards a 'community music' model.

# THE COMMUNITY ARTS MOVEMENT AND COMMUNITY MENTAL HEALTH NURSING

Some comparisons have been made here between music therapy and community music groups which might also inform comparisons between the other creative arts therapies and their corresponding community arts manifestations. Moreover, there is the relationship between the community arts movement and community mental heath nursing. Whether or not a community mental health nurse wishes to become involved in any artistic activity such as those described here, he or she may wish to espouse some of the philosophy of the community arts movement. The key features of this have already been mentioned but are worth reiterating, this time removed from their artistic context. They are: a belief in providing opportunities for individuals and communities, inclusiveness, forging links with community settings, promoting innovation and participation, facilitating access to creativity for people with disabilities, and possibly providing the means for the results to reach a wider audience. Regardless of artistic activity, these would seem to be laudable values for community mental heath nursing, and were nurses to stand by these, community mental health nursing might become a more creative activity.

## CREATIVE WRITING AND STORYTELLING FOR PATIENTS AND NURSES

While music, drama and the visual arts might be considered useful means of facilitating expression, creative writing might be seen as well suited to reflection. I have been involved with creative writing groups in psychiatric day hospitals where the emphasis was not on writing skill but on encouraging patients to express themselves in writing, and to use this as a vehicle for verbalising their thoughts and feelings, generating discussion and giving and receiving feedback from one another. If this is helpful for patients, it seems reasonable that writing and recounting stories might be useful tools for promoting reflection in practitioners.

## REFLECTIVE PRACTICE AND STORYTELLING

At its worst, reflective practice can be regarded as one of those requirements of the nursing establishment, and something which nurses have to dutifully inflict upon themselves. It is this tendency which Bowles (1995) pokes fun at, when he writes of the reluctance of the nursing profession – in the UK especially – 'to approach the serious business of nursing with anything less than scientific or academically acceptable labels' (Bowles 1995, p. 366). Bowles draws attention to the idea of using 'storytelling' as a way of enriching nurses' lives. This seems a very natural suggestion since many would agree that it is the wealth of fascinating human stories that makes community mental health nursing such an interesting job.

Nurses do tell stories, in clinical notes and letters (their everyday documentation), sometimes in the form of reflective diaries, in professional portfolios, in case studies and in clinical supervision. There is nothing wrong with these tools for reflection, but Bowles is critical of 'the attendant jargon and models for implementation' with which we make things more difficult for ourselves (Bowles 1995, p. 366). Storytelling, he suggests, provides the perfect antidote to all 'the confusing and almost elitist rhetoric which surrounds reflective practice' (ibid.). In contrast to the wealth of literature from the United States about the use of storytelling in nursing, there is almost a complete lack of it in the British literature. Bowles takes this as an indication of our reticence about 'unscientific' or 'unacademic' methods, hence the contrast between the narrow reflective techniques used by British nurses and the apparent simplicity of telling stories.

## CASE HISTORIES, NARRATIVES AND TALES

Hippocrates introduced the 'case history' (a description, or depiction, of the natural history of disease), but Sacks argues that:

> there is no 'subject' in a narrow case history; modern case histories allude to the subject in a cursory phrase ('a trisomic albino female of 21'), which could as well apply to a rat as a human being. To restore the human subject at the centre . . . we must deepen a case history to a narrative or tale: only then do we have a 'who' as well as a 'what'.
>
> (Sacks 1986, p. x)

Sacks urges us to 'deepen' our case histories so as to restore the human subject to the centre of the story. If Sacks's concern is with re-humanising the case history (for the sake of the patient at its centre), Bowles believes that storytelling 'is a medium by which personal experience can be communicated to others with immediacy and relevancy and which is capable of effecting personal change in the *narrator* as well as the audience' (Bowles 1995, p. 366). He also believes that the 'loss of identity, and the impoverishment of role models and collegial networks may be mitigated by story telling' (ibid.).

If this is so, it follows that community mental health nurses can use storytelling to enrich their practice. We should tell stories, about our patients, about our work, in our reflective diaries, in professional portfolios, in clinical supervision and, of course, in everyday conversation with each other. Perhaps we should also develop what Bowles calls our 'collegial network' by *writing* more stories, as case studies, articles and books which have a 'who' as well as a 'what'.

## WRITING ABOUT COMMUNITY MENTAL HEALTH NURSING

Earlier, parallels were drawn between the creative arts therapies and community mental health nursing. It seems reasonable when considering writing about community mental health nursing, to draw inferences from writing about music therapy. Ansdell has reflected on basic questions underpinning the reasons why music therapists might write about music therapy (Ansdell 2001), and these same questions could be put to community mental health nurses. They include such considerations as 'who reads our writing, and why? Is its appeal mainly inter- or intra-professional? Could people outside (the discipline) understand our discourse?' (Ansdell 2001, p. 3). Ansdell goes on to ask what kind of genre is this writing, is it mostly technical or narrative in style, is it scientific or artistic, is it interesting or dull? He also raises the question of whether anyone would read it *non*-professionally as, for example, they read Oliver Sacks, and if not why not? Ansdell wonders whether music therapy writing has 'become a "stranded discourse" – detached from the wider cultural and political context we work in' (ibid.). He concludes that these questions may influence decisions about whether to write about our work, and those to whom we choose to show our writing.

# CREATIVE NON-FICTION

One way in which community mental health nurses might avoid their writing becoming what Ansdell terms a 'stranded discourse' and, at the same time, acknowledge Sacks's plea for deepening case history to the level of narrative or tale is by aiming to write 'creative non-fiction'. Gutkind describes creative non-fiction as a literary, cultural and political movement rather than a genre (Gutkind 1997). Creative non-fiction differs from both fiction and journalism. Fiction is literally not totally true, while creative non-fiction aims to be as truthful and factual as possible. In technique, though, creative non-fiction is closer to fiction in that it uses description, dialogue, characterisation, and writing in scenes and from differing 'points of view'. It is story-orientated, i.e. narrative, but the non-fiction element is its substance, in that it seeks to impart information.

Of course, it would be perverse, in a chapter aiming to promote creativity and wider use of creative arts, to be overly prescriptive of how community mental health nurses should express themselves in writing. The idea of creative non-fiction is introduced here simply to provide one way in which nurses, when writing about their professional experiences, might feel more comfortable using 'less than scientific or academically acceptable labels' (Bowles 1995, p. 366).

# CONCLUSION

If community mental health nursing is to be a creative activity, then attention needs to be paid to those psychological factors within the individual and those aspects in the environment that promote creative behaviour. It should be remembered that creativity is not exclusively about acclaimed work or even artistic activity, but includes examples of 'everyday creativity' such as 'being daring', 'unlearning', 'challenging assumptions' and 'making novel associations'. These tendencies could be nurtured through nurse education and, in an ongoing way, through supervision and the promotion of reflective practice.

It has been suggested that storytelling could be encouraged as a tool for producing more reflective practitioners, and could help to mitigate loss of identity, and the impoverishment of role models and collegial networks. Thus, community mental health nurses would develop a greater sense of their own identity and a sense of community with their fellow professionals in what is recognised as potentially isolating and extremely challenging work.

Finally, there are opportunities for community mental health nurses to become actively involved in using the creative arts in their own practice, either by working as co-therapists with professional creative arts therapists or by becoming involved in community arts initiatives. Community mental health nurses can only be enriched by involvement in the creative arts, whether this be through artistic work alongside patients, or through arts activities for their own personal or professional development.

# REFERENCES

Ansdell, G. (2001) 'Music therapist's dilemma', *British Journal of Music Therapy*, 15 (1): 3.

Ansdell, G. and Pavlicevic, M. (2001) *Beginning research in the arts therapies – a practical guide*, London: Jessica Kingsley.

Barker, A. (1995) *Creativity for managers*, London: The Industrial Society.

Bowles, N. (1995) 'Story telling: a search for meaning within nursing practice', *Nurse Education Today*, 15: 365–369.

Bunt, L. (1994) *Music therapy: an art beyond words*, London: Routledge.

Clarke, L. (1999) *Challenging ideas in psychiatric nursing*, London: Routledge.

Cropley, A.J. (2001) *Creativity in education and learning: a guide for teachers and educators*, London: Kogan Page.

Everett, M. (2000) 'Organised chaos', *Mental Health Care*, 3 (5): 154–155.

Gillam, T. (2002) *Reflections on community psychiatric nursing*, London: Routledge.

Gutkind, L. (1997) *The art of creative non-fiction: writing and selling the literature of reality*, New York: Wiley.

Mason, P. (1999) 'Charting success', *Mental Health Nursing*, 19 (1): 30–31.

Sacks, O. (1986) *The man who mistook his wife for a hat*, London: Picador.

Sternberg, R.J. (1988) *The nature of creativity*, New York: Cambridge University Press.

Thomson, M. (1989) *On art and therapy: an exploration*, London: Virago Press.

Warren, B. (ed.) (1993) *Using the creative arts in therapy: a practical introduction*, 2nd edn, London: Routledge.

# FURTHER READING

Cropley, A.J. (2001) *Creativity in education and learning: a guide for teachers and educators*, London: Kogan Page.

More than simply a guide for teachers and educators, a very comprehensive, rigorous and authoritative overview of creativity.

Warren, B. (ed.) (1993) *Using the creative arts in therapy: a practical introduction*, 2nd edn, London: Routledge.

A wide-ranging, inspiring overview which provides a theoretical rationale for creative therapy, followed by practical chapters on various arts therapies including visual arts, dance, drama, storytelling and puppetry.

Bunt, L. (1994) *Music therapy: an art beyond words*, London: Routledge.

A definitive text on music therapy which explains the purposes and techniques and emphasises the need for a strong research base and the synthesis of artistic and scientific processes.

# CHAPTER 25

# WORKING WITH MENTALLY DISORDERED OFFENDERS

*Michael Coffey*

## SUMMARY OF KEY POINTS

- Mentally disordered offenders may be mental health service users who have committed criminal offences ranging from the petty to the serious, or career criminals who develop mental illness while on remand or following sentencing.

- The profession of psychiatry, while having an important role to play in the care and treatment of mentally disordered offenders, should acknowledge the important input provided by other professions.

- Community mental health nurses should recognise and support the role of informal carers and relatives as an important element within the social support networks of these service users.

## INTRODUCTION

Community mental health nurses, of whatever specialism, are frequently called upon to work with people with mental health problems who have come to the attention of the criminal justice system. These service users are the somewhat contentiously titled 'mentally disordered offenders', and for want of a more accurate title I will resort to its use here. Mentally disordered offenders are not a homogeneous grouping, and the service users who might be grouped under this category will suffer from a range of mental health problems, and have committed offences ranging from petty nuisances to more serious offences of violent assault and homicide. As such, the type of service responses required will necessarily vary, as will the demands of therapy versus public safety. Whilst recognising this diversity in the client group, this chapter will focus upon service users convicted for a serious offence who have a mental illness of a degree that requires continuing mental health service support. For community mental health nurses there will be understandable concern about working with 'forensic' patients, a term that invokes no small amount of anxiety in most professionals. It is with this in mind that I will explore what it is we know about these service users, what models of practice are evidenced to work and what demands these might place on community mental health nurses. In doing so I shall cast a critical eye over the process of working with mentally disordered offenders in the community and highlight some research issues for the future.

The Reed Report (Department of Health/Home Office 1992) was largely responsible for the development of modern forensic community mental health services. Its emphasis on providing services of no greater security than justified by the risk posed by the individual essentially paved the way for forensic service development. Since this report was published there has been steady development of medium and low secure services and a consequent rise in the number of forensic community mental health nurses (Brooker and White 1997). This development, while providing support to generic community mental health teams, has also provided an enhanced route for the movement of mentally disordered offenders back into mainstream services.

## WHO IS THE MENTALLY DISORDERED OFFENDER?

A number of questions might reasonably be asked at the outset, including: who are mentally disordered offenders, what and who defines them, is this changing and if so why? The literature gives a number of responses in this regard.

Shepherd (1993) has suggested that the mentally disordered offender is synonymous with the seriously mentally ill. So we might assume that mentally disordered offenders will have complex needs, will require long-term interventions and may be socially disadvantaged in much the same way as anyone with a serious mental illness. While this gives us some help in determining what sort of services these service users might require, it creates its own difficulties. Definition of exactly what is a serious mental illness is fraught with problems, not least because there is no one clear or unambiguous definition. Service responses for the seriously mentally ill are usually focused upon schizophrenia, and while not doubting the importance of providing services to this often neglected group, it remains the case that there is little evidence in support of extending these service responses to other conditions within the possible range of serious mental illness. One example of this is the *Building bridges* (Department of Health 1995) definition of serious mental illness which is so broad it could include service users with dementia and personality disorder. While there is some indication of potentially helpful interventions for personality disorder (see, for example, Norton and Hinshelwood 1996), these do not as yet include what are now becoming accepted as standard interventions for schizophrenia (see, for example, Chapters 19 and 20 in this volume). I say 'as yet' because there may indeed be some value in applying concepts such as stress vulnerability, with the aim of improving coping skills, to other groups. Returning to the issue of a definition of a mentally disordered offender, it has to be noted that much of this lies with who it is who is seeking to define them and for what purpose. There is a plurality here that we would do well to recognise, and, as much as psychiatry is keen to extend itself (for whatever reasons) into other areas of society, it has no monopoly in defining mentally disordered offenders (Webb 1999). So it is the case that many professions – for example, the police, solicitors and probation officers – have contact with people who have mental health problems and have committed criminal offences. What we can be clear about is that mentally disordered offenders are those people who have committed an offence serious enough to attract the attention of the criminal justice system in terms of arrest and arraignment, and who display a mental health problem of such magnitude that it is noticed by non-mental health professionals such that they request (in some liaison service models) the opinion of mental health professionals. This therefore includes career criminals who develop mental health problems as well as those with an enduring mental health problem who commit criminal offences either unrelated to their condition or as a direct result of their symptoms.

It is probably true to say that the make-up of mentally disordered populations seen by community mental health nurses is changing rapidly. Since the Reed Report (Department of Health/Home Office 1992) there has been a sharp increase in the number of medium secure services, and police and court liaison schemes and a consequent increase in the number of professionals in dedicated forensic community teams. This has meant that forensic psychiatry now attracts service users it would previously have been unable to serve. There is, however, another perspective on this process. Rose (1998, 2002) has suggested that the rise of risk thinking has also created a situation in which the net of supervision of offenders has been narrowed to ensure that smaller and smaller fish are caught. The practice of forensic psychiatry can therefore be conceptualised as a form of social control (Cohen 1985) or indeed public hygiene in which supposed deviants are removed from or controlled within the societal body. Whether this is a form of psychiatric imperialism or a case of psychiatry seeking validation by association with perhaps more valued disciplines – for example, law – is open to question. It is certainly true that many mental health services now creak under the burden of providing services to populations that would have been previously dealt with by the criminal justice system. Community mental health nurses will have on their caseloads service users who traditionally might have been considered forensic patients, as well as service users who have not followed a traditional route to mentally disordered offender status.

## AN EMERGING EVIDENCE BASE?

There is a range of data on mentally disordered offenders that provides some evidence of strategies that can be said to help when working with this client group. The evidence, it must be said, however, is limited not only by its depth but also by its range. Most studies of mentally disordered offenders focus on the demands of the profession of psychiatry. Some are interested only in a case-finding strategy, while others seek to follow up known service users and chart their 'outcomes'. In almost all cases the methodologies are quantitative and the theoretical orientation positivist. The evidence base is therefore limited to fixed interpretations of material events and often fails to acknowledge differing perspectives, personal experiences and their impact upon outcomes or indeed the influence of factors such as power within the application and receipt of forensic services.

The array of policy and service responses to service users whom services find difficult is indeed enormous. Conditional discharge, supervised discharge, probation with conditions of treatment, hybrid orders, psychosocial interventions, risk assessment practice, models of practice including specialised and integrated teams, the requirement for multi-agency liaison, the importance of team-working, and Home Office reporting requirements are all evident in this field of practice.

Traditional mentally disordered offenders will be those service users who were placed on a hospital order with restrictions by the courts and who have graduated through lower levels of security before their eventual return to the community. The risk of behaviours prompting recall to hospital among this group is often considered to be low and they are frequently seen to have learnt compliant behaviours. Gibbens and Robertson (1983), for example, conducted a fifteen-year follow-up study of men receiving hospital orders (without restriction) to determine outcomes. Of the 249 men still alive fifteen years later, 42 per cent had no court appearances, 28 per cent had one or two court appearances and 30 per cent had three or more. Offences following discharge included: homicide (n=2), arson (n=1), wounding with intent or grievous bodily harm (n=6) and aggravated bodily harm (n=24). Half of all convictions occurred within twelve months of leaving hospital. Based on this evidence, Gibbens and Robertson (1983) concluded that hospital orders did not fail to protect the public. More recently Home Office figures suggest that service users leaving hospital on conditional discharge have reconviction rates of approximately 12 per cent for any offence and 5 per cent for serious offences (Street 1998). During the study period in question Street found that 25 per cent of those on conditional discharge were recalled to hospital. This figure seems a relatively consistent finding (Dell and Grounds 1995, Kershaw *et al.* 1997) and no doubt has contributed to the low reconviction rates already indicated. Interesting as all of this undoubtedly is, we are no wiser now about what factors actually helped to produce such results, presuming that we can accept that hospital orders with restrictions are only one possible variable which might prevent recidivism. For instance, Pilgrim and Rogers (1999) suggest that it is the conservative discharge policy of the Special Hospital system that creates the illusion of discharged Special Hospital service users being less recidivistic than their counterparts leaving prison. The need for further exploration employing research strategies that transcend counting numbers might therefore be indicated.

So what of the newer clientele, the non-traditional forensic patients if you will? These will include service users who have spent little or no time in high-secure services, ex-prisoners and those subject to conditional bail or probationary licences. Dvoskin and Steadman (1994) argue that they will not have learnt compliant behaviours and are likely to be difficult to follow up and treat. They may regard services as their enemies and as such choose to avoid contact with the community mental health nurse. In these circumstances it has been the standard response of policy-makers to generate departmental guidance (Department of Health 1994) as well as primary legislation (Department of Health 1995) in an attempt to control those service users who, for whatever reason, choose to refuse mental health intervention. So what can CMHNs do about this? Whatever the advantages of assertive community treatment or the concerns that CMHNs are a *de facto* social police force (Coffey 1997, Rose 1998), it remains the case that service users can quite easily avoid contact with services just by refusing to be at home when the nurse calls. Defensive practice is not to be advocated as I believe it tends to narrow treatment options. That said, CMHNs would do well to remain informed of what the expectations are of them in performing their duties and recording what it is they do. Shutting the stable doors, however, can be a lonely experience and establishing meaningfully helpful relationships with service users might be one way of preventing this proverbial horse from bolting.

Many mentally disordered offenders are subject to restrictions and possible recall to hospital should they fail to comply with the conditions imposed upon them (Kershaw *et al.* 1997). This may be seen by some as leverage in securing compliance with treatment decisions, but many forensic community mental health nurses whilst recognising the pragmatic benefits of such legislation, are keen to acknowledge its limitations (Jenkins and Coffey 2002). These nurses have significant experience of supervising mentally disordered offenders in the community. They view the establishment and maintenance of the relationship with the service user, in which negotiation and collaboration are essential elements, as being of prime importance in the success of restriction orders. This is not surprising, as they are first and foremost mental health nurses and the emphasis on relationships is long-established within this field (Peplau 1988). What is surprising is that they seem relatively unaware of the potential effects of restriction orders upon the therapeutic relationships they have with service users (Jenkins and Coffey 2002). This may indicate that concerns about such coercive powers as expressed in the literature (Fulop 1995, MIND 1995, Coffey 1997, Godin and Scanlon 1997) do not have any real impact upon day-to-day clinical practice. More likely, however, it suggests that service users and nurses alike have learned to comply with a number of unspoken rules to facilitate the success of these arrangements. It has to be said that, despite these real concerns about extending more broadly coercive community treatment, conditional discharge seems to work. At least this appears to be the case in terms of reconviction rates, although these in themselves may not be the most accurate way of determining offending (see Abel *et al.* 1987 for a non-mental health example). It remains, however, that what we know about what works with mentally disordered offenders in the community is limited by the insufficient research that has addressed this specific population. A default position is therefore often adopted, and this is to address mentally disordered offenders in terms of serious mental illness. That is, if it works with serious mental illness, it will work with mentally disordered offenders. While this has its advantages, it ignores the many complex contextual issues that result from the combination of barriers to community reintegration that potentially arise for someone with a mental illness and a criminal record. Coupled with this, the yawning chasms of lapse into offending behaviour or relapse of the illness present significant anxieties that the service user must attend to. In addition, mentally disordered offenders as a group are likely to include service users with diagnoses of personality disorder, for which there is precious little research on providing community-based interventions. Service responses that directly address these anxieties, and they will be anxieties for the service user as much as anyone, will be required.

There are now a number of established models of community work with mentally disordered offenders (see Tighe *et al.* 2002). As yet, however, there is little resounding evidence to support any of these approaches, and it seems in many cases that an assertive outreach model, favoured for those with serious mental illness, may be most appropriate (Marshall and Lockwood 2000).

As indicated above, risk assessment and management are often the main focus of care of the mentally disordered offender. This emphasis is such that it is often difficult to find in many forensic texts anything else that could conservatively be described as treatment approaches. While this focus is understandable in the wake of violence perpetrated by the mentally ill, it is also perhaps misplaced (Taylor and Gunn 1999) and has attracted intelligent critique (Rose 2002). Andy Alaszewski offers an erudite reading of risk assessment and management in this volume (Chapter 16) and it has also been covered competently and comprehensively enough by other authors (see Doyle 2000) to allow me the opportunity to focus my attention elsewhere. For while risk assessment and management may be said to be important aspects of the role of CMHNs working with mentally disordered offenders, there are other areas of practice that receive far less attention than they deserve. One such area is that of social support of service users and their informal carers and relatives.

## INFORMAL CARERS AND SOCIAL SUPPORT

The role of informal carers and relatives of mentally disordered offenders may be regarded as a potentially crucial element in the success of returning to, and maintaining tenure in, the community. Perkins and Repper (1996) have likened the social support needs of the seriously mentally ill to the needs of the physically disabled in that both groups require assistance to negotiate the able-bodied world. This essentially advocates a social disability and access model. That is, mental illness or more accurately the consequences of mental illness create social disabilities, and as a result the person experiences social exclusion and requires help to facilitate access to the social world we all enjoy. Mentally disordered offenders, however, are additionally socially disadvantaged by their criminal history. They may, for example, be perceived as doubly deviant. This will restrict their reintegration into the community – for example, in terms of access to employment or, indeed, return to their own communities. Informal carers and relatives of service users can provide many opportunities for reintegration and CMHNs should be prepared to work with them to ensure the successful return and maintenance of community living. This is perhaps the most important element of community mental health nursing of mentally disordered offenders. It is at least as important as any monitoring function that might be perceived to hold precedence.

So what is social support and what can CMHNs reasonably provide? Thoits (1982, p. 147) defines social supports as 'the degree to which a person's basic social needs are gratified through interaction with others'. Basic social needs include affection, esteem or approval, belonging, identity and security. These may be met either by the provision of socio-emotional aid (affection, sympathy and understanding, acceptance and esteem from a significant other), or by the provision of instrumental aid (advice, information, help with family or work responsibilities, financial aid). Tanzman (1993) considered the need for 'material' supports among the mentally ill and suggested that service users themselves are aware that their ability to manage at an optimum level of independence in the community is dependent upon other supports and services. Support for the mentally ill, it seems, should be an inclusive term that incorporates assistance with money management, advice about daytime activities, and emotional support, as well as working with people to achieve their treatment goals. Support such as this is considered to be essential in facilitating recovery from mental illness and the consequences of mental illness (Hatfield and Lefley 1993). For mentally disordered offenders it may provide the element of hope considered fundamental to establishing their recovery (Kirkpatrick *et al.* 2001).

Informal care-givers will often meet many support needs and CMHNs must strive to facilitate the development and maintenance of social support networks in this group. Macinnes (2000) has suggested that problems of burden, coping and personal support of carers by friends and the wider community are important foci for mental health nurses. Informal carers are an important source of social support for mentally disordered offenders and as such CMHNs should focus attention on facilitating and supporting this role. They can do this by offering education to relatives and informal carers on mental illness as well as the factors that support recovery. Formal and informal support groups of carers and relatives should be supported by CMHNs and financed by health and social care services to enable the sharing of experiences and to provide opportunities for learning from each other.

Social support may help mentally disordered offenders to successfully remain in the community; however, Suls (1982) has indicated that social support may also have negative consequences and CMHNs will need to be aware of these (Box 25.1). This is not to suggest that social support should be treated with caution but rather that CMHNs should be mindful that it is rarely value-neutral. Despite the potentially negative elements of social support, there are other benefits to be gained in improving social supports among mentally disordered offenders. There are some data which suggest for instance that social supports may help in reducing violent behaviour among those mentally ill persons who can be a danger to others (Estroff *et al.* 1994). Simply providing an improved social network, however, may not be sufficient. Lazarus and Folkman (1984) have pointed out that the ability to draw on social support is itself a coping skill, and, as such, poor social skills or illness-related symptoms may reduce this ability. We may therefore have to work with service users to enhance their use of these skills.

---

**Box 25.1   Potential negative consequences of socially supportive relationships**

- Creating uncertainty and worry
- Setting a bad example
- Negative labelling
- Giving misleading information
- Discouraging compliance
- Negative social comparisons
- Creating dependence

(Suls 1982)

---

## CONCLUSION

Community mental health nursing services working with mentally disordered offenders have many opportunities for future development. These might include the development of inreach services to prisons to facilitate, among other things, better post-release support to mentally disordered offenders leaving prison. While we might be concerned about the quality of discharge planning in our health services, there is almost a complete absence of discharge planning in relation to prison. This appears to be a combination of mental health services' inflexibility and the prison service's almost obsessive concern with confidentiality as a cover for anxiety about security. Added to this is the tendency for the prison service to routinely move prisoners to prisons many miles away, which further complicates communication and ease of post-release follow-up. One potential response to this may be provided by inreach services, but better liaison with colleagues in the probation service would probably reduce this problem. Mental health services, however, will have to be prepared to act promptly when informed of release, and the flexibility of CMHNs can be seen as a strength in this regard.

An enhanced focus upon the care and treatment of mentally disordered offenders in the pre-registration training of mental health nurses is necessary. This needs to take account of issues of risk but must also examine the role of power, coercion and control within service provision, so that mental health nurses do not adopt uncritically responses to service users which further disempower and reduce their options for the future.

There are numerous opportunities for future research in this area of community mental health nursing. For example, there is little formal study of mentally disordered offenders' experiences of the process of rehabilitation, their recovery or indeed their return to community living under supervision. Coupled with this we know little about their families and carers' experiences and what additional and unique factors might exist for them in supporting their family member. The community care of mentally disordered offenders (as with most mental illness) falls most heavily on families and informal carers. CMHNs should be mindful of this and attempt to adopt strategies that will lessen this burden.

# REFERENCES

Abel, G.G., Becker, J.V., Mittelman, M., Cunningham-Rathner, J., Rouleau, J.L. and Murphy, W.D. (1987) 'Self-reported sex crimes of non-incarcerated paraphiliacs', *Journal of Interpersonal Violence*, 2 (1): 3–25.

Brooker, C. and White, E. (1997) *The fourth quinquennial national community mental health nursing census of England and Wales*, Manchester and Keele: Universities of Manchester and Keele.

Coffey, M. (1997) 'Supervised discharge: concerns about the new powers for nurses', *British Journal of Nursing*, 6 (4): 215–218.

Cohen, S. (1985) *Visions of social control*, Cambridge: Polity Press.

Dell, S. and Grounds, A. (1995) *The discharge and supervision of restricted patients*, Report to the Home Office, London: Home Office.

Department of Health/Home Office (1992) *Review of health and social services for mentally disordered offenders and others requiring similar services* (The Reed Report), London: HMSO.

Department of Health (1994) *Introduction of supervision registers for mentally ill people from 1 April 1994*, HSG(94)5, London: NHS Management Executive.

Department of Health (1995) *Building bridges: a guide to arrangements for interagency working for the care and protection of severely mentally ill people*, London: Department of Health.

Doyle, M. (2000) 'Risk assessment and management', in Chaloner, C. and Coffey, M. (eds) (2000) *Forensic mental health nursing: current approaches*, Oxford: Blackwell.

Dvoskin, J.A. and Steadman, H.J. (1994) 'Using intensive case management to reduce violence by mentally ill persons in the community', *Hospital and Community Psychiatry*, 45 (7): 679–684.

Estroff, S., Zimmer, C., Lachicotte, W. and Benoit, J. (1994) 'The influence of social networks and social support on violence by persons with serious mental illness', *Hospital and Community Psychiatry*, 45: 669–679.

Fulop, N. (1995) 'Supervised discharge: lessons from the U.S. experience', *Mental Health Nursing*, 15 (3): 16–20.

Gibbens, T.C.N. and Robertson, G. (1983) 'A survey of the criminal careers of hospital order patients', *British Journal of Psychiatry*, 143: 362–369.

Godin, P. and Scanlon, R. (1997) 'Supervision and control: a community psychiatric nursing perspective', *Journal of Mental Health*, 6 (1): 75–84.

Hatfield, A.B. and Lefley, H.P. (1993) *Surviving mental illness: stress, coping and adaptation*, New York: Guilford Press.

Jenkins, E. and Coffey, M. (2002) 'Compelled to interact: forensic community mental health nurses and service users relationships', *Journal of Psychiatric and Mental Health Nursing*, 9 (5): 553–562.

Kershaw, C., Dowdeswell, P. and Goodman, J. (1997) *Restricted patients – reconvictions and recalls by the end of 1995: England and Wales*, Home Office Statistical Bulletin 1/97, London: Home Office.

Kirkpatrick, H., Landeen, J., Woodside, H. and Byrne, C. (2001) 'How people with schizophrenia build their hope', *Journal of Psychosocial Nursing*, 39 (1): 46–53.

Lazarus, R.S. and Folkman, S. (1984) *Stress, appraisal and coping*, New York: Springer.

Macinnes, D. (2000) 'Relatives and informal caregivers', in Chaloner, C. and Coffey, M. (eds) *Forensic mental health nursing: current approaches*, Oxford: Blackwell.

Marshall, M. and Lockwood, A. (2000) *Assertive community treatment for people with severe mental disorders* (Cochrane review), in The Cochrane Library, Issue 4, Oxford: Update Software.

MIND (1995) *Care not coercion*, Position Paper, London: MIND.

Norton, K. and Hinshelwood, R.D. (1996) 'Severe personality disorders. Treatment issues and selection for in-patient psychotherapy', *British Journal of Psychiatry*, 168 (6): 723–731.

Peplau, H. (1988) *Interpersonal relations in nursing: a conceptual frame of reference for psychodynamic nursing*, Basingstoke: Macmillan.

Perkins, R. and Repper, J. (1996) *Working alongside people with long-term mental health problems*, London: Chapman and Hall.

Pilgrim, D. and Rogers, A. (1999) *A sociology of mental health and illness*, 2nd edn, Buckingham: Open University Press.

Rose, N. (1998) 'Living dangerously – risk thinking and risk management', *Mental Health Care*, 1 (8): 263–266.

Rose, N. (2002) 'Society, madness and control', in Buchanan, A. (ed) *Care of the mentally disordered offender in the community*, Oxford: Oxford University Press.

Shepherd, G. (1993) 'Case management', in Watson, W. and Grounds, A. (eds) *The mentally disordered offender in an era of community care: new directions in provision*, Cambridge: Cambridge University Press.

Street, R. (1998) *The restricted hospital order: from court to the community*, Research Study 186, London: Home Office.

Suls, J. (1982) 'Social support, interpersonal relations and health: benefits and liabilities', in Sanders, G.S. and Suls, J. (eds) *Social psychology of health and illness*, Mahwah, NJ: Lawrence Erlbaum Associates.

Tanzman, B. (1993) 'An overview of surveys of mental health consumers' preferences for housing and support services', *Hospital and Community Psychiatry*, 44 (5): 450–454.

Taylor, P.J. and Gunn, J. (1999) 'Homicides by people with mental illness: myth and reality', *British Journal of Psychiatry*, 174: 9–14.

Thoits, P.A. (1982) 'Conceptual, methodological and theoretical problems in studying social support as a buffer against life stress', *Journal of Health and Social Behaviour*, 23: 145–159.

Tighe, J., Henderson, C. and Thornicroft, G. (2002) 'Mentally disordered offenders and models of community care provision', in Buchanan, A. (ed.) *Care of the mentally disordered offender in the community*, Oxford: Oxford University Press.

Webb, D. (1999) 'A balance of possibilities', in Webb, D. and Harris, D. (eds) *Mentally disordered offenders: managing people nobody owns*, London: Routledge.

# FURTHER READING

Buchanan, A. (ed.) *Care of the mentally disordered offender in the community*, Oxford: Oxford University Press.

An excellent if limited text on the community care of mentally disordered offenders. It combines real critique with an attempt at comprehensiveness and includes a discussion on the relationship between forensic and generic services. Its main weakness is the absence of any acknowledgement of forensic community mental health nursing or the role of informal carers as central elements of the social support networks of these service users.

Chaloner, C. and Coffey, M. (eds) (2000) *Forensic mental health nursing: current approaches*, Oxford: Blackwell.

This text is written exclusively by forensic nurses for forensic nurses. It covers the main areas of work of forensic mental health nurses and offers many recommendations for the treatment of mentally disordered offenders and suggestions for future research by forensic mental health nurses.

Webb, D. and Harris, D. (eds) *Mentally disordered offenders: managing people nobody owns*, London: Routledge.

For an excellent treatment of the issues from a non-psychiatric viewpoint you could do worse than this book. David Webb and Robert Harris have in this text produced a thoughtful, sensitive and robustly articulated account of the issues involved in providing services for mentally disordered offenders. They take as their guiding hand the influential Hershel Prins, and this book, while an acknowledged homage to their mentor, is a valuable work in its own right. The chapter by Paul Cavadino on diversion is one that I have frequently found particularly useful.

Further resources for forensic nurses: Phil Woods has developed an online resource – The Forensic Nursing Resource Homepage can be found at http://www.fnrh.freeserve.co.uk and includes many useful links to other forensic resources.

# CHAPTER 26

# WORKING WITH PEOPLE WITH COEXISTING MENTAL HEALTH AND SUBSTANCE MISUSE PROBLEMS

*Jeff Champney-Smith*

## SUMMARY OF KEY POINTS

- Coexisting mental health and substance misuse problems are increasing and present a challenge to the community mental health nurse.

- Although evidence of effectiveness in managing this client group is limited, there are a number of interventions that services can adopt.

- Brief, motivational interventions delivered at appropriate times can help individuals to modify their substance use.

## INTRODUCTION

Community mental health nurses (CMHNs) are increasingly coming into contact with individuals who have problems with both their substance use and mental health. Such clients often have poorer outcomes in relation to cessation or reduction of substance use and present workers with more challenges with regard to their mental health. Furthermore, working with dually diagnosed clients may compound feelings of stress and 'burnout' experienced by CMHNs who feel that the substance use problem is outside their expertise (Maslin *et al.* 2001).

The use of diagnostic labels such as dual diagnosis and comorbidity, to describe this group of people, is the subject of some controversy. Manley (1998) points out that, as in practice individuals rarely receive a formal diagnosis of both mental illness and substance misuse, the term 'dual diagnosis' may be considered a 'misnomer'. However, either term (dual diagnosis or comorbidity) is useful at present to identify those individuals whose combination of problems often leads to them being less than adequately served by existing services. The literature on the subject of dual diagnosis is usually written from the point of view of either substance misuse or mental health, and little research into dual diagnosis as a specific diagnostic category has been undertaken. Furthermore, Petersen (1998) argues that if the term is applied carefully and with forethought, closer working relationships between substance use services and general mental health services may be fostered.

In an attempt to describe the nature of dual diagnosis, Zimberg (1999) defines three types of coexisting mental health and substance use problems:

- Type 1 – a primary mental health problem with a substance use disorder which becomes apparent only when the person is experiencing mental ill health symptoms, i.e. the substance is used as self-medication by the client to enable them to cope with or obliterate symptoms.
- Type 2 – primary substance misuse with substance-induced mental health problems; for example, the amphetamine user who develops 'amphetamine psychosis'.
- Type 3 – Mental health and substance misuse problems coexisting in the same individual over a long period of time (considered by Zimberg to be 'true' dual diagnosis).

## PREVALENCE AND INCIDENCE

There is evidence to suggest that the incidence of dual diagnosis has increased over time. A study of two cohorts of admissions to a psychiatric hospital in Nottingham, 1978–80 and 1992–4, noted a particular increase in drug-related psychosis in the later sample (Brewin *et al.* 1997). Smith and Hucker (1993) suggest that the increase may be due to two factors. First, the increased exposure of individuals with mental health problems to illicit drug and alcohol use as a consequence of reduced hospitalisation brought about by community care programmes. Second, the increase in alcohol use and experimentation with illegal drugs in the general population.

Evidence from the Epidemiological Catchment Area Study (ECAS) undertaken in the United States of America (Regier *et al.* 1990) showed an 83 per cent diagnosis of substance misuse in individuals with personality disorder, and 47 per cent in those diagnosed with schizophrenia. The overall rate of substance misuse in those with a mental illness was 29 per cent, estimated to be 2.7 times higher than in the general populace. Rates of mental illness in individuals with substance misuse were found to be similarly high: 53 per cent in drug users and 37 per cent in alcohol abusers, 4.7 and 7 times the rate for the rest of the sample. From these figures it was estimated that substance misusers with a comorbid mental illness made 62 per cent of 56.3 million visits to walk-in psychiatric services.

Another US study showed that up to 53 per cent of psychiatric service users with a diagnosis of schizophrenia have been identified as also having an alcohol-related problem (Drake *et al.* 1990). Nearly half (44 per cent) of amphetamine users in an Australian study showed significant psychological problems. This result correlated highly with an individual's transition from the oral route to the intravenous injection of amphetamine (Hall *et al.* 1996).

## UK STUDIES

There have been few studies published looking at UK populations. A sample of 171 individuals with a psychotic illness in south London revealed a prevalence rate of 36.3 per cent for drug and alcohol problems (Menezes *et al.* 1996). Young males were identified as being the most likely to have substance misuse problems. In the two-year period preceding the study it was found that clients with substance misuse problems spent almost twice as long in hospital as those without such problems.

In a study of mental health and addiction services in East Dorset, Virgo *et al.* (2001) found an occurrence of coexisting serious mental illness and substance abuse or dependence in 12 per cent of both addiction and mental health clients. Notably, however, in the mental health sample dual diagnosis occurred more in younger males. The psychiatric diagnoses tended to differ in the addiction and mental health samples; affective disorders were more prominent in the addiction sample and schizophrenia less. The main drugs of misuse in the mental health sample were alcohol and cannabis. Virgo *et al.* (2001) also noted that those with a dual diagnosis presented with more complex and severe problems. Significant mental health problems were identified in opiate-dependent and amphetamine-dependent attendees at a substance misuse clinic in Cardiff (Barrowcliff *et al.* 1999).

Subject to the type of assessments used and the nature of the research samples, up to two-thirds of individuals with alcohol dependence have been identified as having coexistent psychopathology (Davidson and Ritson 1993). The most common disorders are antisocial personality disorder and affective disorder, with women being more affected by both conditions than men.

When considering prevalence and incidence data it should be remembered that the diagnostic criteria used, and the awareness of, knowledge of and ability to assess both substance use and mental health problems will impact on the reliability of statistics. Statistics also need to be considered in relation to geography and sample type. Urban studies centred on areas of deprivation where social drift and transience are high may show different results to rural or affluent areas and more stationary populations.

## FORENSIC IMPORTANCE

The role of substance use in violent crime is an important one and is often overlooked. Ward and Applin (1998) examined seventeen reports into murders committed by mentally ill individuals in the UK and found that thirteen involved significant substance misuse, though only one mentioned this as a contributory factor in the murder. The failure to recognise the role of substance misuse in these cases demonstrates a failure to give sufficient credence to the existence and the potentially dangerous outcomes of dual diagnoses.

## SUBSTANCES OF MISUSE

Alcohol and cannabis have been shown to be the substances used most commonly by people with mental health problems. Studies of the prevalence of comorbidity show two distinct patterns of substance misuse identified in individuals diagnosed with schizophrenia: one the use of high levels of alcohol and cannabis with little or no other drug use; the other, the use of a number of substances, including alcohol and cannabis, in combination (Cuffel *et al.* 1993). However, it is as well to remember that, as Gournay *et al.* point out:

> there is clearly a great deal of heterogeneity in this area and the types of substances used are obviously determined by availability and cultural variations. Furthermore, there is a need to investigate the similarities and differences between populations who use single drugs, such as alcohol or cannabis, and populations that show multiple use.
>
> (Gournay *et al.* 1997, p. 90)

Recent changes in substance misuse patterns, notably the rise of alcohol, opiate and crack cocaine use, may reflect on future studies. The impact of these increases on both specialist and generic mental health services is certain to further compound the problems faced by nurses. It is imperative that policy-makers are responsive and flexible enough to ensure that adequate provision is made in anticipation of these changes.

Cannabis ingestion, often not considered 'problematic' in society, can have a significant effect on mental health and treatment outcomes, including increase in negative symptoms, more severe symptoms and more likely relapse (Martinez-Arevalo *et al.* 1994). Changes in UK law with regard to cannabis use will almost certainly lead to more social acceptance of the drug. The CMHN will be presented with a challenge when attempting to negotiate reduced cannabis use as a means of reducing symptoms and preventing relapse, particularly with young people suffering from schizophrenia.

The chicken and egg 'which comes first' question needs consideration. Allan (1995) found convincing evidence that alcohol use is likely to be a causative factor in the development of anxiety disorders. However, Davidson and Ritson (1993) suggested caution when interpreting their findings that affective disorders remit after detoxification and subsequent abstinence from alcohol. They argued that confusion over what constitutes a dual diagnosis, and a failure to differentiate between current and lifetime diagnosis of depression have led to an 'overstatement' of the relationship between alcoholism and affective disorder.

Siegfried (1998) notes that dual diagnosis is also associated with increased uptake of services, violence, non-compliance with treatment, involvement with the criminal justice system and social deprivation. Despite the high prevalence and increased morbidity associated with dual diagnosis, detection remains low and both specialist and generic services have failed to adopt flexible responses to the problem. The continued arguments with regard to the appropriateness of terminology do little to address this issue, as Leahy and Hawker contend:

> our concern as mental health workers should not be to debate whether certain people suffer a certain syndrome known as 'dual diagnosis', but rather how we can ensure that individuals with these intensive and complex problems are able to access a service which understands and responds appropriately to their multiple needs.
>
> (Leahy and Hawker 1998, p. 275)

## TREATMENT

Gournay *et al.* (1997) proposed that the current situation in the United States offers a model for the development of UK services, suggesting that the co-existence of mental illness and substance misuse problems is best approached in an integrated manner. The development of a service specifically designed for individuals with coexistent mental health and substance use problems, based in seven community mental health centres (CMHC) in New Hampshire, is described by Drake and Noordsy (1994). The authors suggest a model of care where caseworkers have twenty-four-hour responsibility for a small number of clients. Interventions are delivered both individually and in group settings. A non-confrontational approach is utilised that does not require immediate abstinence. The programme is described as being stepwise, comprising:

* engagement
* persuasion
* treatment
* relapse prevention.

Drake *et al.* (1998) conducted a comparison study of clients involved in the New Hampshire programme. One hundred and fourteen received standard case management (SCM) treatment, 109 assertive community outreach (ACO). ACO differed from SCM in that caseworkers had smaller caseloads (typically twelve). This allowed workers time to engage individuals more often and for longer periods. Interventions included helping with finances, taking people to work, encouraging access to community facilities, etc. Results, evaluated via validated substance use and quality of life measures, suggested little difference in outcome for both groups. However, the researchers noted a reduction in the severity of substance use and a reduction in the necessity for hospitalisation in the ACO group. The model of assertive outreach currently favoured by many mental health services and providing the basis of UK dual diagnosis projects is similarly constituted (Dodd 2001).

Alleviation of the tensions between traditional bio-psychosocial and rehabilitation mental health treatments and the recovery model favoured by some substance misuse services is the underlying principle in treatment programmes for dually diagnosed clients proposed by Minkoff (1989). The process of harmonisation between the philosophies of traditional mental health services and the recovery model employed by addiction services is described. Four treatment stages are identified:

- acute stabilisation
- engagement
- prolonged stabilisation
- rehabilitation

It is argued that, during the four phases, traditional psychiatric and addiction treatments should be offered alongside each other. Harmonisation should be achieved through a process of education of clinical staff in the particular philosophies of each treatment model, constant validation of treatment methods and practical demonstration of treatment efficacy.

Motivation has been identified as a potential source of treatment matching in individuals with schizophrenia and coexistent substance misuse (Ziedonis and Trudeau 1997). It is suggested that low motivation is matched to harm minimisation outcomes and high motivation to abstinence. A residential setting has been incorporated into one approach (Clenaghan *et al.* 1996). An innovative residential treatment programme supplements the principles of integrated services, intensive case management and assertive outreach for dually diagnosed clients.

Of the integrated treatment approaches described thus far, only the New Hampshire model (Teague *et al.* 1995) has been evaluated. A particular strength of the project is the adoption of a bio-psychosocial model. Manley (1998) argues that the adoption of the bio-psychosocial model requires clinicians to understand and be experienced in both mental health problems and alcohol and substance misuse problems.

Gournay *et al.* (1997) believe that the training in case management and psychosocial interventions provided by such training programmes as the Thorn initiative (Butterworth 1994) could be supplemented with specific training in assessment, group methods and motivation enhancement techniques required in the treatment of substance misusers.

## EFFECTIVENESS

A recent Cochrane review of effective interventions for dual diagnosis (Ley *et al.* 2000) found little evidence suggesting the effectiveness of any particular treatment over any other. However, Siegfried (1998) suggests that there is enough consensus to suggest that integrated mental health and substance misuse services offering tolerant, non-confrontational approaches offer the best and most appropriate way forward for those people with a dual diagnosis.

In summary, although evidence of effectiveness in managing this client group is limited, there are a number of options services may consider:

- comprehensive assessment of both mental health and substance use problems;
- shared risk assessment and risk management protocols;
- training for mental health workers in the recognition and management of substance use problems;
- training for substance misuse workers in the recognition and management of mental health problems;
- interventions that are non-judgemental, flexible and take account of the principles of harm minimisation;
- assertive outreach approaches;
- clear understanding of roles and responsibilities;
- good liaison between agencies, clearly identifying which has the lead responsibility;
- development of care pathways and a range of outcome measures.

The importance of early risk assessment and effective risk management cannot be over-emphasised. This client group demonstrates an increase in aggressive behaviour, suicide, self-harm and HIV infection. Many homicides committed by those with a mental illness have a significant substance use component.


## CONCLUSION

It is clear that the increasing coexistence of substance misuse and mental illness presents a challenge to both substance misuse services and generic mental health services. Although evidence for effective interventions is limited, enough consensus exists to suggest that integrated services offer the best way forward in terms of treatment and assessment. The Department of Health (2002) advises that integrated care should be delivered within mental health services supported by specialist dual diagnosis and substance misuse services.

For CMHNs involved with this client group on a face-to-face basis the challenge is to provide appropriate interventions tailored to the needs of such individuals. Use of brief, motivational interventions at appropriate times may impact positively on problem substance use. However, this may not always be possible. Constraints imposed by service philosophies and practical barriers, such as waiting lists, caseload size and complexity, working hours, geography, discharge criteria, etc., can prove difficult to work within.

Practitioners in both mental health and substance misuse services need to increase their knowledge of current research into this problem. Increased knowledge levels may enhance practitioners' confidence in dealing with clients with a dual diagnosis, and work towards improving attitudes. Practitioners should be prepared to question and challenge established practice. It is essential that research into this increasing problem continues. Of particular importance is the continuing evaluation of the effectiveness of treatment programmes. Contemporary developments such as GP and psychiatric liaison services, closer links with the criminal justice system and the current strategic emphasis on partnership working may help pave the way for future change.

# REFERENCES

Allan, C. (1995) 'Alcohol problems and anxiety disorders – a critical review', *Alcohol and Alcoholism*, 30 (2): 145–151.

Barrowcliff, A., Champney-Smith, J. and McBride, A. (1999) 'The Opiate Treatment Index (OTI): treatment assessment with a Welsh sample of opiate prescribed or amphetamine prescribed clients', *Journal of Substance Use*, 4 (4): 98–103.

Brewin, J., Cantwell, R., Dalkin, T., Fox, R., Medley, I., Glazebrook, C., Kwiecinski, R. and Harrison, G. (1997) 'Incidence of schizophrenia in Nottingham: a comparison of two cohorts, 1978–80 and 1992–94', *British Journal of Psychiatry*, 171: 140–144.

Butterworth, T. (1994) 'Developing research ideas from theory to practice: psychosocial interventions as a case example', *Nurse Researcher*, 1: 78–87.

Clenaghan, P., Rosen, A. and Colechin, A. (1996) 'Serious mental illness and problematic substance use', *Journal of Substance Misuse*, 1: 199–204.

Cuffel, B., Heithoff, K. and Lawson, W. (1993) 'Correlates of patterns of substance abuse among patients with schizophrenia', *Hospital and Community Psychiatry*, 44 (3): 247–251.

Davidson, K. and Ritson, B. (1993) 'The relationship between alcohol dependence and depression', *Alcohol and Alcoholism*, 28: 147–155.

Department of Health (2002) *Dual diagnosis good practice guide*, London: Department of Health.

Dodd, T. (2001) 'Clues about evidence for mental health care in community settings: assertive outreach', *Mental Health Practice*, 41 (7): 10–14.

Drake, R. and Noordsy, D. (1994) 'Case management for people with co-existing severe mental disorder and substance use disorder', *Psychiatric Annals*, 24: 427–431.

Drake, R., Osher, F. and Noordsy, D. (1990) 'Diagnosis of alcohol use disorders in schizophrenia', *Schizophrenia Bulletin*, 16 (1): 57–67.

Drake, R., McHugo, G., Clark, R., Teague, G., Xie, H., Miles, K. and Ackerson, T. (1998) 'Assertive community outreach for patients with co-occurring severe mental illness and substance use disorder: a clinical trial', *American Journal of Orthopsychiatry*, 68 (2): 201–215.

Gournay, K., Sandford, T., Johnson, S. and Thornicroft, G. (1997) 'Dual diagnosis of severe mental health problems and substance abuse/misuse: a major priority for mental health nursing', *Journal of Psychiatric and Mental Health Nursing*, 4: 89–95.

Hall, W., Hando, J., Darke, S. and Ross, J. (1996) 'Psychological morbidity and route of administration among amphetamine users in Sydney, Australia', *Addiction*, 91 (1): 81–87.

Leahy, N. and Hawker, R. (1998) 'Re-inventing the wheel', *Mental Health Care*, 1 (8): 275.

Ley, A., Jeffrey, D.P., McLaren, S. and Siegfried, N. (2000) *Treatment programmes for people with both severe mental illness and substance misuse* (Cochrane review), in The Cochrane Library, Issue 1, Oxford: Update Software.

Manley, D. (1998) 'Dual diagnosis: approaches to the treatment of people with dual mental health and drug abuse problems', *Mental Health Care*, 11 (6): 190–192.

Martinez-Arevalo, M., Calcedo-Ordoñez, A. and Varo-Prieto, J. (1994) 'Cannabis consumption as a prognostic factor in schizophrenia', *British Journal of Psychiatry*, 164: 679–681.

Maslin, J., Graham, H., Cawley, M., Copello, A., Birchwood, M., Georgiou, G., McGovern, D., Mueser, K. and Orford, J. (2001) 'Combined severe mental health and substance use problems: what are the training needs of staff working with this client group?', *Journal of Mental Health*, 10 (2): 131–140.

Menezes, P., Johnson, S., Thornicroft, G., Marshall, J., Prosser, D., Bebbington, P. and

Kuipers, E. (1996) 'Drug and alcohol problems among individuals with severe mental illness in south London', *British Journal of Psychiatry*, 168: 612–619.

Minkoff, K. (1989) 'An integrated treatment model for dual diagnosis of psychosis and addiction', *Hospital and Community Psychiatry*, 40 (10): 1031–1036.

Petersen, T. (1998) 'Is "dual diagnosis" a useful term?', *Nursing Times*, 94 (37): 56–57.

Regier, D.S., Farmer, N. and Rae, D. (1990) 'Co-morbidity of mental disorders with alcohol and other drugs of abuse: results from the Epidemiological Catchment Area (ECA)', *Journal of American Medical Association*, 264: 2511–2518.

Siegfried, N. (1998) 'A review of comorbidity: major mental illness and problematic substance use', *Australian and New Zealand Journal of Psychiatry*, 32: 707–717.

Smith, J. and Hucker, S. (1993) 'Dual diagnosis patients: substance abuse by the severely mentally ill', *British Journal of Hospital Medicine*, 50 (11): 650–654.

Teague, G., Drake, R. and Ackerson, T. (1995) 'Evaluating use of continuous treatment teams for persons with mental illness and substance abuses', *Psychiatric Services*, 46 (7): 689–695.

Virgo, N., Bennett, G., Higgins, D., Bennett, L. and Thomas, P. (2001) 'The prevalence and characteristics of co-occurring serious mental illness (SMI) and substance abuse or dependence in the patients of adult mental health and addictions services in eastern Dorset', *Journal of Mental Health*, 10 (2): 175–188.

Ward, M. and Applin, C. (1998) *The unlearned lesson: the role of alcohol and drug misuse in inquiries into homicides by people with mental health problems*, Ware: Wynne Howard Books.

Ziedonis, D.M. and Trudeau, K. (1997) 'Motivation to quit using substances among individuals with schizophrenia: implications for a motivation-based treatment model', *Schizophrenia Bulletin*, 23 (2): 229–238.

Zimberg, S. (1999) 'A dual diagnosis typology to improve diagnosis and treatment of dual disorder patients', *Journal of Psychoactive Drugs*, 31 (1): 47–51.

# FURTHER READING

Gossop, M. (2001) *Living with drugs*, Aldershot: Ashgate.
Well-written and easy to read, a balanced discussion of drug and alcohol use in a social and historical context.

Hussein Rassool, G. (1998) Substance use and misuse, Oxford: Blackwell Science.
A comprehensive overview of substance misuse including treatments and intervention strategies.

Tyler, A. (1995) *Street drugs*, London: Hodder and Stoughton.
Although written by a journalist, this is the drug worker's bible. Highly recommended for an objective view of recreational drugs and their role in society. If you only want to read one book on substance misuse, this should be it.

# CHAPTER 27

# WORKING WITH PEOPLE WITH DEMENTIA AND THEIR CARERS

*John Keady*

---

## SUMMARY OF KEY POINTS

- CPNs in dementia care can work with carers and people with dementia throughout the trajectory of the condition.

- Dementia is included in a policy definition of serious mental illness.

- There is a need to further define the CPN's role boundaries and practice epistemology in dementia care.

---

> People can cope with this disease. But you need time.
>
> (Sterin 2002, p. 9)

## INTRODUCTION

Towards the end of the last century, dementia care began to shake off its medical roots and stigmatising discourses (Pitt 1982) and galvanise itself into a movement for change. This change was propelled forward on a number of fronts and involved advancements in:

- psychosocial interventions for carers of people with dementia (Cooke *et al.* 2001, Pusey and Richards 2001);
- emotion-orientated approaches for the support of people with dementia (Finnema *et al.* 2000);

- pharmacological treatments for early Alzheimer's disease (Matthews *et al.* 2000);
- evidence-based guidelines for primary care practitioners (Palmer 1999);
- principles to address the needs of people with intellectual disabilities affected by Alzheimer's disease and related dementias (Wilkinson and Janicki 2001);
- co-ordinated community care programmes that place the person with dementia at the centre of support (Challis *et al.* 1997);
- person-centred design for the continuing care of people with dementia (Judd *et al.* 1998);
- philosophical and ethical values to underpin practice; values that see beyond 'the dementia' to embrace the person and their efforts to retain a sense of self and personhood (Kitwood 1997, Sabat 2001).

CPNs in dementia care have contributed to this movement and have had their practice value highlighted in a number of reports and policy directives (see, for example, Williams *et al.* 1995, O'Shea and O'Reilly 1999, Audit Commission 2000). However, there is no room for complacency, as the CPN role in dementia care has recently come under criticism for its absence of role clarity and suitable practice models, particularly in its work with carers (Pickard 1999, Pickard and Glendinning 2001, Carradice *et al.* 2002). To ensure that each perspective is addressed fairly, therefore, this chapter will divide itself into three sections. First, an overview of the demographics of dementia will be provided, together with a summary of some recent policy trends. Next, the chapter will discuss the CPN's role in dementia care and will focus on how CPNs, at times with the input of other commentators, have described their practice and professional boundaries. Finally, the chapter will briefly consider some potential developments for CPN work in dementia care and explore some future challenges facing the profession.

## DEMENTIA: DEMOGRAPHICS AND POLICY TRENDS

Within the United Kingdom the Alzheimer's Society has revealed that, at present, some 800,000 people have a dementia (Alzheimer's Society 2000), and that around 500 people per day develop the condition. As a society with an ageing population, by the year 2021 it is estimated that there will be nearly 1 million people living in the UK with a dementia (Alzheimer's Society 2000), a figure that is expected to rise to 1.2 million by 2050 (Department of Health 2001). Moreover, around one person in five diagnosed with a dementia will, at some time, if not from the outset, live on their own with the condition and be at an increased risk of self-neglect, financial abuse and injury (Alzheimer's Society 1994). In situations where a family member is present to provide care (usually a spouse or adult child), studies have repeatedly demonstrated that, compared to other care-giving groups, such carers are prone to increased levels of depression, stress, loneliness and self-injury (for a comprehensive review, see Briggs and Askham 1999). Accordingly, it is not surprising that CPNs in dementia care have seen a role for themselves in alleviating family stress by intervening with carers to augment coping skills and support fractured relationships; this issue will be returned to again later in the chapter.

In recent years the advent of the anti-dementia drugs has provided a challenge to primary care practitioners to identify and diagnose dementia earlier in its course. However, this outcome has not always found favour with general practitioners, for a variety of reasons, including a belief, recorded in the *Forget me not* report (Audit Commission 2000), that 'there is no point looking for an incurable condition' (p. 21). Such negative attitudes need to be challenged, as an earlier diagnosis and communication of this to the person concerned are essential if those living with a dementia are to benefit from a range of psychosocial interventions, such as access to memory rehabilitation (Clare 1999) and early-stage support groups (Yale 1995). Such a paradigm shift has recently led some clinical nurse specialists and CPNs in dementia care to begin to explore their role within a memory clinic setting (see, for example, Royal College of Nursing Institute 1999, Adams and Page 2000) and in leading support groups for people with dementia (Hawkins and Eagger 1999).

This need to start benchmarking national service standards for the mental health care of older people was reflected, in England, in the publication and dissemination of the National Service Framework (NSF) for Older People (Department of Health 2001). Standard 7 of the NSF for Older People specifically addressed 'mental health and older people' with the overarching aim 'to promote good mental health in older people and to treat and support those older people with dementia and depression' (Department of Health 2001, p. 90). As this wording explicitly suggests, Standard 7 is built squarely on the foundations of depression and dementia and, later on in its pages, aligns its recommendations to the cause of younger people with dementia whose needs are frequently overlooked in policy and planning documents (Cox and Keady 1999). Standard 7 also emphasises the need to 'treat and support' older people with mental health needs around a community-orientated model that is underpinned by three key interventions, namely:

1   promoting good mental health;
2   early recognition and management of mental health problems;
3   access to specialist care.

(Department of Health 2001, p. 91)

The chapter will now turn to a consideration of these approaches, and the role that CPNs in dementia care have described as an appropriate service model.

## CPNs: ROLE DESCRIPTION AND PRACTICE DEVELOPMENT

Some time ago now, Simmons and Brooker (1986) indicated that when CPNs specialised with a client group it tended to be 'with elderly mentally ill people' (p. 46), a population that included those with dementia. As methods of recording the specialisms and numbers of practising CPNs became more sophisticated, the fourth quinquennial national CPN census of England and Wales reported that the total number of CPNs in these two countries had increased from 4,000 in 1990 to nearly 7,000 in 1996 (White 1999). However, by 1996, it was reported that CPNs were less likely to specialise in the care of older people, a fate that was also shared with CPNs working with children/adolescents, substance abusers and those with HIV and AIDS.

Arguably, the most significant reason behind this diminished emphasis centred on the UK government's policy push – and, it must be said, that of some influential mental health nurse commentators – to pin the CPN role down to the cause of 'serious mental illness' – a label that all but came to represent working-age adults with schizophrenia. This more targeted focus allowed CPNs a specialist role in case management, psychosocial interventions and brief intervention approaches (White 1999). Moreover, CPNs working with people with schizophrenia and their families could now be supported in their work by new programmes of education gleaned from the results of controlled studies, such as the Thorn initiative (Gournay and Birley 1998). Whilst not wishing to disparage any of this innovative work – indeed similar principles and evidence are required for dementia care nursing – a consequence of the realignment was that 'dementia' became displaced within the CPN profession.

This turn of events could be considered surprising as the Health of the Nation Report *Building bridges* (Department of Health 1995) provided a definition for severe mental illness that focused on the establishment of three key elements, namely: *disability*, *diagnosis* and *duration*, with the addition of two further dimensions, *safety* and the need for *informal* or *formal care*. In developing the notion of 'people suffering from severe mental illness' the report clearly aligns it to individuals who are:

> diagnosed as suffering from some sort of mental illness (typically people suffering from schizophrenia or a severe affective disorder, but including dementia . . .).
>
> (Department of Health 1995, p. 11)

Unfortunately, we do not know how many commissioners of health services, if any, include people with dementia within their own definition of severe mental illness. My experience and cursory reviews of the topical/academic mental health journals would suggest few, but this is anecdotal and could be construed as 'sour grapes'. More to the point, an inhibitory factor to the inclusion of dementia in serious mental illness is that CPNs in dementia care have often failed to adequately define their role, knowledge base, professional boundaries and/or practice efficacy (Keady and Adams 2001a, b). As an example, is the role of the CPN in dementia care about:

- being solely therapeutic and activity-driven? Or should it include some personal care work, such as bathing the person with dementia?
- focusing solely on dementia? Or should the CPN be part of a wider multidisciplinary team that addresses all mental health needs in older people?
- working with the person with dementia on his or her own? Working solely with the carer (as in the Admiral Nurse Service – see Woods *et al.* 1999)? Working with the carer and the person with dementia to the exclusion of

other family/community members? Or working with the family and community as a whole?

- being short term and focused? Or is it about forging a trusting relationship from the point of referral right through to the person with dementia's death, or beyond to work with the family through their transition and adjustment to loss?

There are simply no manuals to turn to that provide answers to any of these points, and the result is that CPN practice in dementia care has developed in a piecemeal and *ad hoc* fashion (Pickard 1999). As intimated earlier in the chapter, there is also public/professional uncertainty about the role. For instance, the Royal College of Psychiatrists' (1997) occasional paper on *Community psychiatric nursing* largely supported a holistic (family-centred) direction by defining the CPN role with older people as one in which the emphasis is on 'support to patients and their families living at home or in accommodation in the community' (p. 16). It was further argued within the report that the operational definition of 'accommodation' should include care within the nursing/residential homes sector, and that the CPN's liaison role with other multidisciplinary team members was particularly important.

In contrast, however, the public information brochure *Who cares?* (Health Education Authority 1997), which is aimed at carers of people with confusion, aligns the role of the CPN in dementia care to the person with dementia, and defines their specialist skills as an ability to help with the person's emotional and behavioural problems. In such a model, more physically based tasks such as attending to the person's needs for bathing, getting out of bed, dressing and so on are seen as the responsibility of the district nurse and/or health visitor. Interestingly, within this information pamphlet carers are advised to seek help for their emotional needs 'primarily with social workers or doctors' (Health Education Authority 1997, p. 30), thus contradicting the more family-centred values propounded by the Royal College of Psychiatrists' (1997) report and other commentators (see, for example, Adams 1989a, b, 1994, 1996a, 1998, Matthew 1990, Keady and Nolan 1994, 1995, Keady and Adams 2001a, b).

To begin to reach a consensus on understanding CPN activity in dementia care, it may prove useful to compile an overview of the role by documenting past/present role descriptions from the literature. The results of this exercise could then indicate how the role is constructed and provide a context for practice. With this outcome in mind an early paper detailing the retrospective role of the 'psychiatric nurse in the community nursing service' was written by John Greene. In this paper Greene (1968) argued that 'psychogeriatric' and 'partially confused' patients required a different approach to services compared to other client groups. Picking up on the practice examples provided in the paper, Keady and Adams (2001a, p. 37) suggested that for the CPN working with people with dementia and their families this early role description encompassed:

- the value of experience in working with people with dementia and their families;
- a knowledge of dementia and its likely course;
- attention to personal care needs;

Table 27.1 CPN and dementia care: selected overview of role attributes and practice domains

| Author(s) | Year of publication | Identified focus for CPN activity in dementia care | Research approach (if any) | Identified role attributes/practice domains |
|---|---|---|---|---|
| Royal College of Physicians | 1981 | Carers/relatives Person with dementia | Commentary on role | Support relatives; advise on medication; help settle and monitor in their own home 'disturbed patients' (original wording, p. 158) |
| Gunstone | 1983 | Family contact Relative support | Reflection on own practice | Starting support groups; co-ordinating with other (primary care) colleagues; flexible management, good liaison and a knowledge of other people's expertise; managing other junior nurses; accessing a consultant psychiatrist; developing a preventative function |
| Adams | 1989a, b | Family | Academic commentary | Need to apply to practice a family-stress model of chronic confusion. Articulated through: assessment; planning; intervention through a problem-solving framework; evaluation |
| Matthew | 1990 | Carers | Questionnaire to carers on CPN caseloads (n=32) Professional/academic sensitivity | Advice and information; gatekeeper to other services; general support, including counselling and listening; using therapeutic approaches, such as recognising the coping strategies of carers and non-judgemental counselling; training; skills exchange; planning of patient care; promotion of the CPN role; social and political awareness |
| Hughes-Roberts and Jones | 1991 | Carers Person with dementia (through specialist team support) | Description of own team practice | Assessment – social, medical and psychological needs; organisation of care packages; acting as case supervisors |
| Parker | 1992 | Carers Person with dementia | Description of own practice | Assessment; liaison; education (including assisting the training of social workers and doctors); administration and monitoring of medication; crisis intervention; advocate; therapist (counselling described as the most important aspect of intervention) |

continued . . . .

| Author | Year | Focus | Method | Findings |
|---|---|---|---|---|
| Rolfe and Phillips | 1995a, b | Advanced nurse practitioner (ANP) – community and unit based. Focus on carer and person with dementia | Action research<br>– interviews with staff (n=42)<br>– reflective interviews with the advanced nurse practitioner | Outreach by maintaining a high community profile; early intervention; open access; non-medical autonomous practice; specialist service provision; health education; liaison and collaboration with other agencies; ability to undertake a range of interventions |
| Williams, Keady and Nolan | 1995 | Carer – younger onset dementia | Single case interview. Professional/academic sensitivity | Promotion, support and facilitation of coping skills; assessment; information provision; empowerment; counselling; networking with other services; consistency of contact |
| Dennis, Furness, Lindesay and Wright | 1998 | Screening to detect early dementia | Consecutive referrals (n=64) to a memory clinic. Screening conducted by a CPN. Blind research trial | Assessment instruments used by the CPN included: ascertaining referral and informant history; conducting 15-item Geriatric Depression Scale and symptom checklist for anxiety, psychosis and mania; physical checklist; ADL (Activities of Daily Living) indicators; MRC (Medical Research Council) extended version of the MMSE (Mini Mental State); clock drawing |
| Gunstone | 1999 | Carers | Case study approach. Observation of one CPN and her practice with 7 carers. Semi-structured interview with the CPN after each session | Socialising; assessing; developing coping strategies; advice; (exploring) family dynamics; liaison; education;* counselling; crisis intervention; loving<br><br>* education seen as a 'significant proportion of the work' and involved education on: the disease process and stage-specific care; stress; stress management and assessments; general health matters; medication |
| Ho | 2000 | Carers | Interviews (n=8) with family carers about the role | Emotional support and advice; liaison and networking; training and information-giving; preventing isolation and loneliness. Personal qualities of CPN valued by carers and seen as important: caring, understanding and attentive; mature; respectful and sensitive; calm; patient; easy-going and helpful; confident; intelligent, knowledgeable, empowered |
| Pickard and Glendinning | 2001 | Carers | Semi-structured interviews with CPNs (n=12) | Education; counselling: advice-giving |

- information sharing with families;
- promotion of autonomy for people with dementia;
- maintaining regular visits and contact;
- establishing trust with both the person with dementia and their family;
- service co-ordination.

Building on this model of CPN work in dementia care, Table 27.1 (see pp. 324–5) provides an overview of some of the key role attributes and/or practice domains that have subsequently been suggested by other authors. Please note that this table is not meant to be representative of all CPN activity in dementia care, only illustrative.

As can be seen from this table, CPN work in dementia care is not homogeneous and, as indicated earlier, one outcome of this individualised activity is practice diversity. Moreover, as Adams (1996b) cogently argues, CPNs' knowledge base in dementia care is drawn predominantly from the psychological, social and health care sciences, but has no dominant paradigm. This is a crucial point, as a lack of focus for CPN activity has recently caused some commentators to begin to question the value of CPN practice in terms of both carer support (Pickard and Glendinning 2001) and the models used to guide their day-to-day work with family carers (Carradice *et al.* 2002). The study by Pickard and Glendinning (2001) presents a timely reminder of this conundrum by suggesting that carers value help with personal care tasks, but that the CPNs in their sample (n=12) failed to provide such a service and generally constructed their usefulness through 'advice and moral support' (p. 8). As these authors go on to explain:

> family carers are unclear as to why and in many cases as to when they first had contact with CPNs, and remain unclear as to their role and purpose.
>
> (Pickard and Glendinning 2001, p. 9)

Whilst applying a generalisation of these findings to all CPN practice in dementia care would be unwise on the basis of what Pickard and Glendinning (2001) themselves readily admit is a 'small-scale qualitative study' (p. 6), there is still an uncomfortable resonance in the quotation. To a significant extent, from the early 1990s onwards, the Admiral Nurse Service in England has attempted to address this dilemma by providing a clear focus and operational base to their community nursing role. Mainly comprising CPNs 'experienced' in dementia care, Admiral Nurses provide community support to carers of people with dementia within an agreed model of assessment and intervention, with nurses having their interventions measured to ascertain the effectiveness of their engagement. It is this emphasis on performance measurement coupled with regular access to structured clinical supervision (see Wills and Woods 1997) that could point a way forward for the CPN service to restructure its activities, albeit with a wider population base that includes the person with dementia.

# DISCUSSION

To date there have only been two reviews of CPN practice: in 1968 through *Psychiatric nursing today and tomorrow*, and in 1994 through *Working in partnership*, a report of the Mental Health Nursing Review Team under the chairmanship of Professor Tony Butterworth (Department of Health 1968 and 1994 respectively). The development of CPN work in dementia care has been overlooked in both reports, and, as someone who believes passionately in the role of nursing in dementia care, it is sometimes difficult to stem a creeping paranoia about its exclusion from current debates on the nature of serious mental illness and its destabilised place within the profession. In my opinion, it is important to return to the *Building bridges* report from the mid-1990s (Department of Health 1995) to recapture an inclusive mental health agenda and bring dementia care back into the mainstream of CPN activity. Such an alignment becomes increasingly important as nurses across the wide spectrum of the profession bemoan the lack of opportunities to learn more about dementia care during both pre- and post-registration courses (Nolan *et al*. 2002). Moreover, general practitioners and other primary care practitioners are seen as requiring specialist training in dementia care (Audit Commission 2000) and CPNs would appear ideally suited to under-take (and evaluate!) this work. However, to achieve this will take commitment and a willingness to develop a strategic and educational agenda.

However, over and above such concerns, there is a real need to consolidate the search for the distinct contribution of the CPN in dementia care, and move away from anecdotal descriptions to ones that embrace structured evaluations of practice efficacy. Coupled to astute political manoeuvring, this development is, in my opinion, the critical next step facing the profession and the challenge we all need to face.

# REFERENCES

Adams, T. (1989a) 'Dementia and family stress', *Nursing Times*, 85 (38): 27–29.

Adams, T. (1989b) 'Growth of a speciality', *Nursing Times*, 85 (40): 30–32.

Adams, T. (1994) 'The emotional experience of caregivers to relatives who are chronically confused – implications for community mental health nursing', *International Journal of Nursing Studies*, 31 (6): 545–553.

Adams, T. (1996a) 'A descriptive study of the work of community psychiatric nurses with elderly demented people', *Journal of Advanced Nursing*, 23: 1177–1184.

Adams, T. (1996b) 'Informal family caregiving to older people with dementia: research priorities for community psychiatric nursing', *Journal of Advanced Nursing*, 24: 703–710.

Adams, T. (1998) 'The discursive construction of dementia care: implications for mental health nursing', *Journal of Advanced Nursing*, 28 (3): 614–621.

Adams, T. and Page, S. (2000) 'New pharmacological treatments for Alzheimer's disease: implications for dementia care nursing', *Journal of Advanced Nursing*, 31 (5): 1183–1188.

Alzheimer's Society (1994) *Home alone – with dementia*, London: Alzheimer's Society.

Alzheimer's Society (2000) *Introduction to dementia*, London: Alzheimer's Society.

Audit Commission (2000) *Forget me not: mental health services for older people*, London: Audit Commission.

Briggs, K. and Askham, J. (1999) *The needs of people with dementia and those who care for them*, London: Alzheimer's Society.

Carradice, A., Shankland, M. and Beail, N. (2002) 'A qualitative study of the theoretical models used by UK mental health nurses to guide their assessments with family caregivers of people with dementia', *International Journal of Nursing Studies*, 39 (1): 17–26.

Challis, D., von Abendorff, R., Brown, P. and Chesterman, J. (1997) 'Care management and dementia: an evaluation of the Lewisham intensive case management scheme', in Hunter, S. (ed.) *Dementia: challenges and new directions*, London: Jessica Kingsley.

Clare, L. (1999) 'Memory rehabilitation in early dementia', *Journal of Dementia Care – Research Focus*, 17 (6): 33–38.

Cooke, D.D., McNally, L., Mulligan, K.T., Harrison, M.J.G. and Newman, P. (2001) 'Psychosocial interventions for caregivers of people with dementia: a systematic review', *Aging and Mental Health*, 5 (2): 120–135.

Cox, S. and Keady, J. (eds) (1999) *Younger people with dementia: planning, practice and development*, London: Jessica Kingsley.

Dennis, M., Furness, L., Lindesay, J. and Wright, N. (1998) 'Assessment of patients with memory problems using a nurse-administered instrument to detect early dementia and dementia subtypes', *International Journal of Geriatric Psychiatry*, 13: 405–409.

Department of Health (1968) *Psychiatric nursing today and tomorrow*, London: HMSO.

Department of Health (1994) *Working in partnership: a collaborative approach to care. Report of the Mental Health Nursing Review Team*, London: HMSO.

Department of Health (1995) *Building bridges: a guide to arrangements for interagency working for the care and protection of severely mentally ill people*, London: Department of Health.

Department of Health (2001) *National service framework for older people: modern standards and service models*, London: Department of Health.

Finnema, E., Dröes, R.-M., Ribbe, M. and Van Tilburg, W. (2000) 'The effects of emotion-orientated approaches in the care of persons suffering from dementia: a review of the literature', *International Journal of Geriatric Psychiatry*, 15: 141–161.

Gournay, K. and Birley, J. (1998) 'Thorn: a new approach to mental health training', *Nursing Times*, 94 (49): 54–55.

Greene, J. (1968) 'The psychiatric nurse in the community nursing service', *International Journal of Nursing Studies*, 5: 175–184.

Gunstone, S. (1983) 'The scope for prevention', *Nursing Times*, 79 (37): 42–43.

Gunstone, S. (1999) 'Expert practice: the interventions used by a community mental health nurse with carers of dementia sufferers', *Journal of Psychiatric and Mental Health Nursing*, 6 (1): 21–27.

Hawkins, D. and Eagger, S. (1999) 'Group therapy: sharing the pain of diagnosis', *Journal of Dementia Care*, 7 (5): 12–14 and 8.

Health Education Authority (1997) *Who cares? Information and support for the carers of confused people*, London: Health Education Authority.

Ho, D. (2000) 'Role of community mental health nurses for people with dementia', *British Journal of Nursing*, 9 (15): 986–991.

Hughes-Roberts, J. and Jones, T.R. (1991) 'A novel remit', *Nursing Times*, 87 (13): 26–28.

Judd, S., Marshall, M. and Phippen, P. (eds) (1998) *Design for dementia*, London: Hawker.

Keady, J. and Adams, T. (2001a) 'Community mental health nursing and dementia care', *Journal of Dementia Care – Research Focus*, 9 (1): 35–38.

Keady, J. and Adams, T. (2001b) 'Community mental health nurses in dementia care: their role and future', *Journal of Dementia Care – Research Focus*, 9 (2): 33–37.

Keady, J. and Nolan, M. (1994) 'The Carer Led Assessment Process (CLASP): a framework for the assessment of need in dementia caregivers', *Journal of Clinical Nursing*, 3 (2): 103–108.

Keady, J. and Nolan, M. (1995) 'A stitch in time: facilitating proactive interventions with dementia caregivers: the role of community practitioners', *Journal of Psychiatric and Mental Health Nursing*, 2 (1): 33–40.

Kitwood, T. (1997) *Dementia reconsidered: the person comes first*, Buckingham: Open University Press.

Matthew, L. (1990) 'A role for the CPN in supporting the carer of clients with dementia', in Brooker, C. (ed.) *Community psychiatric nursing: a research perspective*, London: Chapman and Hall.

Matthews, H.P., Korbey, J., Wilkinson, D.G. and Rowden, J. (2000) 'Donepezil in Alzheimer's disease: eighteen month results from Southampton memory clinic', *International Journal of Geriatric Psychiatry*, 15: 713–720.

Nolan, M., Davies, S., Brown, J., Keady, J. and Nolan, J. (2002) *Longitudinal study of the effectiveness of educational preparation to meet the needs of older people and carers: the AGEIN (Advancing Gerontological Education In Nursing) project*, London: English National Board for Nursing, Midwifery and Health Visiting.

O'Shea, E. and O'Reilly, S. (1999) *An action plan for dementia*, Dublin: National Council on Ageing and Older People.

Palmer, C. (1999) *Evidence-base briefing: dementia – a compilation of secondary research evidence, guidelines and consensus statements*, London: Royal College of Psychiatrists.

Parker, I. (1992) 'Role of the CPN', *Alzheimer's Disease Society Newsletter*, London: Alzheimer's Society, May, p. 5.

Pickard, S. (1999) 'Co-ordinated care for older people with dementia', *Journal of Interprofessional Care*, 13 (4): 345–354.

Pickard, S. and Glendinning, C. (2001) 'Caring for a relative with dementia: the perceptions of carers and CPNs', *Quality in Ageing – Policy, Practice and Research*, 2 (4): 3–11.

Pitt, B. (1982) *Psychogeriatrics: an introduction to the psychiatry of old age*, 2nd edn, London: Churchill Livingstone.

Pusey, H. and Richards, D. (2001) 'A systematic review of the effectiveness of psychosocial interventions for carers of people with dementia', *Aging and Mental Health*, 5 (2): 107–119.

Rolfe, G. and Phillips, L.-M. (1995a) 'An action research project to develop and evaluate the role of an advanced nurse practitioner in dementia', *Journal of Clinical Nursing*, 4 (5): 289–293.

Rolfe, G. and Phillips, L.-M. (1995b) 'The development and evaluation of the role of an Advanced Nurse Practitioner in dementia – an action research project', *International Journal of Nursing Studies*, 4 (5): 289–293.

Royal College of Nursing Institute (1999) *Nursing in memory clinics: resource pack*, Oxford: Royal College of Nursing Institute.

Royal College of Physicians (1981) 'Organic mental impairment in the elderly: implications for research, education and the provision of services. A report of the Royal College of Physicians by the College Committee on Geriatrics', *Journal of the Royal College of Physicians of London*, 15 (3): 141–167.

Royal College of Psychiatrists (1997) *Community psychiatric nursing*, Occasional Paper OP40, London: Royal College of Psychiatrists.

Sabat, S.R. (2001) *The experience of Alzheimer's disease: life through a tangled veil*, Oxford: Blackwell.

Simmons, S. and Brooker, C. (1986) *Community psychiatric nursing: a social perspective*, London: Heinemann.

Sterin, G. (2002) 'Essay on a word: a lived experience of Alzheimer's disease', *Dementia: The International Journal of Social Research and Practice*, 1 (1): 7–10.

White, E. (1999) 'The 4th quinquennial national community mental health nursing census of England and Wales', *Australian and New Zealand Journal of Mental Nursing*, 8 (3): 86–92.

Wilkinson, H. and Janicki, M.P. (2001) *The Edinburgh principles with accompanying guidelines and recommendations*, Stirling: University of Stirling Centre for Social Research on Dementia.

Williams, O., Keady, J. and Nolan, M.R. (1995) 'Younger-onset Alzheimer's disease: learning from the experience of one spouse carer', *Journal of Clinical Nursing*, 4 (1): 31–36.

Wills, W. and Woods, B. (1997) 'Developing a specialist nursing service for family care-givers of people with dementia: dilemmas of role expectation, perceived dependency and control', in Denicolo, P. and Pope, M. (eds) *Sharing understanding and practice*, Farnborough: The European Personal Construct Association.

Woods, B., Wills, W., Higginson, I., Whitby, M. and Hobbins, J. (1999) , London: NHS Executive North Thames R&D Directorate.

Yale, R. (1995) *Developing support groups for individuals with early-stage Alzheimer's disease: planning, implementation and evaluation*, London: Health Professions Press.

# FURTHER READING

Adams, T. and Clarke, C. (eds) (1999) *Dementia care: developing partnerships in practice*, London: Baillière Tindall.

Edited by two respected nurse academics, this book pulls together some key research findings and commentary on the state of the art in dementia care. An essential guide for those entering the profession and more experienced practitioners.

Kitwood, T. (1997) *Dementia reconsidered: the person comes first*, Buckingham: Open University Press.

Written shortly before his untimely death, this book draws together Professor Kitwood's writings on dementia care and charts the importance of personhood and person-centred values. Arguably the most influential text written on dementia care in the 1990s, its impact will stretch long into this century.

Sabat, S.R. (2001) *The experience of Alzheimer's disease: life through a tangled veil*, Oxford: Blackwell.

A recent publication that explores the meaning of self and identity in dementia. Written by a respected authority in dementia care, Professor Sabat's book challenges practitioners to see the meaning of people's actions and their right to assert their identity.

# CHAPTER 28

# WORKING WITH PEOPLE WITH MENTAL HEALTH PROBLEMS AND LEARNING DISABILITIES

*Dave Coyle*

## SUMMARY OF KEY POINTS

- People with learning disabilities are at increased risk of developing mental health problems.

- Assessing the mental health of people with learning disabilities is a complex activity.

- Collaboration between services and practitioners can improve the care of people with learning disabilities and mental health problems.

## INTRODUCTION

Within the past ten years it has come to be accepted that people who have a learning disability may also experience mental health problems. People with a learning disability can and do experience the full range of mental health difficulties, and there is also a recognition that they may be at a greater risk of experiencing such difficulties than the general population (Reid 1982, Raghavan 2000). As people with learning disabilities have many of the vulnerability factors and characteristics associated with people who experience serious and enduring mental health problems, and have additional factors, the identification of risk and appropriate interventions are paramount.

The presence of this chapter in a text that is aimed at mental health practitioners focusing on the practice issues of recognising and responding to the mental health needs of people with learning disabilities makes its relevance clear.

This chapter will examine the underlying trends that have led to an acceptance of the mental health needs of people with learning disabilities. It will discuss the challenges for services in attempting to assess the presence of mental ill health for this group. Finally, it will outline practice issues for community mental health nurses when engaging with people who have a learning disability, their carers and specialist services, in providing support.

Learning disability will be used in this chapter to describe children and adults who have cognitive, social and adaptive impairments to a nature and degree that fall within the World Health Organization's *ICD-10: International statistical classification of diseases and related health problems* definition (World Health Organization 1992).

## RECENT TRENDS IN MENTAL HEALTH AND LEARNING DISABILITIES

The issue of appropriate services for people with learning disabilities has been the focus of successive policy initiatives and strategies within the United Kingdom for over twenty years. Documents such as the *All Wales strategy* (Welsh Office 1983) laid the foundations for more community-based, more inclusive lifestyles for this client group. The resultant shift away from traditional facility-based services with their all-encompassing role has created as many challenges as it has provided opportunities.

The advent of community care and the distinction of health and social care provision radically altered the landscape of care in the 1990s. At the same time, services for people with learning disabilities underwent enormous change, with many health-based facilities shifting towards a more appropriate social model of provision. People with learning disabilities were not ill; they did not require nurses and doctors. Instead, their needs would be best met through a collaborative approach between social, voluntary and generic services with liaison and consultancy with community learning disability teams (Department of Health 1989).

This meant that, instead of specialist provision, people with learning disabilities would access the same services as those used by the general population. Whilst for the majority of people with a learning disability this strategy would be advantageous (some issues would persist about the appropriateness and training of health professionals in those settings, and these will be discussed), those individuals with complex need, and/or challenging behaviours, would find access to some services difficult and continuity problematic (Department of Health 1993, 1999, Welsh Office 1994, NHS Executive 1998).

Those people with either complex challenging behaviour or a superimposed mental health need required more levels of support and comprehensive assessment than could be provided for in generic services. As a result special facilities proliferated in England and Wales. Successive reports highlighted the need for appropriate provision for this client group (Department of Health 1993, Welsh Office 1994). Within learning disability-based health services, units that provided a broad, yet short-term intervention came into existence.

These treatment and assessment units were mostly located within learning disability services and were staffed, again, mostly by qualified learning disability nurses. Whilst these units attempted to bridge the gap in community care, they served to keep mental health and learning disability services separate. Their role encompassed emergency assessment of deterioration of mental health, monitoring medication, review of epilepsy and, at times, emergency accommodation. They remain in many areas the mainstay of accommodation for clients with complex and enduring problems. As such they are fraught with problems of congruence and persistent bed blocking (Cumella *et al.* 1998).

The problems presented by people with mental ill health and learning disability have been clearly highlighted by the Royal College of Psychiatrists (RCP) (1996). Their report recognised the differing approaches to care in the UK for this client group. They articulated the difficulties in organising care when admission to mental health services may be blocked because of the client's underlying learning disability and the limited ability of specialist learning disability services to meet client needs. The RCP recognised that problems of access and equity existed irrespective of the level or degree of disability. The problems of access to services and appropriate treatment were most acute for those people whose learning disability was mild and who had an unclear or atypical presentation.

The focus on social care provision post-community care has arguably made the development of health-based services for the mental health of people with learning disabilities more difficult. The question of how services for this client group should be organised is a challenge.

## PREVALENCE OF MENTAL ILLNESS IN PEOPLE WITH LEARNING DISABILITIES

The prevalence of mental illness in people with learning disabilities is difficult to ascertain. This is due in part to difficulties of assessment and diagnosis. It is also due to some special factors that pertain to this population alone (Gilbert *et al.* 1998). The wide variation in reported incidence is in part due to the different approaches to the studies and their methodological differences. Early studies which reported very high incidences of mental ill health tended to draw upon skewed sample populations (Reid 1972). Other studies have examined referral rates to specialist mental health learning disability community services (Bouras and Drummond 1992). Because of the problematic nature of accurate diagnosis, the underlying level of mental ill health in this population may never be known. Campbell and Malone (1991) reported the variance in incidence studies to range from 14.3 per cent to 67 per cent. Studies such as Lund's (1985) put the figure of morbidity at 28 per cent.

There are similarities that can be drawn between the lives of people with learning disabilities and people who have severe and enduring mental health problems. The risks of isolation, low self-esteem, poor education, low income, reliance on others, and stressful life events with poor autonomy or agency over one's life, combined with a biological predisposition in some instances, make people with learning disabilities most vulnerable. The work of Barrowclough and

Tarrier (1997) and that of Zubin and Spring (1977) create an understanding of how individuals can be at greater risk of experiencing mental health disorder than others without such risk factors. The construct of mental health is inextricably linked to quality-of-life concepts and it is extremely difficult to predict an individual's response to one set of circumstances compared with another. People with a learning disability, however, do appear to have many of the contributory risk factors that may give rise to mental ill health; one might expect, therefore, the prevalence rates in this client group to be far higher than they are.

In addition to the biological, psychological and social vulnerabilities of people with learning disabilities, the effect of the learning disability itself creates a factor both in the prevalence rates and, more importantly, in actually assessing the existence of a mental health problem. This chapter will now focus on the factors that may impede or confuse the process of assessment in adults with learning disabilities. Approaches and tools that can be used will be discussed, with their relevant merits and weaknesses identified.

# ASSESSMENT OF MENTAL HEALTH PROBLEMS IN PEOPLE WITH LEARNING DISABILITIES

Where there are either strong indicators or compelling evidence of mental disorder, psychologists and psychiatrists have attempted to use statistically normative measures as diagnostic instruments. The inadequacies of such tools have long been recognised. Sovner (1986) first identified the difficulties of using statistically normative assessment tools in assessing mental health problems with this client group. The problems he identified hinged on the degree to which such criteria fail to take into account the differences of presentation of psychomorbidity in this group. People with learning disabilities often have an exaggerated baseline of behaviours, such as challenging behaviour, self-injury, or repetitive behaviours. Such behaviours in persons without a learning disability might indicate in themselves a psychological disorder.

Sovner (1986) identified four factors that have significance in the interpretation of the presentation of mental ill health. These are: intellectual distortion, psychosocial masking, cognitive disintegration and baseline exaggeration.

## Intellectual distortion

Where assessment relies on the client's communication, and on the assessment of their thoughts and expression, this deviates significantly from the non-learning-disabled population. Where a person has problems in abstract thinking, it is possible that a misleading conclusion of concrete thinking may be inferred.

A person with a learning disability may have problems in adhering to the rules of communication and with expressing thoughts and feelings. Prosodic (tone, pitch and fluency) and pragmatic (adherence to the rules of communication) verbal disorders may be a usual component of the individual and not a psychological symptom.

The person's voice may be high-pitched and gasping or low and monotone. Their tone and fluency may be unusual in that it might be flattened, slow and full of pauses. This may be indicative of a prosodic disorder and not a symptom of an affective disorder.

## Psychosocial masking

People with a learning disability may have significantly limited experiences in their lives; this factor, combined with difficulties in expressing or being understood, may mean that they present with atypical features of major mental ill health. Sovner (1986) cites Menolascino:

> When the normal person becomes manic, he thinks he's God. When the mentally retarded [sic] person becomes manic, he thinks he's not retarded.

Another example of this might be where an individual with learning disabilities tells their carers that they will be sued. This may be as grandiose or unlikely as delusional statements made by an individual experiencing a manic episode (Weisblatt 1994).

## Cognitive disintegration

This is where the person is said to be vulnerable to cognitive breakdown as a result of the assessment process itself. This phenomenon was thought by Sovner to be brought about through stress. This may result in odd or bizarre behaviour, such as withdrawal and even talking to what might seem like an imaginary friend when responding to questions. Symptoms such as reality testing may also be a feature in someone with a learning disability.

## Baseline exaggeration

People with more severe and profound learning difficulties may express their psychological disorder through behaviour rather than through words (Bouras and Drummond 1992). Behavioural difficulties and unusual patterns of behaviour are often a feature of someone with a learning disability (Moss and Lee 2001) and, as such, may be enduring and persistent over many years. Therefore there is a potential for all behaviour, irrespective of how bizarre or limiting for the individual, to be seen only in terms of the person's usual repertoire.

Equally, where the person's behaviour repertoire possibly includes functional behaviours that are by definition strange or odd, the emergence of additional behaviours indicative of mental disorder may be missed. This creates a double jeopardy for the person with a learning disability in that their behaviour, if seen as functional in its intention (in that all behaviour has meaning and therefore a purpose), may be misinterpreted or its meaning simply missed.

It is not always clear whether challenging behaviour is part of sympto-matology or not. There is a role, here, for the use of behavioural analysis in the assessment of mental health issues (Gilbert *et al*. 1998). The terminology used to describe behavioural problems or challenging behaviour is important here. Russell (1998) makes the point that the diagnosis of behaviour disorder has been little used in the UK. It may, he claims, be of use in trying to separate mental ill health from behaviour problems arising from social and environmental causes and those behaviours that are rooted in the emotional distress of people with a learning disability.

The effects of expressive impairment of communication in a client with learn-ing disabilities will have a significant impact on an assessment interview (Russell 1997, Kroesse *et al*. 2001). With the difficulties of both interpreting and expressing their internal experience, people with learning disabilities may themselves have problems in recognising distress or abnormal behaviours. Communicating their mental health problems is often the single most problematic area for people with learning disabilities, which is compounded as they often rely on a third party (family member or paid carer) to interpret indicators of mental ill health.

The formal process of clinical assessment through a health professional, usually with a structured process or tool, creates the potential for further distortion with the client who has a learning disability. It has been shown that people with a learning disability are more likely to respond to perceived authority figures in suggestible ways. The phenomenon of acquiescence is well documented in people with a learning disability (Sigelman *et al*. 1982, Heal and Sigelman 1995) and raises real practice implications for those interviewing learning-disabled clients. The skill of the interviewer is of great importance in obtaining clear information that will assist in identifying problem areas or psychiatric disorder.

Misinterpretation of the person's presentation or expression as being an integral part of their impairment has been shown to occur with health profes-sionals. The phenomenon known as diagnostic overshadowing (Reiss and Szyszko 1983) may, if not recognised and addressed, significantly reduce the identification of a mental health issue in a person with a learning disability. As a result, mental health issues may remain untreated.

It is important to recognise that the degree and extent of the learning dis-ability will significantly affect the ability to assess the existence of a mental health problem. The less severe the learning disability, the more the presentation of mental health problems will correspond to the non-learning-disabled population. The more severe the learning disability is, the more atypical the presentation of a mental health problem becomes (Fraser and Nolan 1994).

## ASSESSMENT TOOLS

Specific assessment tools to assess the presence of mental health problems in people with learning disabilities have been developed over the past two decades. These have usually been based on, or have been adaptations of, generic criteria from the *Diagnostic and statistical manual of mental disorders (DSM-IV)* (American Psychiatric Association 1994) and/or the World Health Organization's

*International statistical classification of diseases and related health problems (ICD-10)* (World Health Organization 1992).

Adaptations of existing psychological testing batteries have been in existence for some time. Examples include the Zung Anxiety Scales (Lindsay and Michie 1988), the adaptation of the Beck Depression Inventory (Moss 1999) and the Modified Children's Depression Inventory for Adults with Severe Learning Disability (Meins 1996).

Assessment tools for working with people with a learning disability include the Diagnostic Assessment for the Severely Handicapped (DASH) (Matson 1994) which is a DSM (APA 1994) subscale specifically designed for assessment in hospital settings. It is of use for people with severe learning disability as many items relate to observable behaviours. The tool has its merits, although it is unlikely to produce a differential diagnosis. Equally, as the hospital populations are diminishing, the utility of a tool for that area is questionable. Matson (1988) developed an informant and self-report version of the Psychopathology Inventory for Mentally Retarded Adults (PIMRA). The tool seeks to ascertain the degree to which the behaviour and expression of the individual meet a diagnostic threshold. All of these tools attempt to overcome the essential problem of communicating subjective internal experience of people who have learning disabilities. They are all helpful in the process of asking whether an individual has a mental health problem.

The Reiss Screen for Maladaptive Behaviour (Reiss 1988) is of use in identifying and measuring the frequency, intensity and severity of behaviour. It is of help, therefore, in examining the functionality of the behaviour in the person with learning disabilities. Although the Reiss screen has been found to exhibit strong predictive results when used appropriately (Reiss 1999), some doubt must exist in relation to the validity of diagnosis of specific psychological problems.

The Reiss screen can, however, be of use in that another factor pertinent to people with learning disabilities is the high rates of challenging behaviour that are present within the population (Moss and Lee 2001). A significant development in the assessment of mental health disorder in people with learning disabilities is the Psychiatric Assessment Schedule for Adults with Developmental Disabilities (PAS-ADD) (Moss *et al.* 1993). Its development has made it possible to recognise mental disorders more reliably. Its utility, however, remains limited, as the tool has been traditionally restricted to either psychologists or psychiatrists.

The Mini PAS-ADD (Moss *et al.* 1993) has been developed for use by health and social care professionals, such as nurses and social workers. The tool is an eighty-six-item questionnaire which identifies the presence of a problem, significant life events, affective disorder, psychosis, anxiety, and organic or autistic disorder. A four-point scale of the problem's significance is rated over a four-week period. There is in addition a section exploring some of the physiological or biological factors that may present as mental health issues. For example, hypothyroidism presenting as depression or dementia (Prasher and Krishnan 1993). The scores are then combined to identify whether further investigation is required. Although no formal training is required, the authors of the tool suggest that some specialist preparation is given.

The tool is straightforward and provides an indication of whether further investigation is required. In addition to the questionnaire, the Mini PAS-ADD contains an instruction and glossary which are of enormous assistance when attempting to establish what is or might be indicative of a mental health problem and, more helpfully, what is not.

The PAS-ADD checklist has been developed for families of people with learning disabilities or paid carers. The checklist is a simplified version of the Mini PAS-ADD, and is a twenty-eight-item questionnaire using the same categories of investigation.

Both tools show good reliability and validity in indicating a future diagnosis (Moss *et al*. 1998, Prosser *et al*. 1998). The thresholds of clinical significance given in these two shorter subscales are not diagnostic in themselves. They do, however, inform professionals as to whether more detailed investigation is required. Whilst, as with any tool, they should not be the sole measure of assessment, they do provide the care team with an appropriately focused tool to assist their care planning.

# INTERVENTIONS

As in mental health services, there can be an over-reliance on the use of medical approaches in treating and responding to presenting symptomatology (Clarke 1997). The use of medication is undoubtedly a most useful adjunct to the overall care provided in mental health services. In learning disabilities services, because of the difficulties of the client in expressing their internal experiences, or providing direct feedback relating to the efficacy of medication or the experience of potential side effects, the appropriate use of medication is a key issue (Gravestock 1996). Medication with this client group has been said to resemble a 'buckshot approach' (Crabbe 1994). Diagnosis of a psychiatric disorder may have been arrived at retrospectively, and should be a concern.

The importance of distinguishing between a behavioural disturbance and mental ill health is crucial, as, quite apart from the morality of using psychotropic medication as a chemical restraint, there is little or no evidence of such medication having a therapeutic effect (Kroesse *et al*. 2001). Where neuroleptic medication is used, it is of paramount importance that the potential side effects are comprehensively and regularly evaluated using an established tool, such as LUNSERS (Day *et al*. 1995) or DISCUS (Kalachnick 1991).

The use of established mental health treatment or therapeutic approaches with people with learning disabilities is increasingly well documented (see O'Hara and Sperlinger 1997 for a basic discussion). Group-work activities ranging from creative art to drama and dance have all been used as a means of minimising the need for expressive language.

Cognitive–behavioural approaches have been used (Kroesse *et al*. 1997) and modified (Lindsay *et al*. 1993). Adaptations involve minimising the amount of written work (worksheets, homework, diaries and self-report scales). The duration of the sessions is often greatly reduced to accommodate the shorter concentration of the participants, and correspondingly the number of sessions is increased. Psychodynamic approaches have also been used with success with people with learning disability (Waitman and Conboy-Hill 1992). With the strongly interpretive elements of such an approach, its use is clear.

The language used in therapeutic work with learning-disabled people needs to be both clear and unambiguous and, at the same time, cognisant of the phenomena of acquiescence and compliance found with vulnerable client groups. Therefore questions should be phrased in ways that avoid 'yes' or 'no' answers, encouraging the person to find the words themselves. Methods of communication that rely less on language and more on pictorial representation are of use here. Genograms and ecomaps have a role to play in both assessment and formulation for people with learning disability (Dobson 1989).

## SUMMARY

Existing learning disability services can work collaboratively with generic mental health services to assist in the assessment and treatment of service users. Mental health services could also work more in partnership with learning disability services, especially with potential service users with mild or moderate learning disabilities. Certainly it is clear that services for people with learning disabilities who also experience mental health problems should be improved. How this is achieved is more difficult. Services should be local and accessible, avoiding expensive and often inappropriate out-of-county placements. The issues raised by the Mansell Report and other reports (Welsh Office 1994) are still as relevant today as they ever were.

Authors and strategy documents point to the pitfalls and advantages of generic versus specialist services (Piachaud 1999), claiming that local specialist teams may provide the level of support, expert consultancy and clinical practice to meet client need. Research into such teams demonstrated positive outcomes (Allen and Lowe 1995). Simpson (1997) suggested ways in which a specialist learning disability service could provide support for generic services through consultancy and specific intervention, allowing for care and treatment of people with learning disabilities within generic settings.

## REFERENCES

Allen, D. and Lowe, K. (1995) 'Providing intensive community support to people with learning disabilities and challenging behaviour: a preliminary analysis of outcomes and costs', *Journal of Intellectual Disability Research*, 39 (1): 67–82.

American Psychiatric Association (APA) (1994) *The diagnosic and statistical manual of mental disorders (DSM-IV)*, Washington, DC: American Psychiatric Association.

Barrowclough, C. and Tarrier, N. (1997) *Families of schizophrenic patients: cognitive behavioural interventions*, London: Stanley Thornes.

Bouras, N. and Drummond, C. (1992) 'Behaviour and psychiatric disorders of people with mental handicaps living in the community', *Journal of Intellectual Disability Research*, 36: 349–357.

Campbell, M. and Malone, R.P. (1991) 'Mental retardation and psychiatric disorders', *Hospital and Community Psychiatry*, 42: 374–379.

Clarke, D.J. (1997) 'Towards rational psychotropic prescribing for people with learning disability', *British Journal of Learning Disabilities*, 25 (2): 46–52.

Crabbe, H.F. (1994) 'Pharmacotherapy in mental retardation', in Bouras, N. (ed.) *Mental retardation in mental health: recent advances and practices*, Cambridge: Cambridge University Press.

Cumella, S., Marston, G. and Ashok, R. (1998) 'Bed blockage in an acute admission service for people with a learning disability', *British Journal of Learning Disabilities*, 26 (3): 118–121.

Day, J.C., Wood, G., Dewey, M. and Bentall, R.P. (1995) 'A self-rating scale for measuring neuroleptic side-effects. Validation in a group of schizophrenic patients', *British Journal of Psychiatry*, 166: 650–653.

Department of Health (1989) *Needs and responses: services for adults with mental handicap who are mentally ill, who have behavioural problems and who offend*, London: HMSO.

Department of Health (1993) *Challenging behaviours and/or mental health needs of people with learning disabilities*, London: HMSO.

Department of Health (1999) *Facing the facts: services for people with learning disabilities. A policy impact study of social care and health services*, London: Department of Health.

Dobson, S. (1989) 'Genograms and ecomaps', *Nursing Times*, 85 (51): 54–56.

Fraser, W. and Nolan, M. (1994) 'Psychiatric disorders in mental retardation', in Bouras, N. (ed.) *Mental retardation in mental health: recent advances and practices*, Cambridge: Cambridge University Press.

Gilbert, T., Todd, M. and Jackson, N. (1998) 'People with learning disabilities who also have mental health problems: practice issues and directions for learning disability nursing', *Journal of Advanced Nursing*, 27: 1151–1157.

Gravestock, S. (1996) 'Depot neuroleptic usage in adults with learning disabilities', *Journal of Intellectual Disability Research*, 40 (1): 17–23.

Heal, L.W. and Sigelman, C.K. (1995) 'Response biases in interviews of individuals with limited mental ability', *Journal of Intellectual Disability Research*, 39 (4): 331–340.

Kalachnick, J.E. (1991) *The dyskinesia identification system condensed user scale (DISCUS)*, St Paul, MN: Department of Human Services.

Kroesse, B., Dagnan, D. and Loumidis, K. (1997) *Cognitive-behavioural therapy for people with learning disabilities*, London: Routledge.

Kroesse, B.S., Dewhurst, D. and Holmes, G. (2001) 'Diagnosis and drugs: help or hindrance when people with learning disabilities have psychological problems', *British Journal of Learning Disabilities*, 29 (1): 26–33.

Lindsay, W. and Michie, A.M. (1988) 'Adaptation of the Zung rating scale for people with a mental handicap', *Journal of Mental Deficiency Research*, 32: 485–490.

Lindsay, W.R., Howells, L. and Pitcaithly, D. (1993) 'Cognitive therapy for depression with individuals with intellectual disabilities', *British Journal of Medical Psychology*, 66: 135–141.

Lund, J. (1985) 'The prevalence of psychiatric morbidity in mentally retarded adults', *Acta Psychiatrica Scandinavica*, 72: 563–570.

Matson, J. (1988) *The psychopathology inventory for mentally retarded adults*, Worthington, OH: IDS Publishing Corporation.

Matson, J. (1994) *Diagnostic assessment for the severely handicapped revised*, Baton Rouge: Scientific Publishers.

Meins, W. (1996) 'A new depression scale designed for use with adults with mental retardation', *Journal of Intellectual Disability Research*, 40 (3): 222–226.

Moss, S. (1999) 'Assessment of mental health problems', *Tizard Learning Disability Review*, 4 (2): 14–20.

Moss, S. and Lee, P. (2001) 'Mental health', in Thompson, J. and Pickering, S. (eds) *Meeting the health needs of people who have a learning disability*, London: Baillière Tindall.

Moss, S., Patel, P., Prosser, H., Goldberg, D., Simpson, N., Rowe, S. and Lucchino, R.

(1993) 'Psychiatric morbidity in older people with moderate and severe learning disability', *British Journal of Psychiatry*, 163: 471–480.

Moss, S., Prosser, H., Costello, H., Simpson, N., Patel, P., Rowe, S., Turner, S. and Hatton, C. (1998) 'Reliability and validity of the PAS-ADD checklist for detecting psychiatric disorders in adults with intellectual disability', *Journal of Intellectual Disability Research*, 42 (2): 173–183.

NHS Executive (1998) *Signposts for success in commissioning and providing health services for people with a learning disability*, Leeds: NHSE.

O'Hara, J. and Sperlinger, A. (eds) (1997) *Adults with learning difficulties: a practical approach for health professionals*, Chichester: Wiley.

Piachaud, J. (1999) 'Issues for mental health in learning disabilities services', *Tizard Learning Disability Review*, 4 (2): 47–48.

Prasher, V.P. and Krishnan, V.H.R. (1993) 'Hypothyroidism presenting as dementia in a person with Down's syndrome', *Mental Handicap*, 21: 147–149.

Prosser, H., Moss, S., Costello, H., Simpson, N., Patel, P. and Rowe, S. (1998) 'Reliability and validity of the Mini PAS-ADD for detecting psychiatric disorders in adults with intellectual disability', *Journal of Intellectual Disability Research*, 42 (4): 264–272.

Raghavan, R. (2000) 'Cardinal signs', *Learning Disability Practice*, 3 (3): 25–27.

Reid, A.H. (1972) 'Psychosis in adult mental defectives: II schizophrenic and paranoid psychosis', *British Journal of Psychiatry*, 120: 213–218.

Reid, A.H. (1982) *The psychiatry of mental handicap*, Oxford: Blackwell Science.

Reiss, S. (1988) *Reiss screen for maladaptive behaviour*, Worthington, OH: IDS Publishing Corporation.

Reiss, S. (1999) 'Comments on the Reiss screen for maladaptive behaviour and its factor structure', *Journal of Intellectual Disability Research*, 41 (4): 346–354.

Reiss, S. and Szyszko, J. (1983) 'Diagnostic overshadowing and professional experience with mentally retarded persons', *American Journal of Mental Deficiency*, 87 (4): 396–402.

Royal College of Psychiatrists (1996) *Meeting the mental health needs of adults with mild learning disabilities*, London: Royal College of Psychiatrists.

Russell, O. (1997) 'Diagnosis of psychiatric disorder', in Russell, O. (ed.) *Seminars in the psychiatry of learning disabilities*, London: Royal College of Psychiatrists/Gaskell.

Russell, O. (1998) 'Hidden meanings', *Community Care*, 6 (12): 18–19.

Sigelman, C.K., Budd, E.C., Winer, J.L., Schoenrock, C.J. and Martin, P.W. (1982) 'Evaluating alternative techniques of questioning mentally retarded persons', *American Journal of Mental Deficiency*, 86: 511–518.

Simpson, N. (1997) 'Developing mental health services for people with learning disabilities in England', *Tizard Learning Disability Review*, 2 (2): 35–42.

Sovner, R. (1986) 'Limiting factors in the use of DSM-III-R criteria with mentally ill mentally retarded persons', *Psychopharmacology Bulletin*, 22 (4): 1055–1059.

Waitman, S. and Conboy-Hill, A. (1992) *Psychotherapy and mental handicap*, London: Sage.

Weisblatt, S.A. (1994) 'Diagnosis of psychiatric disorders in persons with mental retardation', in Bouras, N. (ed.) *Mental retardation in mental health: recent advances and practices*, Cambridge: Cambridge University Press.

Welsh Office (1983) The *All Wales strategy*, Cardiff: Welsh Office.

Welsh Office (1994) *Challenges and responses: a report of adults with mental handicaps with exceptionally challenging behaviours, mental illnesses or who offend*, Cardiff: Welsh Office.

World Health Organization (1992) *ICD-10: International statistical classification of diseases and related health problems* (10th revision), Geneva: World Health Organization.

Zubin, J. and Spring, B. (1977) 'Vulnerability: a new view of schizophrenia', *Journal of Abnormal Psychology*, 86: 103–126.

## FURTHER READING

Hollins, S. (1997) 'Counselling and psychotherapy', in Russell, O. (ed.) *The psychiatry of learning disabilities*, London: Royal College of Psychiatrists/Gaskell.
This text provides both case studies and principles in using counselling approaches with learning-disabled individuals. It is of use to anyone contemplating counselling with this client group.

Kroesse, B., Dagnan, D. and Loumidis, K. (1997) *Cognitive-behavioural therapy for people with learning disabilities*, London: Routledge.
This text is an excellent resource for CBT with people who have a learning disability.

Moss, S. and Lee, P. (2001) 'Mental health', in Thompson, J. and Pickering, S. (eds) *Meeting the health needs of people who have a learning disability*, London: Baillière Tindall.
This chapter is a thorough discussion of mental health issues in relation to people with learning disabilities across the life-span.

# CHAPTER 29

# CURRENT APPROACHES TO WORKING WITH CHILDREN AND ADOLESCENTS

*Richard Williams and Fiona Gale*

---

## SUMMARY OF KEY POINTS

- The development of child and adolescent mental health services (CAMHS) in the UK has been slow and uneven. However, renewed attention is now being paid to CAMHS, and strategies and frameworks promise improvements in the overall quality of services.

- Evidence-based approaches to CAMHS require services that are provided in a collaborative, multi-agency and multidisciplinary manner.

- Opportunities for nurses to work at all CAMHS tiers exist, including opportunities in specialist community CAMH services.

---

## INTRODUCTION

We begin this chapter with a brief historical summary. Although we present a challenging picture, our intention is to orientate readers to an exciting and rapidly emerging specialty. Later, we draw attention to issues which pose challenges for effective service design that supports clinical practice of rising quality. Towards the end, we review growth areas for nursing.

# THE HISTORICAL CONTEXT

Relative to many other branches of health care, child and adolescent mental health remains a very young specialism. Over the last eighty years, child and adolescent mental health services (CAMHS) have emerged as an identifiably separate component of health care in the UK. Since the 1920s, development has been increasingly powerful yet slow and uneven, and despite service developments in the 1970s and 1980s, which were uncoordinated, geographically uneven and unrelated to need, there were significant setbacks in the later 1980s and 1990s.

Legislation, implemented in 1974, brought a public health approach to planning health services, substantial reorganisation of services and disciplines, and their reallocation between the NHS and the local authorities. Nonetheless, in the last fifteen years, direct involvement of many local authorities in providing specialist mental health care for young people has declined. Arguably, a key influence on this process was the increasing pressure on social services departments to deal effectively with rapid increases in recognition of abuse. In parallel, the abilities of educational psychologists to invest time in working closely with other mental health care practitioners and directly with pupils in need also declined. This reflects rising demand from parents and schools and 'Statementing' challenges that stem, at least in part, from the Education Act 1980. Consequently, increased demands for assessment and therapeutic activities have passed to the NHS and voluntary sectors, but, perhaps paradoxically, these unco-ordinated changes have contributed to the rising importance of nursing.

Until the mid-1990s, much of what had been delivered depended on the inspiration of the professions rather than explicit policy. Predictably, the NHS Health Advisory Service (HAS) report *Together we stand* showed that CAMHS in England and Wales were very patchy (Williams and Richardson 1995). Despite the evident energy and commitment of their staff, there were problems with the availability and accessibility of services, limited standardisation and replication of their work, and the priority given to young people in need varied greatly across services in adjacent areas.

In 1999, the Audit Commission reported on the NHS contribution in its follow-up to the work of the HAS (Audit Commission 1999). It found that the responses of the authorities in England and Wales to the needs of children and adolescents were extremely variable. Expenditure per child on CAMHS varied by a ratio of 7: 1, the mix of staff employed varied substantially, and there was restricted access to Specialist CAMHS and an incoherent response from those services in direct contact with the public. The report verified the pressure under which many Specialist CAMHS are operating. There were long waiting lists in around a third of services. In many instances, this related to the increase in the prevalence of mental disorder in young people (Rutter and Smith 1995). The cases referred to Specialist CAMHS were increasingly complex, with many young people and their families facing multiple problems.

Significantly, a national thrust towards coherent service planning and commissioning has only arisen after completion of the thematic review by the HAS in 1995. With the benefit of hindsight, it is arguable that the generally laudable and groundbreaking changes of 1974 unwittingly contributed to decline of the child guidance approach to service delivery, left a vacuum in service models that was not filled until 1995 by the tiered strategic approach to service design, and contributed to reduction of direct engagement of many local authorities in Specialist CAMHS.

CAMHS are substantially community-orientated and the great majority of patients who use them do so solely as out-patients. In most areas, nurses played little part in the former child guidance services and nursing was not a key discipline until adolescent in-patient units were developed. In the late 1960s and early 1970s, in response to widespread and persisting concern about admitting young people to adult mental illness beds, in-patient units for young people grew in number and the role of nurses emerged. Initially, the majority of nurses worked in the child and adolescent psychiatric in-patient units, and the English National Board courses 600 and 603 were developed to support them. Yet, despite undesirable reductions in the number of places for young people in purpose-specific adolescent psychiatric units during the last two decades, the role of nursing in child and adolescent psychiatric practice has grown.

Child and adolescent community psychiatric nursing first became a visible entity at national level in the 1980s. In the last twenty years, it has grown enormously in size, diversity of role, impact and importance. Nurses now play an important part in delivering high-quality mental health services that are sensitive to the needs of children and families. Set against the backdrop of a rapidly changing and challenging field, mental health nursing is now a vital force with a very positive future.

In the last generation, advances have been remarkable in the academic disciplines relating to child and adolescent mental health and the evidence base that should inform the development of policy, design of services and practice. The scope of practice and training of practitioners in some disciplines has developed rapidly. However, these advances in the potential capabilities of practitioners and services have been accompanied by much slower, sporadic increases in service capacity. This imbalance, together with greater need and demand, has resulted in widening gaps between the potential for services to intervene effectively in evidence-based ways and their capacity to do so. This became apparent to practitioners, policy-makers and health care strategists in the 1980s and brought child and adolescent mental health on to the political agenda in the early 1990s. Contrary to the predictions of many at the time, that position has been sustained.

Indeed, the National Assembly for Wales published its inclusive strategy for CAMHS in 2001. As we write, the English and Welsh governments are engaged in developing National Service Frameworks for children's health containing mental health modules. These are likely to assure continuing political priority for CAMHS in England and Wales and suggest that the challenges may well be tackled. Consequently, we take an upbeat and excited stance about the future.

Our view is that the future of nursing will be extremely important to the success of initiatives to develop CAMHS in the opening years of the twenty-first century. But, while the recent expansion of posts for nurses has been rapid, there remain some major challenges. Not the least of them is the absence of clear criteria for qualifying nurses in the child and adolescent mental health field and the paucity of training that is targeted towards the real and changing jobs of nurses. Now, the gradual creation of nurse consultants in the field is giving the possibility of real life to nurse postgraduate training in CAMH. Implementation of the Welsh

Strategy began in 2002 and it includes an important initiative to tackle the deficit in nursing staff numbers and their training.

# CHALLENGES TO PROGRESS

## The size of the problem

In 2000, the Office for National Statistics (ONS) published the results of its survey into the prevalence of mental disorders in children and young people in Britain (Meltzer *et al.* 2000). It showed that 10 per cent of Britain's child population suffer a disorder in one of three of the many possible categories. Other work suggests that another 20 per cent or more of the child population may suffer less severe problems (National Assembly for Wales 2001). Overall, the prevalence of all mental disorders in community samples is reported to be around 20–30 per cent of school-age children, and there is reasonable agreement that around 15 per cent may have a more serious disorder.

The prevalence of child and adolescent mental health problems and disorders is clearly linked to deprivation, disadvantage, poverty and social exclusion. The ONS showed that, as family income fell from the top economic groups to the lowest, prevalence rose threefold. Abused children, looked-after children, asylum seekers, refugees and homeless children may be particularly vulnerable. Children with diagnosable disorder are more likely to have experienced: poorer physical health; special educational need; learning difficulties; parents with mental health problems; family discord; greater frequency of punishment by their parents; and a number of stressful life events. Substance use by adolescents is also related to indicators of deprivation, alienation and exclusion, and young people who misuse substances are two to three times more likely to have a mental disorder. Mental disorders are three to four times more common in children with learning disabilities than in the general population.

## Burden

Research has shown that there are many more children in our population who fail to receive services than those who do, though their symptoms are similar (Rutter and Smith 1995). It appears that there is more at work than the degree or nature of a young person's symptoms when determining who is referred.

The burden experienced by adults when dealing with problematic children is a more powerful indicator of who gets referred than the extent and severity of their symptoms (Angold *et al.* 1998, Wu *et al.* 1999). So, epidemiology and distribution of disorder in local communities provide only a partial picture of potential need, as the subjective experiences of the population have a greater impact on patterns of demand and service usage.

Research into the effectiveness and costs of intervening in different locations with children who have behaviour disorders (Harrington *et al.* 2000) has shown that changing ideologies in CAMHS have supported, first, community-based service developments, then development of hospital-based services, followed, more recently, by a return to an accent on the community. The researchers hypothesised that children with behavioural disorders would gain significantly more from community-based interventions and that they would be less costly than hospital-based interventions. Their conclusions do not support the hypothesis and their view is that service location is without effect. They advise that greater attention is paid to factors other than location when planning services. For example, they found that the presence or absence of psychiatric conditions in the children's parents had a much greater impact on compliance with treatment and its effectiveness than any of the other factors they examined.

The health economic work of Knapp and colleagues has shown that when conduct-disordered children become adults they have more broken cohabitations, a greater incidence of depression and anxiety disorder, more problems with alcohol, a greater likelihood of antisocial problems, including criminality, and high utilisation of a number of services (Knapp *et al.* 1999).

## Collaboration

The 'CAMHS Concept' (National Assembly for Wales 2001) expresses the view that the best way to reach the high numbers of children in need is for all services that engage with young people to acknowledge what they do already with respect to mental health and play their part in a much broader, better integrated and more mental health-sensitive approach.

Lack of training and time leads many primary-level practitioners to feel discomfort in engaging with young people with mental health problems. The view of the NHS Primary Care R&D Centre is that:

> developing and expanding the expertise of primary care and community practitioners in child and adolescent mental health offers an opportunity to improve access to services that are acceptable to their children and their families, leaving specialists free to work with children and families who have complex and severe needs.
>
> (Macdonald and Bower 2000)

This reveals a huge agenda to identify the roles that a wide variety of professionals in existing services can play and the training and supervision they need to do so. In this regard, development of primary mental health workers is beginning to play a significant part.

The 'CAMHS Concept' raises the importance of achieving better collaboration between agencies and between departments within agencies. This aspiration is not merely ideological but also evidence-based, and the extent of our knowledge is now such that no one discipline can attempt to hold all the knowledge and skills that are now appropriate to delivering effective mental health care for children and young people.

Work by the Dartington Social Research Unit (DSRU) in Devon suggests that problems of integration across agencies are related to: differences in the theoretical bases and organisational structures of agencies; differences in professional perception of need, risk and the intentions of services; differences in perception of effectiveness and good outcomes; and difficulties in agreeing which of the vulnerable client groups should be given greatest priority (Bullock and Little 1999). An overriding feature is that we lack a common language between agencies. Recently, the Welsh Institute for Health and Social Care published a three-dimensional approach to improving collaboration (Williams and Salmon 2002).

## The workforce

A long-term, coherent workforce development plan will be critical to the success of all of the enterprises we identify here. Crucially, CAMHS require more staff and there is a big training agenda. This demands good strategic and operational leadership.

> Any organisation . . . looks to a leader for reassurance, for support, for guidance – but also for a challenge to make it go beyond what it believes it can do, to aim for excellence. . . . Corporate leaders succeed by freeing the creative drive that exists in the best leader elements of the organisation, by letting these people stretch their wings and . . . try new . . . approaches. Yet, at the same time, leaders need to have their eye on the whole, on the strategic direction they have determined and on the goals they have set.
>
> (Maucher 1999)

Our opinion is that the environment provided by organisations that deliver services and leadership will be a key factor in moving forward. Clinical governance could be a principal driver. It is defined by the UK government as:

> a framework through which NHS organisations are accountable for continuously improving the quality of their services and safeguarding high standards of care by creating an environment in which excellence in clinical care will flourish.
>
> (NHS Executive 1999)

While regulation, quality monitoring and risk reduction are important ingredients of clinical governance, there is evidence to support this definition's recognition of the critical importance of organisational culture and climate. An organisation's flexibility; the sense of responsibility of employees to the organisation; the standards that people set for themselves; positive feedback on performance; the clarity that staff have about the intent and values of the organisation; and their level of commitment to a common purpose are vitally important to quality (Goleman 2000). The Bagshaws draw attention to 'a new concept of the organisation itself being a learning, evolving organisation' in which 'status traditionally given to people who know a lot needs to be shifted to people who share a lot' (Bagshaw and Bagshaw 1999). Other authors consider how best to educate and support practitioners to cope well with decision-making in the demanding environment of modern health care services (Downie and Macnaughton 2000, Williams 2002).

# FACING THE FUTURE

## National Service Frameworks and strategies

The governments in England and Wales are working on their National Service Frameworks for children and each will include a CAMHS module. In Wales, the CAMHS module is likely to be based on its national CAMHS strategy (National Assembly for Wales 2001), which proposes to deal with the issues that we have discussed in this chapter.

### Aim, objectives and principles

The Welsh strategy has three clear aims at its core:

1   Relief from current suffering and problems with the intention of improving, as soon as possible, the mental health of children, adolescents and their families.
2   Longer-term interventions to improve the mental health of young people as they grow up and when they become adults, and, thereby, to positively influence the mental health of future generations.
3   Partnership with families, substitute families and all those who care for young people.

The Welsh strategy identifies fifteen objectives and eight principles to underpin and guide its implementation of this strategy. Each principle is capable of translation into standards. The principles are that services should be: child-centred; respectful and protecting; lawful; equitable and responsive; comprehensive and appropriate; integrated; competent and accountable; and effective, efficient and targeted.

The four-tier strategic framework is now policy in both England and Wales. It is more a design tool than a structural approach to service delivery. There is anecdotal evidence that the tiers have been interpreted with variations across the UK since the HAS published them in 1995, but, here, we cite their application in Wales (National Assembly for Wales 2001).

### Tier 1: Primary or direct contact services

Regardless of sector, Tier 1 describes the frontline of service delivery, i.e. all professionals who have day-to-day contact with children. By virtue of their direct contacts with, and continuing responsibilities for young people and/or their families, staff in frontline services are well placed to recognise, assess and intervene with children's mental health problems. Although not necessarily trained as specialists in mental health, these professionals require basic skills in assessment and intervention practices. In order to discharge their responsibilities, professionals at Tier 1 also require training, consultation and support from Tier 2 and ease of access to it.

### Tier 2:  Services provided by individual Specialist CAMHS professionals

Tier 2 is the first line of Specialist CAMHS. The staff include members of health service Specialist CAMHS, the staff of the education support services (educational psychologists and specialist teachers), and specialist children's social workers as well as some staff of voluntary organisations.

Usually, families are directed to Tier 2 by staff working in Tier 1, though this does not have to be the case. Often, families may meet single members of staff from each agency that is involved. While effective liaison between service components is important and potentially time-consuming at Tier 2, this factor in itself does not define such a service as a Tier 3 service.

### Tier 3:  Services provided by teams of staff from Specialist CAMHS

Services at Tier 3 are more specialised. Some young people and their families may require access to them as a consequence of the complexity of their need, the concentration of skill required, or the crucial nature of the inter-service and/or inter-agency planning required to deliver a targeted programme of interventions and care. It may not be efficient or appropriate to provide all modalities of such specialised care in each locality, but each service at Tier 2 requires access to a definable range of Tier 3 services. Many NHS-based Specialist CAMHS are now moving towards working on a 'hub and spoke' model with Tier 2 and some Tier 3 functions delivered locally, and more specialised Tier 3 activities provided at central but accessible locations.

Generic services at Tier 3 include those delivered by specialist multi-disciplinary teams. Still more specialised services at Tier 3 include a variety of focused clinics, day-care services, special units in certain schools, specialist fostering, and social services-led specialised family intervention centres.

### Tier 4:  Very specialised interventions and care

Very specialised services, which need not be available in each district but to which the local Specialist CAMHS require predictable access, are termed Tier 4 functions. They include very specialised clinics that are only supportable on a regional or national basis, in-patient psychiatric services for children and adolescents, residential schools and residential social care.

## THE AGENDA FOR ACTION

So far, we have identified the requirement to: respond to high levels of need and demand; orientate our services to the experiences of young people and their families; recruit, better train, sustain and lead a larger, more plural workforce; and create environments in provider organisations that are capable of working across boundaries and creatively supporting all these developments. The Welsh vision includes: a radical agenda for service development; using the four-tier strategic framework to bind services together; creating and delivering a challenging work-force plan; and tackling the requirements for improved multidisciplinary, multi-agency collaboration.

Consequently, the strategy recognises the need to expand services in all four tiers. Tier 1 requires particularly great development, which, inevitably, requires substantial additional training of many people who work in health care, education and social service settings, with the aim of early recognition of certain child-hood psychiatric problems and attention to the risk factors. Earlier recognition, coupled with greater availability of simple interventions lying within the enhanced capability of non-specialists, could reach out to respond to the needs of many more children and young people. Additionally, work to increase the resilience of the population of young people at large could have a preventative impact, and this requires greatly enhanced delivery of mental health promotion programmes. The evidence is beginning to show the way forward; for example, it is now becoming plain that much could be achieved by cross-agency approaches to parent training.

This requires much greater support from Tier 2 specialists for non-specialist staff in primary-level services, through training, advice and responsive consul-tation, provided by staff in specialised services. A second key function of Tier 2 is provision of prevention programmes targeted at young people who are identified as being most at risk. The third main function of Tier 2 is provision of direct patient care services through application in each local area of short-term therapeutic programmes for those with identified problems.

The intention is that the bulk of present specialist community services will become focused on delivering Tier 2 and Tier 3 functions. Creating greater capacity and capability in Tier 1, backed by necessary Tier 2 functions, requires new investment and creation of new services at both tiers. This could have an impact on Tier 3 services by changing the profile of referrals to them; referral of children with more minor problems could well decline, but referral of young people with more serious problems is likely to increase as access is made available to a greater proportion of the population in need. So, any agenda for service development must envisage greater investment in Tier 3 too. Many current Tier 3 services need to be consolidated, and as expertise continues to grow, more specialised services should be created to offer focused interventions to young people whose problems have not remitted through their engagement elsewhere in the system. Tier 4 describes those very specialised services; they may be relatively small in volume but much greater and more predictable access to them is required.

Cross-cutting with this plan is recognition that certain groups of young people are more at risk of mental disorder than is the general population, while others are disadvantaged by the low level of availability of particular services. Additionally, the considerable impact of parents' mental disorders on their children has been recognised in recent years, as has the potential for interrupting the continuities between young people's problems and psychiatric disorder in their adulthood. Each of these themes has led to the Welsh strategy identifying a list of client groups and services that will require particular attention across all four tiers.

Throughout, the Welsh strategy recognises the significance of wider social conditions to the mental health of young people, and it thereby sets an agenda for action well outside the mental health care domain. Further impetus to this broad approach has been given by the Carlile Review (National Assembly for Wales 2002).

## FUTURE PATTERNS OF NURSE EMPLOYMENT AND TRAINING

Our survey frames an exciting agenda for CAMHS within which the experience and role of nurses will be crucial. The growing body of knowledge and skill and government commitments now provide profound opportunities for nurses to become involved in some of the most innovative programmes at all tiers of CAMHS. Nurses could have enormous influence in shaping new ways of helping children with mental health needs and contributing to developing comprehensive services built on the evolving evidence base. As the children's National Service Frameworks are developed, many more opportunities are likely to arise. Nurses should be integral to all four tiers, and the functions of each present opportunities for their development in diverse ways. This highlights the importance of defining the qualities required for the expanding roles of nurses and ensuring that they receive adequate preparation.

Greater involvement of nurses at Tier 1 will assist greatly in preventing mental health problems and ensuring prompt earlier intervention. This calls for key (general) nurses to be identified within primary care settings. They will require: knowledge and skills in child mental health; assistance with integrating new abilities into their roles in working with children and families; and formalised networks between them and professionals within Specialist CAMHS. This requires managers in health visiting, school nursing, child health and Specialist CAMHS to take a strategic approach which identifies: lines of accountability; clinical supervision; competencies; and training, for primary care nurses in child mental health.

The roles of specialist practitioners at Tier 2 are emerging. They include defined tasks (e.g. triage, assessment and intervention) performed by CPNs (community psychiatric nurses) and clinical nurse specialists working in community out-patient teams. These increasingly diverse activities require experienced, autonomous practitioners. Other roles for nurses include those in territories that have been uncharted until recently, such as the Youth Offending Teams, work with looked-after children, partnerships with social workers and fostering agencies, and work with young people who misuse substances. In the UK, some Specialist CAMHS have had liaison schemes, provided by Specialist CAMHS nurses and other staff, which offer advice and support, and many more are enhancing their support for primary care professionals. In 1995, the HAS recommended that new posts for primary mental health workers (PMHWs) be established and large numbers have been developed in the UK since.

PMHWs are Tier 2 staff working at the interfaces between Tier 1 and Specialist CAMHS. Although appointments may be open to a range of professionals, nurses are well placed to carry them out. The role offers a range of enhanced practice opportunities, which correspond to those of the clinical nurse specialist, but in a unique way. The principal aim is to enhance provision of CAMHS by non-specialists in Tier 1. There is increasing opinion that a combination of consultation, liaison, supervision, training and joint working with primary care professionals in structured and legitimised partnerships enables this process. The results are likely to be greatly increased contributions of Tiers 1 and 2 to, and preventing more severe mental health need, identifying earlier those children who require intervention, providing effective non-specialist services for children with less complex mental health problems, while also increasing the knowledge and confidence of practitioners at Tier 1 in planned ways.

At Tier 3, nurses have been, and are, developing as therapists and specialists providing input to programmes for specific mental health needs, such as early-onset psychosis, self-harm, eating disorders, autistic spectrum disorders and ADHD (Attention Deficit Hyperactivity Disorder). This tier provides opportunities for nurses to become involved with developing: multidisciplinary resource centres that offer sessional and day-care interventions to a range of children and young people; assertive outreach teams; and peripatetic forensic teams.

Many nurses have developed expertise in in-patient settings, at Tier 4, especially with adolescents. Other very specialised commitments in this tier include those within in-patient forensic mental health teams.

Consultant nurses have recently entered the nursing career pathway and their role in CAMHS is emerging in a number of places in the UK. It provides a long-awaited strategic direction for advanced practice, education and research, from which developments in nursing practice can progress. All posts have academic components that integrate services with the universities. Overall, nurse consultants should better harmonise excellence in practice with training, research and development, which is likely to contribute greatly to retention of expert practitioners, while promoting local agendas. Thus, some of the tasks they take on focus on particular specialist clinical activities, while others enhance nursing departments at all levels by leading on the strategic direction of services. This requires recruitment of nurses with specialist clinical expertise who meet the requirements for academic appointment and are capable of: autonomous clinical decision-making; developing partnerships and working collaboratively with professionals from other agencies; understanding the strategic fit between agencies; and training and supervising others.

The 'CAMHS Concept' calls for identification of common and specialist competencies to guide the development of services. Within this approach, nurses require training that enables them to make meaningful transitions from theory to evidence-based practice, and it is vital for the profession to clarify the components of each role and design a framework to guide and strengthen its contribution.

Presently, pre-registration nursing curricula include little coverage of child and adolescent mental health. Also, there is limited access to post-registration child and adolescent training for CAMHS nurses (ENB 603 and 603 Higher Award). Evaluation of the number of mental health nurses holding such a qualification has shown that just 34 per cent of 87 services employed nurses so qualified (Davies *et al.* 2002), and, often, nurse lecturers lack adequate preparation or expertise in CAMH. Many post-registration courses fall short on preparing nurses for more extended roles, such as those that include consultation and multi-agency collaboration, and this can restrict nursing careers (Limerick and Baldwin

2000). For example, there are only a small number of nurses who are qualified for appointment as consultants in CAMHS, and attention must be given to developing candidates. It is particularly important to include the high-level skills, qualities and expertise required within the suites of postgraduate training courses for nurses that are under construction now.

Expert leadership and management for nursing teams are important, as are clear accountability and clinical supervision frameworks, to aid nurses' continuing professional development and their recruitment and retention. Nurses require access to a range of practice experiences to equip them with the specialist knowledge and skills they require to create high-quality services and meaningful career pathways. Nurse managers should consider a programme of secondments and placements for nurses at all levels within the different service components. Further development of nursing academia is also necessary to enable cultivation and dissemination of good practice through defined and planned research and education.

Overall, post-graduate training plans should give nurses greater access to career opportunities and produce a partnership approach to education in which universities come together with services to enable them to cultivate their own practitioners (Gale and Vostanis, in press).

# REFERENCES

Angold, A., Messer, S.C., Stangl, D., Farmer, E.M.Z., Costello, E.J. and Burns, B.J. (1998) 'Perceived parental burden and service use for child and adolescent psychiatric disorders', *American Journal of Public Health*, 88: 75–80.

Audit Commission (1999) *Children in mind: child and adolescent mental health services*, London: Audit Commission.

Bagshaw, M. and Bagshaw, C. (1999) 'Leadership in the twenty-first century', *Industrial and Commercial Training*, 3 (6): 236–239.

Bullock, R. and Little, M. (1999) 'The interface between social and health services for children and adolescent persons', *Current Opinion in Psychiatry*, 12: 421–434.

Davies, J., Cresswell, A. and Hannigan, B. (2002) 'Child and adolescent mental health services: rhetoric and reality', *Paediatric Nursing*, 14 (3): 26–28.

Downie, R.S. and Macnaughton, J. (2000) *Clinical judgement – evidence in practice*, Oxford: Oxford University Press.

Gale, F. and Vostanis, P. (in press) 'Developing the primary mental health worker role within child and adolescent mental health', *Clinical Child Psychology and Psychiatry*.

Goleman, D. (2000) 'Leadership that gets results', *Harvard Business Review*, March–April, pp. 78–90.

Harrington, R., Peters, S., Green, J., Byford, S., Woods, J. and McGowan, R. (2000) 'Randomised comparison of the effectiveness and costs of community and hospital based mental health services for children with behaviour disorders', *British Medical Journal*, 321: 1047–1050.

Knapp, M.K., Scott, S. and Davies, J. (1999) 'The cost of antisocial behaviour in younger children: preliminary findings from a pilot sample of economic and family impact', *Clinical Child Psychology and Psychiatry*, 4 (4): 457–473.

Limerick, M. and Baldwin, L. (2000) 'Nursing in outpatient child and adolescent mental health', *Nursing Standard*, 15: 13–15 and 43–45.

Macdonald, W. and Bower, P. (2000) 'Child and adolescent mental health and primary care – current status and future directions', *Current Opinion in Psychiatry*, 13: 369–373.

Maucher, H. (1999) 'Introduction', in Jonassen, J.R. (ed.) *Leadership – sharing the passion*, Alresford, Hants: Management Books Ltd.

Meltzer, H., Gatward, R., Goodman, R. and Ford, T. (for the Office for National Statistics) (2000) *Mental health of children and adolescents in Great Britain*, London: The Stationery Office.

National Assembly for Wales (2001) *Everybody's business – child and adolescent mental health services strategy document*, Cardiff: National Assembly for Wales.

National Assembly for Wales (2002) *Too serious a thing – the Carlile Review*, Cardiff: National Assembly for Wales.

NHS Executive (1999) *Clinical governance – quality in the new NHS*, London: Department of Health.

Rutter, M. and Smith, D.J. (1995) *Psychosocial disorders in young people*, Chichester: Wiley.

Townley, M. (2002) 'Mental health needs of children and young people', *Nursing Standard*, 16(30): 38–45.

Williams, R. (2002) 'Complexity, uncertainty and decision-making in an evidence-based world', *Current Opinion in Psychiatry*, 15: 343–347.

Williams, R. and Richardson, G. (1995) *Together we stand: the commissioning, role and management of child and adolescent mental health services*, London: HMSO.

Williams, R. and Salmon, G. (2002) 'Collaboration in commissioning and delivering child and adolescent mental health services', *Current Opinion in Psychiatry*, 15: 349–353.

Wu, P., Hoven, C.W., Bird, H.R., Moore, R.E., Cohen, P., Alegria, M., Dulcan, M.K., Goodman, S.H., Horwitz, S.M., Lichtman, J.H., Narrow, W.E., Rae, D.S., Regier, D.A. and Roper, M.T. (1999) 'Depressive and disruptive disorders and mental health service utilization in children and adolescents', *Journal of the American Academy of Child and Adolescent Psychiatry*, 38 (9): 1081–1090.

# FURTHER READING

Dogra, N., Parkin, A., Gale, F. and Frake, C. (2002) *A multidisciplinary handbook of child and adolescent mental health for frontline professionals*, London: Jessica Kingsley.

National Assembly for Wales (2001) *Everybody's business – child and adolescent mental health services strategy document*, Cardiff: National Assembly for Wales.

Williams, R. and Richardson, G. (1995) *Together we stand: the commissioning, role and management of child and adolescent mental health services*, London: HMSO.

# PART 3

## EDUCATION AND RESEARCH

### INTRODUCTION

In the opening chapter of this third and final section, Michael Coffey and Ben Hannigan begin by emphasising the importance of education and training for the community mental health nursing workforce. They then provide an overview of the development of courses for community mental health nurses, and air some old and some new debates. Here, they highlight the strengths and the weaknesses of both 'specialist practice' and more skills-oriented courses, and suggest that a new approach is needed.

Drawing on their experiences of developing and leading a skills-based psychosocial interventions course, Norman Young and Ian Hulatt show the importance of project management and of forging alliances in order to successfully develop innovative mental health education programmes. Norman and Ian write of the particular importance of sustaining new alliances over time, and of continuing support for newly-qualified course completers.

Quantitative research has generated important knowledge relating to the outcomes of community mental health care, and detailed information concerning the characteristics of the community mental health nursing workforce. In his chapter, Kevin Gournay draws on a number of key studies to demonstrate the value of quantitative approaches, and the ways in which findings from quantitative research have been used to drive forward changes in mental health nursing policy and practice.

A strength of qualitative research is its capacity to generate rich, descriptive accounts of people's experiences, and to set these in particular contexts. In the final chapter of this section, Ian Beech outlines some key principles of non-positivist qualitative research, and demonstrates the importance of studies of this sort for community mental health nursing. Ian also points to the value of participatory approaches to the design and execution of research studies.

# CHAPTER 30

# EDUCATION AND TRAINING FOR COMMUNITY MENTAL HEALTH NURSES

*Michael Coffey and Ben Hannigan*

---

## SUMMARY OF KEY POINTS

- Education and training for the mental health professions is a priority area. However, the education and training of community mental health nurses has frequently been subject to the whims of service provision.

- A variety of post-qualifying courses are available for CMHNs, including 'specialist practice' programmes and skills-based courses such as those in 'psychosocial interventions'. Criticism of specialist practice courses often fails to acknowledge the breadth of CMHN practice which these programmes are attempting to address.

- There are a number of potential alternatives available which remove 'specialist practice' CMHN education from its inappropriate co-existence with other branches of community nursing, including pre-registration preparation as CMHNs and generic mental health worker preparation.

---

## INTRODUCTION

Education and training for the mental health professions is a priority area. At a national policy-making level, attention in recent years has turned to how best to prepare the mental health workforce to deliver long-term strategies such as England's *National service framework for mental health* (NSF) (Department of Health 1999). For example, since the publication of the NSF, considerable work has been completed with a view to mapping the skills, knowledge and values required of mental health practitioners working in a 'modernised' health service. Work has also been completed on the capacity of universities to meet this educational need. Education and training also remains high on the professional nursing agenda. There is, for example, a growing debate over the degree to which nurses at a pre-qualifying level should be prepared as 'generalists' or as 'specialists' (Beech *et al.* 2002). Within mental health nursing, there is considerable interest in the idea of inter-professional education, and also in the development of education and training which more strongly reflects the needs and aspirations of mental health service users. Over the last decade, interest within the field of mental health nursing has also grown in the construction of training programmes which prepare practitioners to provide specific evidence-based interventions (Gournay and Sandford 1998).

This chapter focuses on these, and other, current issues and debates in community mental health nursing education. The chapter opens with a brief overview of the historical development of education programmes for community mental health nurses (CMHNs) in the UK. The chapter then addresses a range of contemporary issues related to the education of CMHNs, and sets these in a current policy and professional context. Finally, we consider some potential alternatives to the current provision of education and training to community mental health nurses.

## THE EARLY DEVELOPMENT OF EDUCATION COURSES FOR CMHNs

Drawing on records maintained by the Department of Health and the Community Psychiatric Nurses' Association, and drawing also on first-hand accounts provided by individuals who were personally involved in the earliest initiatives, White (1990) has traced the first course for CMHNs to developments at Chiswick Polytechnic in the early 1970s. Initially running for a period of just thirteen days over nine weeks, the syllabus for this pioneering programme included teaching in psychology, sociology and social administration, along with the principles and practice of psychiatric nursing in the community. Writing at the time, one of those associated with this pilot course described it as 'a landmark in the progress of prevention and care in mental illness', and praised 'home visiting' as a valuable means of promoting early discharge from hospital and reducing re-admission (Cole 1971, p. 16).

This first short course at Chiswick was soon expanded into a year-long programme (White 1990). This, in turn, became one of the first courses to be approved under the new *Outline curriculum in community psychiatric nursing for registered nurses* (clinical course number 800) developed by the Joint Board of Clinical Nursing Studies (JBCNS). Courses approved under these regulations were aimed at both mental health and learning disability nurses, and were designed to:

> prepare a Registered Mental Nurse (RMN) or a Nurse of the Mentally Subnormal (RNMS) to work effectively in a multidisciplinary team in

order to give psychiatric nursing care and therapeutic and habilitative or rehabilitative support to the patient in the community, taking into account his family and all relevant contacts.

(JBCNS 1974, cited in White 1990, p. 285)

Over the years, '800 series' courses approved first by the JBCNS and then by the English National Board for Nursing, Midwifery and Health Visiting (ENB), and equivalent courses approved by the other UK national boards, came to be seen as the 'gold standard' in CMHN education (Brooker and White 1997). The development of these courses reflected wider trends in nursing education, with the academic level at which programmes were offered rising from certificate to undergraduate diploma level, and beyond (Bowers 1996). However, despite lobbying from educators (see, for example, White and Brooker 1990), securing long-term financing for these courses proved difficult. In addition, post-qualifying courses preparing mental health nurses for practice in the community were never made mandatory in the UK – unlike, for example, the preparation required for practice in health visiting. Quinquennial surveys of the CMHN workforce have repeatedly found that only a minority of practitioners have undertaken an '800 series' or equivalent course. In 1996, for example, just under one-third of CMHNs working in England and Wales taking part in that year's survey reported that they had completed an education programme of this type (Brooker and White 1997).

## 'SPECIALIST PRACTICE' IN COMMUNITY MENTAL HEALTH NURSING

Community mental health nursing is now recognised as one of eight 'specialist practice' areas of community nursing (United Kingdom Central Council for Nursing, Midwifery and Health Visiting (UKCC) 2001). Courses preparing 'specialist practitioners' in community mental health nursing are required to follow 'specialist practice' guidelines, which the UK's new Nursing and Midwifery Council (NMC) has, thus far, continued to endorse. Programmes of this type have superseded the now-discontinued '800 series' courses. These newer programmes are offered at bachelor's degree level or higher, and are run over a full-time academic year of at least thirty-two weeks, or the equivalent period part-time. Half of the time allotted to specialist practice courses is devoted to the study of 'theory', with the remaining half devoted to work in a clinical area under the supervision of an experienced practice teacher. The learning outcomes which courses are required to address are widely-drawn (UKCC 2001). The result is curricula which tend to be broad-based, drawing on aspects of the social and behavioural sciences, as well as on material more precisely tailored towards clinical nursing practice. Courses tend to vary from institution to institution, reflecting local interpretation of UKCC (and now NMC) guidance, local educational needs, and curriculum designers' interests. This variation between courses is one of the factors which have given rise to the criticism of a lack of coherence and focus in CMHN education programmes of this type.

There is a tension in 'specialist practice' programmes between the policy-driven demands for specific emphasis in courses (such as an emphasis on training in psychosocial interventions, as discussed in more detail below) and the demands of the differing interest groups within the family of community mental health nursing. For example, specialist practice CMHN courses attract nurses from diverse areas such as elderly services, child and adolescent mental health services, substance misuse services and forensic services, as well as adult acute services. Coupled with the expectation that courses should meet the educational needs of all of these practitioners, specialist practice courses are also expected to contain an element of generic community nursing preparation. This can vary from one-third to two-thirds of the total course content. This generic content is essentially fashioned around the needs of non-mental health disciplines, and there is a tendency among CMHNs to perceive this input as largely irrelevant. In trying to meet these separate agendas it may be argued that CMHN education is being drawn towards the centre and failing to satisfy its main customers, CMHNs themselves and the trusts they work for. More pointedly, however, this lack of specialist mental health input in courses may in turn fail to meet the needs of service users.

We offer this critique of specialist practice education from the viewpoint of pathway co-ordinators for specialist practice CMHN courses in separate institutions. Our critique is reflective of the tension that we experience in our everyday working lives. Attempting to offer specialist courses (which may not be 'specialist' enough) which conform to expectations laid down by the registration body, while countering criticism that these courses do not meet certain highly specific needs (such those of nurses who work with the seriously mentally ill), remains a difficult balancing act. In addition, there is a tendency within mental health services and from some mental health nurse academics to advocate and prioritise solely skills-based courses, such as those fashioned around, potentially amorphous, psychosocial interventions. This creeping reductionism inherent in the demand for skills-based courses only seems to obviate the need for 'education' in favour of 'training'. The concern we have is that the specific skills training being offered is non-transferable and is applied uncritically to suit the mantra of 'fidelity to the model'. Practice situations may then be approached as if the nurse and service user are engaged in a controlled experiment in which variation is to be avoided lest it distort the intervention.

The experience we have of offering courses for CMHNs is reflected in the findings of surveys of course leaders throughout the UK. Over the years, surveys of the leaders of post-qualifying courses for CMHNs have generated data relating to the structure and uptake of courses (see, for example, Bowers 1997, Hannigan 1999). More recently, attempts have been made to generate data regarding the specific content of programmes. In the most recent survey, which took place in the 1998–9 academic year, CMHN course leaders were asked to provide information about course aims and educational philosophy, key areas of content, assessment strategies used and initiatives employed to advertise and market programmes (Hannigan et al. 2001). Table 30.1 summarises responses from course leaders relating to the educational philosophies and aims of their programmes, whilst Tables 30.2 and 30.3 summarise responses relating to course content.

*Table 30.1* 'Specialist practice' courses for CMHNs: educational philosophies and aims

---

*Educational philosophy and aims*

---

Courses underpinned by student-centred, adult learning philosophies

Developing intellectual and academic abilities

Promoting lifelong learning

Meeting required learning outcomes prescribed by the UKCC and/or the degree-awarding institution

Developing teaching skills

Promoting equality for all students

Facilitating a range of experiences

Providing education for balanced and rounded CMHNs

---

Source: Hannigan *et al.* 2001; reproduced by kind permission of Elsevier Science

*Table 30.2* 'Specialist practice' courses for CMHNs: areas of content identified by course leaders related to the development of skills and knowledge associated with professional practice

---

*Area of course content*

---

Developing clinical nursing skills

Developing nursing knowledge and theory

Implementing and co-ordinating care

Promoting health in individuals, families and communities

Reflective practice and self-awareness

Assessing the needs of service users

Assessing and managing risk

Managing information

Providing high-quality services

Developing nursing values

Focusing on working with people with severe mental health problems

Working as an autonomous practitioner

Skills associated with mentorship, preceptorship and clinical supervision

---

Source: Hannigan *et al.* 2001; reproduced by kind permission of Elsevier Science

*Table 30.3* 'Specialist practice' courses for CMHNs: areas of content identified by course leaders related to the preparation of nurses to work in contemporary community mental health settings

---

*Area of course content*

---

Collaborating with users and carers

Managing care and leading services

Developing innovative, change-oriented practitioners

Preparing nurses to work in inter-professional settings

Developing research-based practice

Developing awareness of political and cultural contexts of practice

---

Source: Hannigan *et al.* 2001; reproduced by kind permission of Elsevier Science

Course leaders, from their responses in this survey, appeared to value both the educational *process* associated with their courses and the educational *outcomes*. Tables 30.2 and 30.3 also confirm that specialist practice courses tend to address a wide breadth of material. However, as we have already suggested in this chapter, this breadth has made programmes of this sort vulnerable to criticism. We have suggested elsewhere that the original vision underpinning the design of specialist practice courses was to develop a 'unified discipline' of community nurses (Trenchard *et al.* 2002). As we have noted above, the design of 'specialist practice' courses reflects this, in that shared learning between groups of CMHNs and groups of other community practitioners (for example, health visitors, district nurses, community children's nurses and community learning disability students) is mandatory. However, it is questionable how far contemporary mental health policy and practice support this original vision. A more appropriate version of shared learning for CMHNs might involve work with other mental health professional groups, such as mental health social workers, mental health occupational therapists, psychologists, psychiatrists, service users and carers.

# TRAINING IN 'PSYCHOSOCIAL INTERVENTIONS'

The claim of ENB 800 series courses, and their specialist practice successors, to be the 'gold standard' in CMHN education came to be increasingly challenged from the early 1990s onwards. Gournay (1994), for example, characterised 'traditional' courses for CMHNs as being 'anachronistic', and out-of-step with new trends in mental health practice, policy and research. Over recent years, policy has increasingly urged practitioners and services to focus their energies on meeting the needs of people identified as experiencing 'severe', or 'serious', mental health problems. Throughout all areas of the health service, interest has also grown in evidence-based practice. Reflecting both these trends has been the development of 'psychosocial interventions' (PSI) courses, which have proved increasingly popular with both mental health practitioners and service managers. Arguably, the term 'psychosocial interventions' is a rather loose one, though in common usage in contemporary mental health settings the phrase has come to be a shorthand for a constellation of evidence-based interventions and models of service delivery for people with serious mental illnesses such as schizophrenia. Brooker (2001) has identified the following as core components of PSI: outcome-orientated assessment; behavioural family work; psychological management strategies; case management; early intervention; and psychopharmacology. By far the best-known of the PSI courses are those developed under the umbrella of the Thorn initiative. Thorn courses are now available throughout many parts of the UK. Although members of any of the mental health professions are welcome to apply to Thorn programmes, the majority of Thorn course completers are mental health nurses.

# EDUCATION AND MENTAL HEALTH POLICY

England's National Service Framework for Mental Health (Department of Health 1999) was developed with the aim of improving and 'modernising' mental health care. Education of the mental health workforce is key to the success of the NSF in England, and its equivalent elsewhere in the UK. For example, following the production of the NSF, the Workforce Action Team (WAT) was set up with a remit to consider not only education and training for the mental health professions, but also issues related to recruitment and retention, pay, public understanding of the role of mental health workers and workforce planning (Department of Health 2001). An important piece of work completed on behalf of the WAT was *The capable practitioner* document (Sainsbury Centre for Mental Health 2001). This set out to identify the constellation of 'capabilities' required by mental health practitioners of all disciplines who work with adults with mental health problems (including nursing, psychiatry, psychology, social work and occupational therapy). These 'capabilities' are widely-conceived, and include: ethical dimensions; knowledge of mental health and of mental health service provision; capabilities associated with the process of care, which include working with individuals and families and with different professional groups and agencies; specific 'bio-psychosocial' mental health interventions; and capabilities relating to the application of all of these elements in particular service contexts.

Initiatives such as *The capable practitioner* are important, and it is clear that CMHN education will have to accommodate new developments as current mental health policy is reviewed and extended in this way. As we write, a new draft mental health bill has been published (Department of Health 2002). The emphasis on compulsion inherent within this potential replacement for the current Mental Health Act for England and Wales will have to be addressed directly by CMHN educators, practitioners and those responsible for providing services. If CMHNs are likely to be formally involved in the process of compulsory admission to hospital for the first time, it is clear that courses will have to expand their treatment of issues of compulsion, coercion and use of power within therapeutic relationships. The extension of powers of nurse-prescribing to mental health nurses will also need highly specific educational input.

# A FUTURE AGENDA FOR CMHN EDUCATION

There is a perennial question that confounds much of the discussion of education and training of mental health nurses. It goes something like this: is mental health nursing to create a separate professional identity, or should mental health nurses accept Morrall's (1998) conclusion that we are essentially handmaidens and therefore remain subjugated to psychiatrists? Whilst this is an important debate, it appears that efforts to solve the dilemma occupy us so much that we fail to develop coherent plans for the future preparation of CMHNs. Some would argue that it is the failure to reconcile the dilemma inherent in this debate that so disables thinking about the educational preparation of CMHNs. CMHN education has been something of a football in a game of polemic for a number of years now.

Criticisms of CMHN education alluded to above have been addressed in some courses in so far as the tensions discussed allow. Here we intend to contribute an outline rationale for the education and training of CMHNs that recognises and to an extent engages these polemics while also reflecting the realities of CMHN practice.

As a starting point it is our contention that generic nurse preparation, at either pre- or post-registration level, is designed to serve the needs of users of general hospital and community services and not the needs of service users with mental health problems. We suggest that a number of alternatives to this educational model exist, one of which would be to design pre-registration programmes in mental health education and training leading directly to qualification as a community mental health nurse. This training should be broad enough to prepare CMHNs to work competently with all groups of service users who currently require mental health services. We would envisage this type of CMHN training to comprise content on: the origins of, and political perspectives on, community mental health nursing; sociology of health and the social context of care; mental health policy and the legislative frameworks governing practice; mental health problems through the life-span; skills in multi-agency working, developing evidence and researching practice; concepts of risk assessment; and mental health promotion. Specific specialist skills modules for working with service users with particular needs should also be included and would address adults with serious mental illness, mental health problems in primary care, child and adolescent mental health, elderly mental health, substance abuse, personality disorder and forensic mental health care, as well as issues related to the prescription and administration of psychiatric medication. All of this content should be informed by service users' experiences of the receipt of care. Moreover service users and their representatives should be involved in the development and preparation as well as the delivery of this material. It remains the case that many service users' experience of mental health services is one of disempowerment and being subject to a degree of coercion and control that most other citizens rarely experience. Despite the rhetoric of recent years, service users' involvement in mental health services remains tokenistic, and this is probably true of mental health nurse education. Rudman (1996), however, offers an example of service users' involvement which, if not a model, at least provides a clear account of the potential to be gained in being open to service users' experiences. We suggest that it is a fundamental and moral obligation that the recipients of services which emphasise a strong interpersonal element should have a say in the training of those who will be caring for them. The rhetoric of mental health services (Department of Health 1994) has been to promote partnerships with service users. The reality is that much work is to be done (Campbell 1999) and programmes of CMHN education should address this.

Shared education and training for CMHNs may have much to recommend it, and we believe that this should be with professionals training in the other mental health disciplines, rather than with other community nurses, as is currently the case. Many mental health nurses and the services for which they work reject this latter type of training, especially those working in the adult acute sector, and many appear to prefer mental-health-only education courses. CMHNs spend the bulk of their professional lives working with psychiatrists, psychologists, social workers and occupational therapists, and it follows that it is with these groups that CMHNs should share their education and training. In our view, generic mental health worker education would be preferable to generic nursing preparation.

CMHNs completing pre-registration training in community mental health could access further specialist courses at post-registration level – for example, to prepare them as specialists or as advanced practitioners in working with specific groups of service users, such as the elderly with mental health problems. It is unrealistic in our view to propose that all CMHNs now divert their attention to only one group of service users, such as the loosely-defined seriously mentally ill. Primary care services still demand and value the input of CMHNs despite a decade of this refocusing, and considerable mental health need is known to exist in primary care settings. It follows, therefore, that a need is perceived within these services, and many CMHNs still provide such input. Plans to employ an army of psychology graduates and other 'primary care mental health workers' (Secretary of State for Health 2000) to address short-term mental health problems do not obviate the need for experienced CMHNs. CMHNs will still be required to supervise this work and to see service users with more complex or unremitting mental health needs.

CMHN education and training should be informed by a fundamental mental health nursing ethos which is steeped in the tradition of humanism, while recognising the limitations of such approaches (see Clarke 1999). We would regard Rogerian approaches, for instance, as necessary elements in working with those with mental health problems rather than as sufficient to enable change. Reflective practice, critical thinking and skills in self-directed learning are central to the training and education of CMHNs. It is these elements that are likely to produce the 'knowledgeable doers' that are required in the complex clinical situations seen in modern community mental health settings.

# CONCLUSION

In this chapter we have reviewed the origins and development of CMHN education, and aired some old and some new debates. We have argued for a move away from the type of education that assumes that the needs of mental health nurses are similar enough to the needs of other groups of nurses to justify courses having a large shared learning component. We have also argued that purely skills-based courses are limited. Instead, we have argued for a new approach to CMHN education which combines the best of what is currently available. This would include education which is soundly based in the social, behavioural and clinical sciences, and which is underpinned by a strong mental health nursing ethos. We are in favour of sharing education with other mental health practitioner groups, and are in favour of programmes of study which begin and end with a strong commitment to the needs and interests of mental health service users. We argue, too, for the kind of educational experience that promotes the development of inquisitive, self-sufficient and reflective practitioners.

However, we recognise that, just as we are arguing for a greater commitment to specialisation within nursing and in nursing education, others are arguing in favour of increased genericism. This is a debate that mental health nurses need to engage with, and our view is that the idea of the 'generalist nurse' is one that should be resisted. Mental health nurse educators also need to make strong links with individuals and organisations outside of their usual circles: educators and practitioners from other disciplines, service users and user organisations, and so on. Our experiences are that making and keeping these kinds of alliances often requires a major effort, and many institutional, organisational and attitudinal barriers need to be overcome. We suggest that urgent attention needs to be paid to the (arguably now-outdated) idea of the 'specialist practitioner' course. Finally, we argue for a clear emphasis on the kind of educational experience that is more than simply 'training'.

# REFERENCES

Beech, I., Coffey, M. and Hannigan, B. (2002) 'The case for specialist mental health training', *Nursing Times*, 98 (15): 40–41.

Bowers, L. (1996) 'Community psychiatric nurse education in the United Kingdom: 8 years of surveys and the issues raised', *Journal of Advanced Nursing*, 23: 919–924.

Bowers, L. (1997) 'Community psychiatric nursing courses: take up, content and course leaders' views', *Psychiatric Care*, 4: 26–29.

Brooker, C. (2001) 'A decade of evidence-based training for work with people with serious mental health problems: progress in the development of psychosocial interventions', *Journal of Mental Health*, 10 (1): 17–31.

Brooker, C. and White, E. (1997) *The fourth quinquennial national community mental health nursing census of England and Wales*, Manchester and Keele: Universities of Manchester and Keele.

Campbell, P. (1999) 'The future of the mental health system: a survivors' perspective', *Mental Health Practice*, 3 (1): 12–17.

Clarke, L. (1999) *Challenging ideas in psychiatric nursing*, London: Routledge.

Cole, E. (1971) 'Community psychiatric nursing course', *Nursing Mirror*, 132 (20): 16.

Department of Health (1994) *Working in partnership: a collaborative approach to care. Report of the Mental Health Nursing Review Team*, London: HMSO.

Department of Health (1999) *National service framework for mental health: modern standards and service models*, London: Department of Health.

Department of Health (2001) *Mental health national service framework (and The NHS Plan) workforce planning, education and training underpinning programme: adult mental health services: Final report by the Workforce Action Team*, London: Department of Health.

Department of Health (2002) *Mental health bill: consultation document*, London: The Stationery Office.

Gournay, K. (1994) 'Redirecting the emphasis to serious mental illness', *Nursing Times*, 90 (25): 40–41.

Gournay, K. and Sandford, T. (1998) 'Training for the workforce', in Brooker, C. and Repper, J. (eds) *Serious mental health problems in the community: policy, practice and research*, London: Baillière Tindall.

Hannigan, B. (1999) 'Education for community psychiatric nurses: structure, content and trends in recruitment', *Journal of Psychiatric and Mental Health Nursing*, 6: 137–145.

Hannigan, B., Burnard, P., Edwards, D. and Turnbull, J. (2001) 'Specialist practice for UK community mental health nurses: the 1998–99 survey of course leaders', *International Journal of Nursing Studies*, 38 (4): 427–435.

Morrall, P. (1998) *Mental health nursing and social control*, London: Whurr.

Rudman, M.J. (1996) 'User involvement in the nursing curriculum: seeking users' views', *Journal of Psychiatric and Mental Health Nursing*, 3 (3): 195–200.

Sainsbury Centre for Mental Health (2001) *The capable practitioner*, London: Sainsbury Centre for Mental Health.

Secretary of State for Health (2000) *The NHS Plan: a plan for investment, a plan for reform*, London: The Stationery Office.

Trenchard, S., Burnard, P., Coffey, M. and Hannigan, B. (2002) 'Education for community mental health nurses: a summary of the key debates', *Nurse Education Today*, 22: 258–264.

United Kingdom Central Council for Nursing, Midwifery and Health Visiting (UKCC) (2001) *Standards for specialist education and practice*, London: UKCC.

White, E. (1990) 'The historical development of the educational preparation of CPNs', in Brooker, C. (ed.) *Community psychiatric nursing: a research perspective*, London: Chapman and Hall.

White, E. and Brooker, C. (1990) 'The standing advisory group for community psychiatric nursing: grasping the nettle?', *Nurse Education Today*, 10: 63–65.

# FURTHER READING

Clarke, L. (1999) *Challenging ideas in psychiatric nursing*, London: Routledge.
There is much to recommend in this text, not least the persistent contrariness of the author; however, the chapter '1999: a nursing odyssey' presents a particular viewpoint on mental health nursing that will resonate with many within the profession.

Tilley, S. (ed.) (1997) *The mental health nurse: views of practice and education*, Oxford: Blackwell Science.
This edited collection includes a range of fascinating and lively personal insights into mental health nursing, and into nursing education and practice.

# CHAPTER 31

# DEVELOPING COURSES IN PSYCHOSOCIAL INTERVENTIONS

*Norman Young and Ian Hulatt*

---

## SUMMARY OF KEY POINTS

- Psychosocial interventions training is an essential component within the whole systems approach to mental health and social care.

- The development of a psychosocial interventions course benefits from a project management approach.

- The key to enduring success is the creation of enduring partnerships that will support and sustain the implementation of psychosocial interventions in routine practice.

---

## INTRODUCTION

The development of courses in psychosocial interventions (PSI) could be considered one of the success stories of recent times. Since the original Thorn initiative of 1992 (Gamble 1995) there has been a year-on-year increase in the number of courses available at higher education institutions. This has culminated in the national provision of approximately thirty courses ranging from diploma to master's degree level (Brooker *et al.* 2002). Some 600 students have now received training in PSI, and new courses are continually being developed. Nationally the provision of training shows a patchy distribution, with a 'Londoncentric' over-provision and Wales waiting ten years for its first diplomates at the authors' institution.

This chapter will consider the drive for such enthusiastic educational developments and the processes necessary to not only develop such a course but also sustain the graduates in their new-found role.

Why then has there been such a favourable response to courses offering training in PSI? First it must be acknowledged that such courses are a response to a clearly expressed need. A government beleaguered by claims that its policy of community care for the mentally ill was not so much in trouble as fundamentally flawed articulated this need. The care received by individuals with serious and enduring mental health problems was considered to be patchy at best and at worst woefully inadequate. Importantly, it was also recognised that the carers and families of such individuals were overburdened to the point of detrimental effects to their own health.

In response to these clear needs the Department of Health (1998a, b) declared an agenda to change the services received by clients and their carers, one that included greater investment in 'evidence-based' staff training. This evidence-based training is described under the broad term of PSI. What, then, are the usual components of such a scheme of training?

Brooker (2001) acknowledges that the term has changed in its descriptive power over the last ten years but is currently used to describe a scheme containing 'outcome based assessment; behavioural family work; psychological management strategies for individuals (including cognitive behaviour therapy and coping strategy enhancement); case management; and early intervention'. Medication management, whilst appearing outside of the term PSI, is increasingly becoming an integral component of such programmes, and is consistent with the principle of developing programmes to meet issues of concern in relation to maximising the benefits of medication in the community (Kemp *et al.*, 1997, 1998).

In many areas there exist gaps in providing PSI training to diploma, degree or master's level. Unless an institution makes a franchise arrangement then a course will need to be developed locally. How may this best be carried out and the institution's aim of providing a PSI programme be realised? The following section will illustrate elements of this process through the authors' experience of developing the first Thorn course for Wales. An overview of this process is given in Figure 31.1.

# GETTING STARTED: THE VISION

A new initiative needs to take people to a different position, an improved situation compared to the one they are in now. This will be achieved through a clear and well-articulated vision, allied to strong leadership and the support of key stakeholders, people with power and influence within organisations. Once this critical mass of people is in place, a 'chain reaction' of events will occur, sufficient to carry the project forward.

If the components are not in place, or just lack ignition, then the critical event can take years. The latter appeared to be the case for us. South Wales has a long tradition in schizophrenia family work stretching back to the STEP project (initiated in 1986 but now terminated; Hughes and Abbati-Yeoman 1995, Hughes

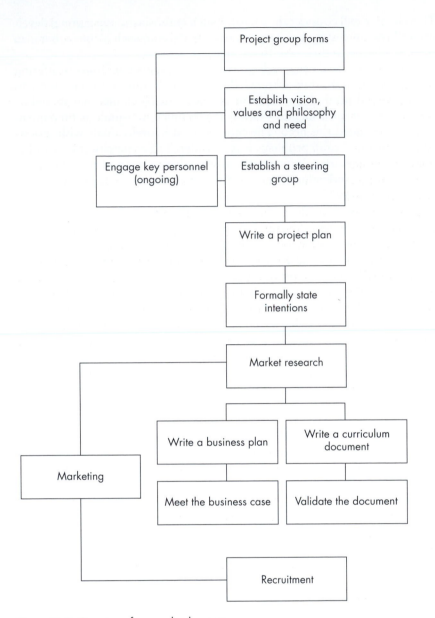

*Figure 31.1* Overview of course development

*et al.* 1996), the Pisces project, and a University of Wales College of Medicine diploma module in behavioural family therapy for schizophrenia, running from 1996 onwards. The expertise in PSI work was available; however, surprisingly, not until 1999 did a full PSI course start to develop.

Perhaps for us a deciding moment was an approach to Professor Kevin Gournay (Professor of Nursing at the Institute of Psychiatry) and colleagues at a Network for Psychiatric Nursing Research conference. He was asked if a small group of people could meet and discuss the process of setting up a Thorn satellite site in Cardiff. The prominence of the meeting in London drew together a number of influential and energetic individuals. Of note were their varying views on mental health education, in particular the Thorn initiative, but they were willing to resist polarisation and to work towards the common goal of skills-based inter-professional training for psychosis.

As our small project group began to form we needed to spend more time addressing the core values and philosophy that would underpin the PSI course. Important questions such as: what level of award is needed? In what way do we describe and value evidence-based practice? What do we understand by multi-disciplinary training? To what extent do we embrace service users and carers in education planning? How far do we consider educational outreach into clinical settings as important?

Establishing core values and philosophy will underpin all your work and provide a point to return to as the project passes key stages and when it is challenged. We were able to come to a consensus and from there we questioned whether we should write a new course or adopt one of the many PSI courses throughout the UK. We had already established and maintained strong links with the Thorn initiative, in particular with Gloucester (Rolls *et al.* 2002), and had been able to dispel the unhelpful image of the Thorn practitioner as a technician. The Thorn initiative's values and philosophy fitted with ours and were what we wished to aspire to, and so we took steps to become a satellite site. With a clear vision, and explicit values and philosophy, our intentions were now much easier to communicate. The task of moving a speculative project to one that would be widely supported was now upon us.

## COMMUNICATING INTENTIONS, AND ENGAGING STAKEHOLDERS

Universities will differ in the way that they apply for consent to develop a new course. Generally this will be achieved through a letter of intent. The purpose of the letter is to seek university approval for the venture, i.e. it meets its strategic aims and objectives. The content of such a letter does not need to be too detailed, but it needs to state the potential market, level of the award, resources required, duration of the course and when it is likely to run. Such details will be expanded on in your business case.

The small project team will be responsible for the majority of tasks throughout the course development; however, a larger steering group will be required in order to provide expert opinion and direct its work. Your letter of intent can be reworded and used to invite members to the steering group; within it you will need to explain your expectations of them. For Thorn courses the steering group needs to consist of a range of mental health professionals, service users and carers. Alongside this the steering group will need to identify another Thorn site that will agree to offer help and advice throughout your course's development.

Good local knowledge of those with influence and interest in PSI training will prove invaluable in identifying key people. It is always wise to write to organisational heads, particularly within hierarchical structures. This will assist you in gaining representation from groups in which you have not identified a person, top management support for the steering group member, and generally raising interest in the development.

## MANAGING A STEERING GROUP

When the steering group meets for the first time it will be necessary to elect a chairperson. The importance of this role can never be overstated. Traditionally steering groups elect a chairperson who has significant experience and influence, with the steering group directing the work of smaller working groups with co-opted members. However, this does not need to be the case, and for small projects it may disadvantage the work due to the higher priority afforded to other more prestigious demands. For us, one of the authors (Norman Young) was elected as chair and also served on the curriculum working group.

With such a small project the chairperson often takes on a significant amount of work. They will need good chairing skills so that meetings are kept to time and matters are effectively covered. Meetings work best when they are short, well-prepared, and have a clear agenda, with work prepared beforehand so that clear tasks are identified and delegated. From the earliest stage it is wise to keep all records of correspondence and take minutes of meetings. Such attention to procedure will allow work to be tracked and support documents when they are presented for scrutiny. It is worthwhile being clear about what types of information are faxed, e-mailed, telephoned and posted. Not all people are familiar with e-mail and letters may seem more personal or official.

In keeping work manageable always question whether someone else can perform the task in hand – remember what you do and do it well. It was an immense help when the steering group secured secretarial help in recording, writing and distributing the minutes of meetings. Such tasks can be quite labour-intensive and demand a good knowledge of etiquette.

## WRITING A PROJECT PLAN

Following consultation and the establishment of a steering group you will be in a position to map out the critical tasks for the project and the dates when these need to be completed. Project management is a term applied to such an approach and has been traditionally used in the manufacturing industry. Many of the skills can be usefully applied to the development of a PSI course, in particular the use of a Gantt chart.

The Gantt chart was developed as a production control tool in 1917 by Henry L. Gantt, an American engineer and social scientist. In the creation of the chart you are required to list all the tasks for the project chronologically so that you can link each one that is dependent on another, and define other relationships. The process of allocating time, resources and relationships to tasks helps in planning each element of the project, calculating overall slippage when one part of the plan is behind, prioritising work and communicating the work plan to others. An example is given in Figure 31.2. Software to assist project work is available at varying costs; however, some can be obtained on a trial basis which may be useful if you do not engage in much project work. Spreadsheets can offer a limited alternative.

Draft Medication Management Project Time Line
Project Curriculum development of a Level III Credit Module of 40 Cat Points

Page 1 of 1 28/12/01

| Start Date | End Date | TASK |
|---|---|---|
| 11/1/02 | 7/2/02 | Budget & Market Research |
| 17/2/02 | 17/2/02 | Letter of Intent |
| 3/3/02 | 4/5/02 | Appoint External Examiner |
| 22/2/02 | 20/9/02 | Project Group Meetings |
| 5/5/02 | 25/8/02 | Marketing |
| 12/7/02 | 9/8/02 | Submit Draft Documents |
| 13/9/02 | 13/9/02 | Final Document |
| 1/11/02 | 8/11/02 | Candidate Interviews |
| | | |
| 20/3/02 | 22/11/02 | PSI Steering Group Meetings |
| 23/8/02 | 31/10/02 | Validation Meetings (Subject to confirmation) |
| 10/1/03 | 10/1/03 | Course Start Date |

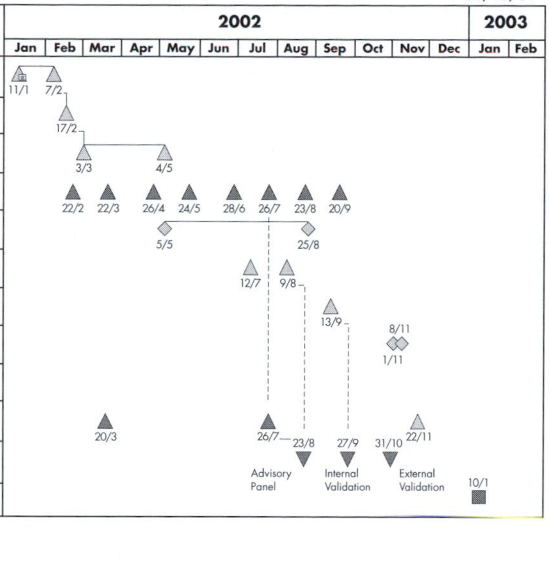


*Figure 31.2* An example of a Gantt chart for a medication management module

# CLARIFYING THE NEED FOR TRAINING: MARKET RESEARCH

In the introduction the need to train mental health practitioners in PSI was made clear. However, such evidence does not necessarily translate into local demand or commitment. It is essential to inform the project plan by writing a business case for the course, and identifying the market for such an initiative, the true cost and the cost that the market will bear.

Need can be identified and supported by the literature, but a failure to conduct some market research can lead to the creation of a white elephant. In order to develop links with those who are budget holders for training in health and social services, the course should be discussed with them in relation to their strategic plan for training and service development. This also underpins contracting for places.

Alongside your research into the commitment to PSI training at a strategic level, you will need to establish whether the workforce itself has an interest in professional development and learning more effective ways of caring. It is worth bearing in mind that there are many pressures that draw those in the caring professions away from spending time on their personal and professional development.

Our market testing showed a strong initial interest and commitment from senior NHS trust management; however, it later became clear that, in one area, understanding, support and interest in the training were poor. We later attributed this to a lack of awareness of the Thorn course, and a poor commitment to training by the workforce for reasons that were not clear. Overall this illustrated an original failure to survey those on the ground, and impacted significantly on our recruitment projections.

## WRITING A BUSINESS CASE

The business case will prove to be the driving document. It will be required to gain support from budget holders and in identifying and gaining resources. The format of a business proposal will be familiar to many and generally follows the pattern below (Finch 2001):

- Introduction
  - Background to the proposal
  - Supporting literature
  - Aims and philosophy
  - Fit with strategic aims and objectives of the college

- Market summary
  - Need for the new course (market fit)
  - Opportunities
  - Competition
  - Market research

- Financial plan
  - Including start-up costs, recurring costs and fit with existing and future pricing structures
  - Other resources

- Work plan
  - Project team
  - Timeline
  - Key tasks
  - Critical dates

- Risks and rewards
  - Including the management of risks

- Summary of key points

The Thorn course is recognised as labour-intensive. This is due to the high staff-to-student ratio required for clinical skills rehearsal, clinical supervision and the review of clinical materials. Hence two lecturers will teach on study days, giving rise to one whole-time equivalent (WTE) lecturer for the course supported by 0.5 of a WTE administrator.

From our business plan we were able to argue for additional resources to train a lecturer in psychosocial interventions as well as recruit a PSI practitioner to work on the course. Without a robust business case it would not have been possible to convince those who held budgets, who were principally aware of only the adult nursing agenda.

# WRITING A CURRICULUM DOCUMENT

Your steering group's main concern in the development of the course will be to scrutinise the work of the curriculum working group. This group needs to be small, diligent and task-focused. It is essential that it is made up of people with knowledge about PSI work and curriculum development. They will need to organise meetings well in advance and bring with them a laptop computer so that work is dealt with there and then.

The steering group will need to periodically scrutinise the curriculum document as progress is made. The steering group should be directed to see themselves as critical friends, and they will appreciate having the document three weeks prior to a meeting. Your steering group members will be busy people, so encourage those who are unable to attend to send constructive comments. Also remember that by now you should have engaged an external examiner for the course and they too should be consulted as the document progresses.

If you know the institution that will be validating your course, then to a certain extent your task is made that much easier. The relevant department, either registry or a quality assurance department, should have supplied you with clear guidance as to their desired format for the submission document, and, if necessary, supporting information. If this is not supplied, then you must obtain it before you proceed with your planning and document construction.

A typical document will contain the items listed in Box 31.1. When the document is finished it will be ready to pass through the university validating procedures. We found that two members of the working group were best placed to oversee this (those who eventually delivered the course).

---

**Box 31.1   General items required for a curriculum document**

- Background to the course
- Philosophy
- Aims and objectives
- Mode of course delivery
  - The length of the course
  - Where it will be delivered
  - The breakdown of course time into taught, clinical and self-directed study
  - How many CAT (Credit Accumulation and Transfer) points are to be awarded

---

- Student support throughout the course
  - Tutor and pastoral support
  - IT and libraries

- Purpose and principles of assessment
  - The rationale for assessing clinical and academic work and how this will be achieved

- Progression through the course
  - Submission dates
  - Rights of appeal

- Entry criteria and selection criteria

- Quality assurance

- Module details
  - Learning outcomes
  - Indicative content
  - Teaching strategies
  - Assignments and other assessments
  - Recommended reading

- Curriculum document references

## VALIDATING A COURSE

What then can you expect at a validation event and who should you choose to represent your planning team? An obvious point here, and one that the authors found useful to observe, is to have a member of the planning team who is familiar with this process present at the event. It is an even stronger position to be in if that person has experience of course delivery as well as planning.

Validation panels sometimes show interest in how you intend to address certain issues that may arise as the proposed course actually comes to life in its delivery. Both parties' best approach to a validation event is to view it as a collegiate consideration of a proposed course rather than a combative event. It is an opportunity for you as the proposer of the course to demonstrate the careful thought you have given to this venture, whilst the panel will equally demonstrate their seriousness in ensuring that they safeguard and promote the institution's academic standards.

Be prepared to carefully (and patiently) explain areas that the panel wishes to have clarification on, and also have a coherent rationale for any aspect of the proposal that may be outside of the panel's normal range of validation experience. It is also equally essential to have considered before the meeting which part of the document you as the proposers will each accept questions on. You therefore need to identify appropriate experience within your group, and also ensure that all of you take part.

This will avoid any embarrassing situations at the validation event, or delays if the institution will not accept what they consider to be a non-standard submission. An important point to make here is that departments such as these are there to support your endeavours not thwart them. Remember it is just as much in their interest to successfully validate your course as it is in yours.

Similarly, are you clear about which parts of the proposed document you consider negotiable, and which are not? Are there areas that you consider so essential to not only the ethos of this course but also its delivery that you would defend them vigorously?

If any panel member seems rather too inquisitorial in his/her questioning, remember it is the role of the validation panel's chairperson to address such issues, not you! All questions are best dealt with patiently, but if you feel that the answer you provide is repeatedly not that required, it is probably best to enquire what exactly the panel member wants to know.

You should leave the event with a clear indication of whether your work has been successful. You will probably be provided with a verbal summary from the panel chairperson, indicating recommendations (things you may like to consider) or additional requirements (things you must do). If the above sounds daunting, be reassured that validation events can actually be quite enjoyable! You are provided with an opportunity to publicly demonstrate the hard work and careful thought that you and your colleagues have put into your proposed course. Seize that opportunity in a planned, systematic manner, and success should follow.

# THORN COURSE VALIDATION

One form of external validation of PSI courses is recognition by the Thorn initiative. If you wish to externally validate your course in this way, then you will need to contact the Thorn steering group early on in your curriculum development process (see recommended further reading at the end of this chapter). They will link you up with a nearby Thorn site who will help you progress through the validation process. Again, as with internal validation, the aim is to help you succeed but at the same time make sure that the course is of high quality. Box 31.2 illustrates the requirements for validation by the Thorn initiative.

# MAINTAINING MOMENTUM

Whilst the skills acquired by PSI graduates are gained on an individual basis, they are expressed within the context of the services they work in. Follow-up studies of PSI graduates would seem to support the view that the skills acquired are finding little expression in routine everyday practice. This has been noted in studies that follow up students who have undertaken training in family intervention (Kavanagh et al. 1993, Fadden 1997), where a low implementation rate of family work was noted.

**Box 31.2   Thorn initiative evaluators' checklist**

1   Is the course supported by a recognised academic institution?
2   Does it meet with outlined criteria and does the stress vulnerability model underpin the overall curriculum?
3   Have the course organisers received appropriate, ongoing support from TSG (Thorn Steering Group) members?
4   Have the local course organisers communicated regularly and coherently with TSG members?
5   Does the curriculum focus on people who experience psychosis?
6   Do the curriculum and teachers involved reflect the multidisciplinary nature of the work?
7   Are the learning outcomes, their relevance and applicability to clinical practice clear?
8   Is the structure of the programme logical and coherent and does it allow for evidence-based acquisition of clinical skills?
9   Are reading lists multidisciplinary, up-to-date and commensurate with the qualification?
10   Is clinical supervision provided as part of the course programme?
11   Is clinical competence directly assessed?
12   Content: is appropriate weighting given to the following components?

   a   User and carer involvement and participation
   b   Assertive care management
   c   Family intervention
   d   Medication management
   e   Management of distressing symptoms
   f   Relapse prevention
   g   Issues of social inclusion and stigma
   h   Meaningful daily activity
   i   Service survival for practitioners
   j   Comprehensive and systematic assessment:

      i   Global measures of need
     ii   Symptomatology
    iii   Social functioning
    iv   Medication side effects
     v   Carer and user satisfaction
    vi   Carer need and burden
   vii   Risk

Notwithstanding the sometimes difficult nature of engagement with this client group there are many other factors that impact upon implementation. Hughes *et al.* (1996) noted benign neglect rather than active opposition regarding the STEP programme in Cardiff, and the request to reduce caseloads in order to either undertake the PSI training or implement it upon completion may face such indifference.

If we are to value and promote psychosocial interventions, then the factors that facilitate its promotion and maintenance need to be more fully understood. Some answers may be found from the wider literature on establishing new work practices. This is dominated by diffusion of innovations research, in particular the work of Everett Rogers. Rogers's model of diffusion (Rogers 1995) proposes that the rate of adoption of innovation is determined according to the following five variables:

1    The perceived attributes of the innovation – this includes how complex the innovation is, what advantage it has over others, whether a sample or trial is possible before adoption, how visible it is, and how compatible it is with the adopter.
2    The type of innovation decision – this describes whether the adopter is free to make the decision to adopt, whether it is a collective decision or enforced.
3    Communication channels – this refers to how the innovation is promoted, ranging from promotion through the mass media, to word of mouth.
4    The social system – this describes the customs, traditions and norms of the social group.
5    The nature of change agents.

Such factors can be used to stimulate an analysis of your local environment, which will lead to strategies that may help overcome the barriers to adoption and implementation of PSI in routine care. An example of this is given in Table 31.1. This review can be developed further, and moved from analysis to action, by weighting each strategy for impact versus effort, prioritising each item and then placing the strategies on a timescale for action. By doing this you will be taking a robust and managed approach to implementation.

One important resource you will have developed during the setting up of the course is your steering group. Once the course has been developed, it is vital that you do not lose its membership, as the group can now refocus and attend to maintaining momentum and exerting influence (akin to the PSI forum mentioned in Table 31.1). This was a strategy employed by ourselves, amongst others, from Table 31.1; as our first cohort finished, we recognised a real need to continue to support and maintain novice PSI practitioners as they attempted to integrate these new skills into their practice.


# CONCLUSIONS

Developing a new training initiative can be a highly enriching and rewarding experience, and one which continues as the initiative grows. Those tasked with this process need to appreciate the 'whole systems' approach to mental health and social care. Education and training are essential components of this system, and educators can enhance their unique position in health and social care by reaching out and participating in governance, practice development, supervision, leadership and the management of change. The partnerships required to achieve this will lead to increased support for practitioners in the workplace, stimulate innovation, and promote research and the development of practice.

*Table 31.1* Applying Rogers's model to the adoption of psychosocial interventions

| Variable | Restraining factors | Strategies to overcome barriers |
| --- | --- | --- |
| The perceived attributes of the innovation | • Psychosocial interventions are often perceived as time-consuming, complex and intensive interventions, which require training and supervision to support their practice<br>• The impact of the interventions in routine practice takes time and is not compatible with contact-driven rather than quality-driven services<br>• The work of practitioners using psychosocial interventions is not particularly visible<br>• The cost of training can be high and length can range from one to two years | • Promote research into reducing the complexity of interventions<br>• Reduce time to train<br>• Train close to the workplace or as required<br>• Reduce cost of training and implementation<br>• Make supervision and support more accessible<br>• Make clear that PSI work reduces work strain |
| The type of innovation decision | • Community practitioners are autonomous, with little monitoring of the type, quality and outcome of their clinical interventions<br><br>• The innovation decision is made predominately on an optional basis set against the directive to utilise evidence-based practice | • Managed care<br>• Clear PSI standards<br>• Ensure that PSI features in integrated care pathways<br>• Monitoring and audit |
| Communication channels | • Whilst good practice is communicated through professional journals, websites and the clinical effectiveness programme, these are not widely read, or are seen as 'not possible here, or with my caseload' | • Integration of PSI into public education programmes<br>• Greater use of web-based information and support, i.e. clinical resources online<br>• Network of PSI good practice<br>• Clinical exchange programmes<br>• Raise consumer awareness of PSI<br>• Conferences and newsletters |
| The social system | • The NHS and social services have traditionally been seen as slow adopters of new innovations<br>• Mental health continues to battle against a public perception of 'big and dangerous', is poorly resourced and is unable to recruit and retain the best staff<br>• National concerns about the NHS reflect inconsistencies in practice and the utilisation of accepted best practice | • Review the organisation's internal and external networks, communication paths and strategy<br>• Ensure that psychosocial interventions are represented in each element of governance<br>• Gain commitment throughout the organisation, from trust board or social services executive through to grassroots<br>• Crystallise commitment in an action-focused PSI forum, which is |

*Table 31.1* continued

| Variable | Restraining factors | Strategies to overcome barriers |
| --- | --- | --- |
| | • There are numerous professions each with their own agendas, and often separately line-managed | tasked with raising standards, audit, training and supporting staff<br>• Assist managers to accommodate PSI as they manage change by engaging them in the PSI forum and/or running PSI for managers workshops<br>• Link PSI into the training and education strategy<br>• Create PSI-supportive work environments, in particular easily accessible, high-quality clinical materials |
| The nature of change agents | • Clinical leadership is a concern for the NHS, with poor retention of skilled and senior staff<br>• The number of people trained in psychosocial interventions is increasing but remains small<br>• Those in positions of influence are unlikely to have experience of psychosocial interventions | • Perform an organisational analysis to identify those with influence and power, internally and externally<br>• Engage opinion leaders and change agents<br>• Gain support for an action-orientated PSI forum with broad representation<br>• Ensure that PSI is incorporated into mental health and social care leadership programmes<br>• Maintain strong links with those trained in PSI, involve them in practice development, supervision, training and leadership |

# REFERENCES

Brooker, C. (2001) 'A decade of evidence-based training for work with people with serious mental health problems: progress in the development of psychosocial interventions', *Journal of Mental Health*, 10 (1): 17–31.

Brooker, C., Gournay, K., O'Halloran, P., Bailey, D. and Saul, C. (2002) 'Mapping training to support the implementation of the National Service Framework for mental health', *Journal of Mental Health*, 11 (1): 103–116.

Department of Health (1998a) *A first class service: quality in the new NHS*, London: The Stationery Office.

Department of Health (1998b) *Modernising mental health services: safe, sound and supportive*, London: Department of Health.

Fadden, G. (1997) 'Implementation of family interventions in routine clinical practice following staff training programs: a major cause for concern', *Journal of Mental Health*, 6 (6): 599–612.

Finch, B. (2001) *How to write a business plan*, London: Kogan Page.

Gamble, C. (1995) 'The Thorn nurse training initiative', *Nursing Times*, 9 (15): 31–34.

Hughes, I. and Abbati-Yeoman, J. (1995) *A S.T.E.P. forward: a guide for people working with schizophrenia sufferers and their families*, Cardiff: Shadowfax.

Hughes, I., Hailwood, R., Abbati-Yeoman, J. and Budd, R. (1996) 'Developing a family intervention service for serious mental illness: clinical observations and experiences', *Journal of Mental Health*, 5: 145–159.

Kavanagh, D.J., Piatkowska, O., Clarke, D., O'Holloran, P., Manicavasagar, V., Rosen, A. and Tennant, C. (1993) 'Application of cognitive behavioural family intervention for schizophrenia in multidisciplinary teams: what can the matter be?', *Australian Psychologist*, 28: 181–188.

Kemp, R., Hayward, P. and David, A. (1997) *Compliance therapy manual*, London: Maudsley Publications.

Kemp, R., Kirov, G., Everitt, B., Hayward, P. and David, A. (1998) 'Randomised controlled trial of compliance therapy: 18-month follow up', *British Journal of Psychiatry*, 172: 413–419.

Rogers, E.M. (1995) *Diffusion of innovations*, 4th edn, New York: The Free Press.

Rolls, L., Davis, E. and Coupland, K. (2002) 'Improving serious mental illness through interprofessional education', *Journal of Psychiatric and Mental Health Nursing*, 9 (3): 317–324.

## FURTHER READING

http://www.thorn-initiative.org.uk
The Thorn website provides a gateway to many other PSI-related links, and resources and information about PSI training, including our own website: http://www.uwcm.ac.uk/study/nursing/thorn

Baker, S. and Baker, K. (2000) *The complete idiot's guide to project management*, New York: Alpha Books.
Project management is not likely to feature heavily on everyone's reading list; however, this publication provides a good overview and quick reference.

# CHAPTER 32

# THE CONTRIBUTION OF QUANTITATIVE APPROACHES TO COMMUNITY MENTAL HEALTH NURSING RESEARCH

*Kevin Gournay*

---

## SUMMARY OF KEY POINTS

- Quantitative research in community mental health nursing spans two decades.

- Evidence supports use of skills in CBT and psychosocial interventions.

- Evidence supports expanding of CMHN role in several areas.

- There are seven major arguments to support a shift by nursing researchers to quantitative methods.

---

## INTRODUCTION

Perhaps the most important point to make at the outset is that this chapter is not about quantitative versus qualitative research. It is my view that both methods have their place in this area of health care. In areas where we require new knowledge, it is important to integrate the two approaches. It is also worth noting that many of the quantitative studies carried out in the area of mental health and mental health nursing have been preceded by qualitative enquiry. Another point that I wish to make at the outset is that I have no objection to qualitative research in principle. What I object to is poor-quality research – be it of a qualitative or quantitative nature.

This chapter will examine a range of quantitative research studies, which, it is argued, have made a major contribution to the development and improvement of community mental health nursing. Following this overview, the chapter will continue by looking at seven major arguments for shifting the emphasis in mental health nursing research towards the quantitative end of the spectrum. Finally, the chapter will conclude by examining the implications of the Medical Research Council Framework for Complex Health Interventions and suggesting a template for future research activities.

## THE CONTRIBUTION OF QUANTITATIVE RESEARCH TO CURRENT CMHN PRACTICE

In order to examine the impact of quantitative research on community mental health nursing one needs to begin more than twenty years ago when Paykel and Griffith (1983) conducted a study which showed that CMHNs (community mental health nurses) were as effective as psychiatrists in a role of continuing care. Unfortunately, this excellent study, which included an economic analysis, was not followed up by further research into CMHN effectiveness.

Throughout the 1980s and 1990s, community psychiatric nursing under-went rapid growth and development, which has been well described (Brooker 1990, Brooker and White 1993, 1995). Although developments by CMHNs were at that time unevaluated in high-quality quantitative studies, Marks (1985) carried out an evaluation of nurse behaviour therapists working in primary care, which showed that they were significantly more effective in clinical and economic terms than a waiting list condition or continuing GP care, for a range of anxiety disorders. Although, strictly speaking, these nurse therapists were not generally included in the population called, at that time, CPNs (community psychiatric nurses), they were psychiatric nurses working in the community. In later years their evidence-based training has become much more relevant to the practice and education of today's CMHNs.

During the 1990s, the Mental Health Nursing Review (Department of Health 1994) stated that CMHNs should focus their efforts on people with serious and enduring mental illness. This focus was in contrast to the rather *ad hoc* and disorganised developments which had seen CMHNs set themselves up as 'specialists' in primary care and a range of other specialities away from work with people with serious and enduring mental illnesses – i.e. people with schizophrenia and other psychoses. The central recommendation of the review was influenced mainly by an emerging body of research directly related to the CMHN practice referred to in detail below.

The Mental Health Nursing Review took place within the context of growing public disquiet at the fate of patients in 'community care'. High-profile incidents, such as the stabbing to death of Jonathan Zito at Finsbury Park underground station by Christopher Clunis, demonstrated that considerable resources were needed to manage the most seriously ill individuals and that they should become a priority for CMHNs. The results of quantitative research underpinned the change in policy and then led to the developments which have produced today's models of CMHN practice.

One study (Gournay and Brooking 1994, 1995) examined the work of CMHNs working in six health centres in north London with a total of thirty-six GPs. One hundred and seventy-seven patients with a range of problems – mainly adjustment disorders and anxiety and depression – were randomly allocated to one of eleven CPNs or to standard GP care. The study showed that the intervention of the CPN, which was largely 'counselling', produced no clinical benefits for the patient, and the economic analysis demonstrated that the interventions were very expensive, with much lower return of improvement in quality of life than when CMHNs were working with people with schizophrenia. The study also highlighted the problems of working with common mental disorders, in so far as the study population seemed to have a high rate of spontaneous remission, with problems resolving in the majority of cases, whether or not the person received any professional intervention. Although this study received a great deal of criticism, those arguing for continuing similar involvement of CPNs in primary care failed to provide any evidence of effectiveness. At that time, one particular argument by the authors was somewhat overshadowed by the general debate. In this, Gournay and Brooking (1994) argued that, apart from work with people with serious and enduring mental illnesses, it was reasonable for CMHNs to work in primary care, providing they used evidence-based interventions for those patients with conditions known to be responsive to treatment. This argument was underpinned by a suggestion by Marks (1985) that there was probably a need for some 1,800 nurse behaviour therapists in the UK. This continued shortage of nurse therapists is now recognised as a grave deficit and, coupled with the parallel shortage of clinical psychologists, leads to enormous problems in meeting the aspirations of the National Service Framework for Mental Health (Department of Health 1999), which demands access to high-quality psychological treatments in primary care.

The second important study which influenced CMHN developments was that of Brooker et al. (1994), who demonstrated, within a quasi-experimental design, that CPNs could be trained to develop family interventions. This study examined the work of eight community psychiatric nurses who were trained to deliver family interventions to patients with schizophrenia and their families. Brooker et al. concluded that both the positive and the negative symptoms of schizophrenia improved significantly to twelve-month follow-up, as did a global measure of social functioning. Brooker et al. also stated that there was tentative evidence that family intervention reduced in-patient episodes and that the benefits for patients included a decrease in minor psychiatric morbidity and an increase in knowledge about neuroleptic drugs. This study was important for two reasons. First, it provided the first real test of training for CMHNs, an area which is still greatly under-researched (Gournay and Thornicroft 2002), and this training became central to the development of the Thorn Programme, an initiative which has now been disseminated to universities across the United Kingdom and which focuses on providing CMHNs with skills in assertive community treatment, psychological interventions and family interventions. Thorn-trained nurses are now practising within an evidence-based framework and, ten years on, Thorn has been developed in other guises (e.g. masters' programmes, the COPE initiative in Manchester, etc.), and is arguably the most positive development in the history of community mental health nursing.

A corollary to the development of Thorn concerns the current government policy focus on providing intensive community-based support for the most seriously ill population, who at one time spent the majority of their lives in hospital, or at least as 'revolving door patients'. An important quantitative study underpinning this approach concerned an evaluation of an intensive community care service, called the Daily Living Programme, based at the Maudsley Hospital in London (Audini *et al.* 1994, Knapp *et al.* 1994, Marks *et al.* 1994). This study, although mixed in its results, arguably provided an impetus for developments in assertive community treatment (ACT), a method shown to be effective in the 1970s and 1980s in Madison, Wisconsin and Sydney, Australia (Stein and Test 1980, Hoult *et al.* 1983). Perhaps the major lessons for this study came from the wide range of problems encountered, which included hostile responses from the general public (and some mental health professionals), high levels of stress in the treatment team, and the logistical problems of running a highly responsive service. Although there is some controversy about the relative merits of ACT (Rosen and Teesson 2001), it is clear that this approach is here to stay and will be central to CMHN activity for many years to come. However, one must note that one of the authors of the Daily Living Programme study, Dr Matt Muijen, currently Director of the Sainsbury Centre for Mental Health, showed convincingly that merely reconfiguring CMHN services into new community mental health teams provided no benefit over standard care (Muijen *et al.* 1994). Simply put, ACT, home treatment, crisis resolution, and all the other buzz phrases of current policy amount to nothing, unless these service developments are supported by decent and robust training of the staff involved.

Thus, the early 1990s saw the shape of the CMHN workforce change considerably as a direct response to quantitative evidence. It could be argued that these quantitative research approaches have had, on their own, a much greater impact than all of the qualitative research carried out in community mental health nursing in the 1980s and 1990s.

In considering the impact of quantitative research on community mental health nursing, it is also worth noting that the quinquennial surveys carried out by Ted White and Charlie Brooker, and widely reported (e.g. Brooker and White 1997), have served to provide a picture of community mental health nursing across the United Kingdom. Although the headcounting and detailed collection of data relating to day-to-day practice may not have the appeal of some of the more esoteric enquiries, this work has been valuable in providing government with a very clear picture of CMHN practice and provides the opportunity to project various workforce developments. In parallel to White's extensive surveys, the nurse therapy workforce has been followed up in similar fashion some twenty-five years after the initial development (Newell and Gournay 1994, Gournay *et al.* 2000). These surveys have added to the arguments for the development of therapeutic roles for mental health nurses, although at the present time these developments are compromised by the lack of funding for the intensive training necessary to produce skilled practitioners.

This overview of quantitative research would perhaps not be complete without mentioning two other areas. The excellent work of Anna Waterreus (1993) does not immediately come to mind when one considers community mental health nursing. Waterreus examined the efficacy of CMHN intervention with elderly people with depression in the setting of the larger Gospel Oak Depression Study. Waterreus showed quite clearly that the CMHN role with the elderly could be extended, with associated benefits to the elderly person. However, because of the lack of emphasis on the needs of elderly people with functional mental health problems, Waterreus's work has not been properly recognised, nor extended as it deserved. The limitations of the National Service Framework for Mental Health have served to compound the neglect of the elderly by emphasising the focus on adults of working age.

The second strand of work which deserves further comment belongs to Joanna Bennett (Bennett *et al.* 1995). Bennett is, by professional background, a general nurse and midwife who became interested in the work of community psychiatric nursing because of the illness of her brother, Rocky, and because of the apparently poor standards of care that he received. In the course of her Ph.D., Joanna set about examining CMHN skills and then developed a rating scale to assess the side effects of antipsychotic medication to assist with CMHN practice. This work began in the late 1980s, when her brother had already been ill for some years. At this point, the reader should be told that eventually mental health services failed Rocky Bennett in the most catastrophic way. Rocky died following a restraint incident in the year 2000 and, at the time of writing, the public inquiry into his death is still to be launched. The jury at Rocky's inquest returned a verdict of accidental death, aggravated by neglect – a finding which needs to continue echoing in all our minds. Notwithstanding these tragic events, Joanna's work demonstrated, first of all, that the CMHNs selected for her study initially had a low level of skill in medication management, but a simple medication management training programme helped them acquire these skills.

Joanna's work has directly influenced a major programme of quantitative research commenced at the Institute of Psychiatry in 1996, where a training programme in medication management for CMHNs was developed and, eventually, subjected to randomised trial (Gray *et al.* 2003). This study, which is currently being replicated in a national definitive trial in England, and a five-country European Union funded study, shows quite clearly that eighty hours of training in medication management leads not only to substantial changes in CMHNs' skills and knowledge but also, and obviously more importantly, to very substantial clinical changes in the patient. This training programme has underpinned further developments in the aforementioned Thorn Programme and may yet be influential on the subject of mental health nursing prescribing, currently under consideration by the Department of Health and now widely enshrined in psychiatric practice in the USA (Gournay and Gray 2001).

This overview does not purport to provide a definitive account of quantitative research carried out in community mental health nursing. It does, however, demonstrate by reference to some selected studies that the quantitative research approach has produced very valuable new knowledge, which has influenced practice by developing different skill sets in CMHNs and by making a fundamental impact on mental health policy.

# SEVEN ARGUMENTS FOR A SHIFT TO QUANTITATIVE METHODS

It needs to be said once more that mental health nursing research in general has been characterised by a great imbalance in favour of qualitative research. I believe that there are seven major arguments for mental health nursing research (and probably nursing research in general) to shift to a greater emphasis on quantitative methods.

The first argument is that qualitative research on its own is of very limited utility, unless it is linked to clear outcomes. Nursing journals are full of studies which give accounts of the individual perceptions of health professionals and patients, but these studies are very seldom linked to any outcome data. Surely, if we are to provide accounts of how people perceive their interventions, we should also be able to say whether these interventions are successful or not. For example, in the Gournay and Brooking (1994) study we linked qualitative data with outcome data (Devilly and Gournay 1995), including measures of symptoms, social function, satisfaction and health economics. From this we obtained results that were complex and, in some ways, contradictory. For example, some patients, while perceiving their CMHNs as warm, caring and easy to talk to, had poor clinical outcomes and, after the CPN intervention, remained very distressed and disabled. This, of course, was not the picture of every patient in our study, but it certainly helped us to see that not only does one need to examine changes in different domains of function, but one also needs to examine the process and the outcome of care together.

The second argument regarding the shift to quantitative methods is that qualitative findings need to be used as the basis for developing quantitative instruments. A classic example of such a development is found in the work of my colleagues, Graham Thornicroft, Mike Slade, and others (Phelan *et al.* 1995). This research team was inspired by a number of famous qualitative studies, which concluded that patients felt that their needs for care were not being properly met. The researchers used qualitative findings to begin the development of a valid and reliable measure of need – the Camberwell Assessment of Need. This is a simple-to-use instrument, which allows the patient, their carer and their keyworker to quantify met and unmet needs. It has now been translated into many languages and is used across the world as both a clinical and a research tool. For patients with psychosis, who one may expect will only achieve modest outcomes (in terms of symptoms) with the best treatment available today, meeting needs for housing, occupation and various aspects of daily living is perhaps the most important objective of intervention. Thus, this simple measure allows staff, patients and their carers to quantify their needs for care over time.

The third argument regarding the need to move towards quantitative methods concerns the obvious requirement to quantify the cost of what we do. Even in other European countries, which spend nearly double the percentage of gross domestic product on health we spend in the UK, there is a need to make hard choices about what care and treatments the system can afford. Currently, in the UK, the National Institute for Clinical Excellence makes, at times, controversial decisions about who should receive, for example, anti-influenza drugs, beta interferon or fertility treatment. Every day, local managers have to decide whether additional monies coming into their budget should be used for the reduction of waiting lists or for improving the services to people with cancer. Such decisions should be based on hard data concerning not just the cost of treatment, but how valuable that treatment is in terms of improving quality of life. As previously mentioned, Julia Brooking and I looked at the costs and benefits of community psychiatric nursing within the context of a large randomised controlled trial (Gournay and Brooking 1995) and our data suggested very strongly that CMHNs could do much more about improving quality of life for patients with schizo-phrenia than for patients with common mental disorders. This finding, in itself, raises a number of issues beyond the scope of this chapter. However, when it comes to deciding on the provision of one treatment versus another, we do need to have as much information on quality of life as possible. Sadly, cost is a factor that has to be considered, and it could be argued that every health professional makes rationing choices – whether consciously or unconsciously. Nurse researchers therefore have a clear interest in health economics studies.

The fourth argument regarding the need for a shift to quantitative methods concerns the evaluation of education and training. Although a great deal of educational research has been carried out, very little has attempted to assess the impact of training on patients. Research has generally focused on the attitudes and satisfaction of the nurses, who are trained using methods such as focus groups or semi-structured interviews. The obvious question needs to be asked: 'Does training make any difference to the outcome of the patient who is the recipient of the intervention delivered by the "trained" nurse?' There have been several studies where patient outcome has been assessed, following the provision of training in specific interventions to small numbers of staff, and compared in a randomised trial with outcomes after interventions by staff without such training. However, until very recently, there have been no efforts to assess the outcome of training in relation to the patients of ordinary clinical staff employed in ordinary clinical (rather than research) settings. As noted before, Brooker et al. (1994) were probably the first to attempt to assess the impact of training on a reasonable number of ordinary CMHNs. More recently, researchers at the Institute of Psychiatry have completed three randomised controlled trials, assessing the impact of training for medication management, and the detection and management of mental health problems by practice nurses and, in dual-diagnosis interventions, by case managers from various professional backgrounds (Gournay et al. 2001). Obviously, there is a great need to assess the outcome of training programmes across a wide range of areas of health care provision as we cannot assume that simply providing training will improve clinical outcomes for patients. One further area, which is obviously ripe for research, is to follow up trainees after training in order to examine whether they remain effective and to see how their practice varies. A study from Australia (Kavannagh et al. 1993) followed up workers who had received family intervention training, and showed that trainees, at follow-up, were seldom using the interventions in which they had been trained, or, if they were using these interventions, used them in a very modified fashion. The issue of refresher training is also important in health care, and a recent survey (Lee et al. 2001) shows that, while in the area of management of violence refresher training is widely recommended as essential, it is seldom provided.

The fifth argument for shifting the emphasis of mental health nursing research into the quantitative area concerns the presence of nursing within multidisciplinary research groups. Within the British university system, nursing researchers are often isolated from their research colleagues. This isolation is a phenomenon which obviously has complex roots. One factor may be the continuing pressure from within nursing to improve the status of nursing science and, with it, the autonomy of nurse researchers. While this view is understandable, given the low status of nursing compared with other professions and, indeed, the (until recently) very poor funding of research training for nurses, the point needs to be made that health outcomes are seldom attributable solely to one professional group. Rather, the health gains which patients experience are attributable to a combined effort across the whole system. The health service has become very outcome-oriented in its nature and, hence, the research agenda is based on quantitative approaches. Nursing, therefore, needs to see itself as part of a multidisciplinary endeavour and to move into interdisciplinary groups. In one or two centres, mental health nurses have joined with their professional colleagues within health service research groupings; at the Institute of Psychiatry, for example, nurses have become the beneficiaries of the 'five stars' gained in the last Research Assessment Exercise – a truly collective endeavour where all of the professions at the Institute contributed to one entry into the exercise, rather than adhering to tribal boundaries.

The sixth argument for an increase in the emphasis on quantitative research in mental health nursing concerns the need to critically examine our interventions in the same way as other health care providers. There is no doubt that evidence-based medicine is here to stay and that the general public are increasingly demanding evidence from quantitative research to justify the treatment which is used. Very simply, mental health nursing researchers need to move into the mainstream with other health care professionals to be judged by the same standards.

The seventh, and final, argument for mental health nursing to move into the more quantitative areas is a very pragmatic one. The relatively small amount of research money provided by the government and funding councils is now the subject of great competition. The rules of the competition are set by the funders, and these funders all agree that quantitative approaches should be the primary method of assessing benefits. In turn, quantitative methods must underpin areas outside of effectiveness research – for example, epidemiology. If research into mental health nursing is to develop, these researchers will need to simply follow orthodoxy in order to survive.

So far this chapter has focused on past research, of a quantitative nature, which has influenced the work of CMHNs. What seems clear from the overview is that research is piecemeal and meagre in quantity. Indeed, Lewis *et al.* (1997), in examining the evidence for interventions in mental health care, concluded that, while the literature in many areas of medicine was complete, mental health care was, by contrast, a veritable desert. The task of developing a significant evidence base was deemed, aptly, 'Herculean'. What then should the future approach to mental health research, and community mental health nursing research in particular, be? I am of the very firm view that for many reasons, some of which are outlined above, mental health nursing needs to become inextricably linked with other professional groups within health service research departments. This will not represent a loss of identity, rather it will strengthen the approach to those subjects at the heart of community mental health nursing practice. In turn these health service research departments need to work in collaboration with other groups. The new National Institute for Mental Health in England probably provides a good example of the way forward in its proposition for a research network spearheaded by two centres of excellence (the Institute of Psychiatry and the University of Manchester). This policy shift recognises that attempting to spread out the finite research funds available across, literally, scores of university departments will yield little impact, whereas a concentration of the best researchers in centres of excellence, working together, should provide the most effective way forward. Such networks also have the benefit of supporting researchers through a process of training and development, by ensuring access to a comprehensive range of supports and services.

Recently, the Medical Research Council issued a framework for complex health interventions. This structural framework provides a helpful outline of what is needed to guide researchers and policy-makers (Figure 32.1).

Bindman *et al.* (2002), in a paper based on a thematic review of research priorities for the English Department of Health, considered this framework and concluded that a large majority of studies in mental health research are completely atheoretical and, thus, the pre-clinical part of this framework is poorly served by

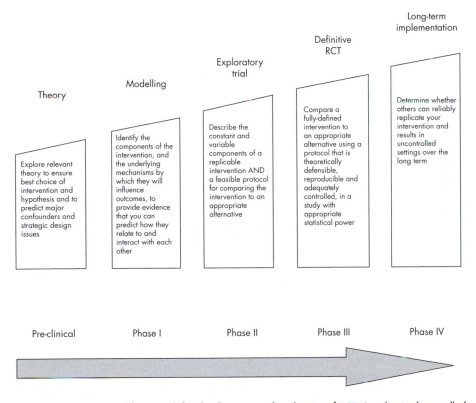

*Figure 32.1*   A structural framework for development and evaluation of RCTs (randomised controlled trials) for complex interventions to improve health
Source: Campbell *et al.* (2000)

research in mental health. As a corollary of this, it could be argued that many of the authors in mental health nursing research, who are excited by one model or other of nursing, are focusing their efforts on the first theory box of this framework, while completely ignoring the need to carry out modelling, exploratory and definitive trials, and long-term implementation studies. What evidence we have in mental health care, and this needs to be replicated, is very sparse and concentrated in the area of trials, many of which have characteristics of an exploratory trial and some of a definitive trial – but rarely conforming to the highest standards of clinical trials. Studies on long-term implementation are currently notably absent. We still have little knowledge of how even well-defined interventions, such as cognitive behaviour therapy for neurotic problems – a subject which has been researched extensively in, literally, hundreds of trials – fare when delivered by nurses and psychologists, working in routine settings under the considerable constraints of today's services.

## CONCLUSIONS AND WAY FORWARD

In conclusion, I argue that quantitative research has produced substantial new knowledge relevant to community mental health nursing research, but, having said that, our knowledge base at the present time is poor. I also strongly believe that mental health nurses who are interested in this area, or indeed any area of research, are best located within multidisciplinary health service research teams, located in centres of excellence. This is the only way that the research discipline within mental health nursing will grow. In turn, therefore, this is the only way that research into topics relevant to community mental health nurses will be properly focused.

## REFERENCES

Audini, B., Marks, I., Lawrence, R., Connelly, J. and Watts, V. (1994) 'Home based versus outpatient/inpatient care for people with serious mental illness. Phase 2 of a controlled study', *British Journal of Psychiatry*, 165: 204–210.

Bennett, J., Done, J., Harrison-Read, P. and Hunt, B. (1995) 'Development of a rating scale/checklist to assess side effects of anti-psychotics by community psychiatric nurses', in Brooker, C. and White, E. (eds) *Community psychiatric nursing: a research perspective*, vol. 3, Cheltenham: Stanley Thornes.

Bindman, J., Thornicroft, G., Goldberg, D., Huxley, P. and Gournay, K. (2002) *A thematic review of research to support the National Service Framework*, Report to Department of Health, London.

Brooker, C. (ed.) (1990) *Community psychiatric nursing: a research perspective*, Cheltenham: Stanley Thornes.

Brooker, C. and White, E. (eds) (1993) *Community psychiatric nursing: a research perspective*, vol. 2, Cheltenham: Stanley Thornes.

Brooker, C. and White, E. (eds) (1995) *Community psychiatric nursing: a research perspective*, vol. 3, Cheltenham: Stanley Thornes.

Brooker, C. and White, E. (1997) *The fourth quinquennial national community mental health nursing census of England and Wales*, Manchester and Keele: Universities of Manchester and Keele.

Brooker, C., Falloon, I., Butterworth, A., Goldberg, D., Graham-Hole, B. and Hillier, V. (1994) 'The outcome of training community psychiatric nurses to deliver psycho-social intervention', *British Journal of Psychiatry*, 165: 222–230.

Campbell, M., Fitzpatrick, R., Haines, A., Kinmonth, A.L., Sandercock, P., Spiegelhalter, D. and Tyrer, P. (2000) 'Framework for design and evaluation of complex interventions to improve health', *British Medical Journal*, 321 (7262): 694–696.

Department of Health (1994) *Working in partnership: a collaborative approach to care. Report of the Mental Health Nursing Review Team*, London: HMSO.

Department of Health (1999) *National service framework for mental health: modern standards and service models*, London: Department of Health.

Devilly, G. and Gournay, K. (1995) 'Community psychiatric nursing with non-psychotic patients: relating process to outcome', *Australian and New Zealand Journal of Mental Health Nursing*, 4: 53–60.

Gournay, K. and Brooking, J. (1994) 'Community psychiatric nurses in primary health care', *British Journal of Psychiatry*, 165: 231–238.

Gournay, K. and Brooking, J. (1995) 'An economic analysis of the work of mental health nurses in primary care', *Journal of Advanced Nursing*, 22: 769–778.

Gournay, K. and Gray, R. (2001) *Should mental health nurses prescribe?*, Maudsley Discussion Paper No. 11, London: Institute of Psychiatry.

Gournay, K. and Thornicroft, G. (2002) 'A UK perspective of case management', Letter in *Australian and New Zealand Journal of Psychiatry*, 36 (5): 701.

Gournay, K., Denford, L., Parr, A. and Newell, R. (2000) 'British nurses in behavioural psychotherapy: A 25-year follow-up', *Journal of Advanced Nursing*, 32: 343–351.

Gournay, K., Plummer, S. and Gray, R. (2001) 'The dream team at the Institute of Psychiatry', *Mental Health Practice*, 4 (7): 15–17.

Gray, R., Wykes, T. and Gournay, K. (2003) 'The effect of medication management training on community mental health nurses' clinical skills', *International Journal of Nursing Studies*, 40(2): 163–169.

Hoult, J., Reynolds, I. and Charbonneau-Powis, J. (1983) 'Psychiatric hospitals versus community treatment: a randomised trial', *Australian and New Zealand Journal of Psychiatry*, 17: 160–167.

Kavannagh, D., Clark, D. and Piatkowska, O. (1993) 'Application of cognitive behavioural family interventions for schizophrenia', *Australian Psychologist*, 28: 1–8.

Knapp, M., Beecham, J., Koutsogeorgopoulou, V., Hallam, A. and Fenyo, A. (1994) 'Service use and costs of home based versus hospital based care for people with serious mental illness', *British Journal of Psychiatry*, 165: 195–203.

Lee, S., Wright, S., Sayer, J., Parr, A., Gray, R. and Gournay, K. (2001) 'Physical restraint training for nurses in English and Welsh psychiatric intensive care and regional secure units', *Journal of Mental Health*, 10 (2): 151–162.

Lewis, G., Churchill, R. and Hotoph, M. (1997) 'Editorial: Systemic reviews and meta-analysis', *Psychological Medicine*, 27: 3–7.

Marks, I. (1985) *Nursing in behavioural psychotherapy*, London: RCN.

Marks, I., Connelly, J., Muijen, M., Audini, B., McNamee, G. and Lawrence, R. (1994) 'Home based versus hospital based care for people with serious mental illness', *British Journal of Psychiatry*, 165: 179–194.

Muijen, M., Cooney, M., Strathdee, G., Bell, R. and Hudson, A. (1994) 'Community psychiatric nurse teams: intensive support versus generic care', *British Journal of Psychiatry*, 165: 211–217.

Newell, R. and Gournay, K. (1994) 'British nurses in behavioural psychotherapy: a 20 year follow-up', *Journal of Advanced Nursing*, 20: 53–60.

Paykel, E. and Griffith, J. (1983) *Community psychiatric nursing for neurotic patients*, London: RCN.

Phelan, M., Slade, M. and Thornicroft, G. (1995) 'The Camberwell assessment of need', *British Journal of Psychiatry*, 167: 589–595.

Rosen, A. and Teesson, M. (2001) 'Does case management work? The evidence and abuse of evidence based medicine', *Australian and New Zealand Journal of Psychiatry*, 35: 731–746.

Stein, L. and Test, M. (1980) 'Alternatives to mental hospital treatment: conceptual model treatment programme and clinical evaluation', *Archives of General Psychiatry*, 37: 392–397.

Waterreus, A. (1993) 'The CPN and depression in elderly people living in the community', in Brooker, C. and White, E. (eds) *Community psychiatric nursing: a research perspective*, vol. 2, Cheltenham: Stanley Thornes.

# FURTHER READING

Brooker, C. (ed.) (1990) *Community psychiatric nursing: a research perspective*, Cheltenham: Stanley Thornes.

Brooker, C. and White, E. (eds) (1993) *Community psychiatric nursing: a research perspective*, vol. 2, Cheltenham: Stanley Thornes.

Brooker, C. and White, E. (eds) (1995) *Community psychiatric nursing: a research perspective*, vol. 3, Cheltenham: Stanley Thornes.

These three books cover the majority of the most significant research findings concerning CMHNs over the past two decades. The books contain data from randomised trials, quasi-experimental studies, literature reviews, surveys and other research reports. For anyone interested in CMHN research, these three volumes are a *sine qua non*.

Department of Health (1999) *National service framework for mental health: modern standards and service models*, London: Department of Health.

This document, which, in a sense, sets out a ten-year plan for mental health services in England, is essential reading for anyone with an interest in mental health. Certainly all practitioners should at least have read the Executive Summary, if not the entire document.

Marks, I. (1995) *Nurse therapists in primary care*, London: RCN.

This research report provides an account of the study carried out in the early 1980s in a general practice in south-east London. It provides food for thought regarding the issue of which skills are important in primary care. Although the world has moved on a great deal since the publication of this book, it contains many messages relevant to the contemporary scene.

Thornicroft, G. and Szmukler, G. (eds) (2001) *Textbook of community psychiatry*, Oxford: Oxford University Press.

This textbook is the most comprehensive account of community psychiatry in the British literature and includes chapters from the leading authorities on every area of community psychiatry, both in the United Kingdom and in other parts of the world. CMHNs, researchers, teachers and policy-makers will find something to interest and inform.

# CHAPTER 33

# THE CONTRIBUTION OF QUALITATIVE APPROACHES TO COMMUNITY MENTAL HEALTH NURSING RESEARCH

*Ian Beech*

## SUMMARY OF KEY POINTS

- Qualitative research can be underpinned by a number of different philosophical and methodological ideas.

- There are at least three approaches to non-positivist qualitative research: descriptive, interpretive and discourse analysis.

- Participatory research approaches facilitate the empowerment of people traditionally seen as the subjects of research.

## INTRODUCTION

Within this chapter there will be a discussion of what constitutes qualitative research and in particular how some types of qualitative research may be positivist, whereas others may not. There will naturally be a discussion of some of the different types of qualitative research. In spite of the fact that there has been a debate within psychiatric and mental health nursing about the research methodology of choice, qualitative or quantitative, this chapter will not discuss this since the arguments have been exhaustively rehearsed elsewhere (e.g. Beech 1997, Gournay and Ritter 1997, Burnard and Hannigan 2000). There will, however, be a discussion of the relevance and value of qualitative approaches to community mental health nursing.

# THE NATURE OF QUALITATIVE RESEARCH

Someone approaching qualitative research for the first time encounters a confusing array of philosophical and methodological descriptions and arguments concerning the nature of qualitative research and the philosophical underpinnings of the same. It would seem therefore useful to consider negotiating a path through some of this confusion.

It is not uncommon for quantitative research to be characterised as positivist and qualitative research to be characterised as non-positivist in terms of their philosophical foundations (Streubert and Carpenter 1995). So let us commence by considering the ideas of positivism and non-positivism.

Streubert and Carpenter (1995) considered positivism to be characterised by a belief in a single reality that can be captured and represented by research so that generalisations may be made. In other words, a finding about, for example, the behaviour of people with a diagnosis of schizophrenia in Croydon in the UK may be generalised to the behaviour of people with a diagnosis of schizophrenia in Adelaide in Australia. The findings are deemed to be objective and free of any value being ascribed to the data by the researcher. While there are a variety of different meanings to the term positivism (and it has changed over time), the main thing to take away from ideas of positivism as a grounding philosophical stance to research is that research that is qualitative is not necessarily non-positivist (Crotty 1998).

So how might a qualitative piece of research be positivist in its foundation? The answer to this is simply that if the researcher has a view both that there is a true reality underlying the research data and that that reality can be theorised and modelled in some way, and then chooses a qualitative method to achieve this, then the research can be both positivist and qualitative (Ashworth 1997a). This is often seen in qualitative research when researchers seek to demonstrate reliability and validity in their research findings. By so doing the researchers are attempting to show that reality can be represented by, for example, approaching the research using a number of different methods and arriving at the same point (triangulation of method). An example of this can be seen in the following quote from Marrow:

> To have used interviews alone would only have represented the participants' viewpoint.
>
> (Marrow 1996, p. 45)

What we see here is an undervaluing of personal viewpoints and experiences as a means of representing a single reality. It is indeed the case that individual experiences and viewpoints can give access to the reality of the person having the viewpoint or the experience, but not to some general truth. So, generally speaking, when the researcher is attempting to demonstrate that the research has captured some aspect of a universally accepted truth or a law of cause and effect, qualitative methods fair poorly in comparison with quantitative methods because of the accusation that the research merely reflects people's personal experiences and viewpoints. Ashworth (1997a) provided us with some considerations that researchers employing positivist qualitative research might take into account in order to provide reliability and validity. Such considerations include: awareness of presuppositions that might influence results; awareness of the two-way process of such things as interviews and observation (that the interviewer or observer is as much a part of the interview or observation as the interviewed or observed); consideration of reliability checks such as asking colleagues to independently analyse the same data; and consideration of validity checks such as providing field notes and interview transcripts to colleagues.

Where qualitative research of a non-positivist turn has an unrivalled role is in the exploration of people's experiences and viewpoints without making claims that these are universalisable. It is to these types of qualitative research that we shall confine ourselves for the rest of this chapter.

# TYPES OF NON-POSITIVIST QUALITATIVE RESEARCH

Ashworth (1997b) indicated that there are at least three approaches to non-positivist qualitative research: descriptive; interpretive; and discourse analysis. Confusion often reigns because researchers do not make clear the nature of the research being carried out. For example, Crotty (1996), Walters (1995) and Paley (1997) have all been critical of nurses who claim to be carrying out phenomenological research, because the nurses have wandered between the descriptive and the interpretive without being clear about what it is they are doing.

When qualitative research is descriptive in nature it has to be understood that the description is not of some external truth but of the experience of the participant in the research. Such research is phenomenological in approach, but, as I have demonstrated elsewhere (Beech 1999), a distinction should be drawn between this empirical type of research and phenomenological philosophy. Empirical research has its roots in the philosophy of Husserl but traces a more direct lineage through the work of psychologists at Duquesne University in the USA, most notably Giorgi (1970, 1985). When carrying out such research one of the first principles is the technique known as bracketing. In bracketing, the researcher acknowledges and then puts to one side all that they know about the phenomenon under investigation in order to enter into the life-world of the other person unencumbered by their own experiences of the phenomenon under investigation. From the descriptions obtained, care should be taken over claims to have obtained any essential structure of the phenomenon. In effect what has been obtained is a collection of descriptions of the phenomenon as it appeared in the life-worlds of the interviewees at the time the interview took place. It cannot be claimed that 'this is the experience of the interviewees', as opposed to 'this was the experience of the interviewees', because the act of engaging in the interview process will have caused the interviewees to reflect on the phenomenon and so has affected their experiences. Researchers should also be wary of searching for themes in the data, as such an endeavour militates against the ability of the researcher to approach the data in a way that enables entry into the life-world of the other.

It may be asked, therefore, what the use of phenomenological research might be to community mental health nurses. If the research can offer entry into the life-world of another person in order to gain access to how that person experiences a phenomenon, but each piece of data stands alone, how might such research be of use to the wider community? The answer to this is in terms of both the stories that are told and the resonance they have with the lives of people. Van Manen (1990) refers to the 'phenomenological nod' as an indication of good phenomenological research having taken place. By this he means whether or not the reader can nod to a piece of research as being resonant of the experience of the reader. Chris Stevenson and I have written elsewhere (Stevenson and Beech 2001) of the value of research being in its use to people in addressing local problems with local solutions. An example of this is the work of Hagan and Green (1994). In this project phenomenological research was employed to establish the experience of mental health service users of community mental health services in Wakefield. As a result of the research, commissioned by Wakefield Healthcare NHS Trust, local services were designed to meet local needs.

As previously stated, qualitative research may not be descriptive, it may be interpretive. Such research would trace its philosophical lineage to the work of Heidegger. In this type of research the technique of bracketing is held to be neither desirable nor indeed possible. In such research the researcher is encouraged to explore his or her understanding of the phenomenon under investigation and to take this as the starting point for the research. From this point the research progresses with the researcher gathering data. These data are analysed and then become part of the researcher's overall understanding of the phenomenon, which is then applied to the next set of data to be analysed. In other words, understanding becomes a circle of pre-understanding that becomes informed by the research which then becomes the next pre-understanding. This is known as the hermeneutic circle (Morrison 1992). In this type of research, therefore, a thematic analysis is possible (Leonard 1994), but it is still not to be taken as a snapshot of the 'real world' – rather a systematic interpretation of the co-creation of the worlds of the people involved in the research process.

Graham (2001) used a phenomenological interpretive approach to clarify what it was that nurses in a community mental health centre in the north of England were doing in their practice. Such a piece of research may be accused of being philosophical navel-gazing, but its value is in doing what it says in the title of the research paper, 'clarifying meaning'. In a profession which, as Clarke (2001) pointed out, has failed to define what it actually does, this clarification could be very important in helping people in the care of nurses.

Pejlert et al. (1998) and Berg and Hallberg (2000) both employed hermeneutic approaches to investigate the meaning of working with people with psychiatric problems in in-patient settings. The methods employed in both studies could easily be applied to community settings.

Discourse analysis has been seen by Ashworth (1997b) as an extension of the interpretive phenomenological method in interpreting data as expression of culturally available discourses. Discourse is taken to mean any spoken or written interaction. Within this method, therefore, there are assumptions made that there is social discourse between members of a discourse community within which meaning is taken for granted (Tilley et al. 1999). Within research using this method discourses are addressed in terms of uncovering what might constitute the dominant discourse in a community – for example, the discourse of illness and wellness

in people diagnosed as suffering from schizophrenia. Other, perhaps less dominant, discourses are also analysed. For example, a researcher addressing the
discourse community of CPNs might conceivably discover a dominant discourse
of medically orientated illness and wellness when discussing people diagnosed
with schizophrenia, but may discover other discourses based on social inclusion/
exclusion, or consumerism, and perhaps others as well (Tilley *et al.* 1999).

The value of discourse analysis is to provide nurses with the tools with which
to analyse their own language. The language used by a discourse community
creates the reality for that community. As an example let us take the oft-used word
'transference'. This is a word taken from psychoanalysis and means the removal
of an emotion such as love or hatred from the original object of the emotion,
e.g. the person's mother or father, and transferring the emotion to a substitute
object, e.g. the therapist. Originally the word was used to describe a mechanism
theoretically taking place within the particular discourse community of psychoanalysts. It is common nowadays to hear nurses talk about transference occurring
within the nursing relationship with people in care. But the term has become
reified. In other words transference has become so much part of the language that
there is an assumption that it exists as some entity. Yet there is an argument
that transference cannot possibly occur. If we take the example of hatred of one's
mother being transferred to hatred of the nurse, at some point the hatred must
become disconnected from the mother and connected to the nurse, so there
must be a point where the hatred has no object. The idea of a general hatred of
nothing in particular seems inconceivable (van den Berg 1972). This discourse,
however, has become marginalised. By examining the discourses employed within
nursing we can question the taken-for-granted assumptions that hinder effective
practice. An example of the value of this sort of exercise is seen in the work
of Tilley *et al.* (1999) who used discourse analysis to investigate the discourses
prevalent in the ways people in care are talked about by nurses, and how such
discourses may or may not facilitate the empowerment of such people.

Whether the researcher is using a descriptive, interpretive or discourse
analysis, as we have seen, the researcher is not laying claim to representation of
a single reality. The advantage of qualitative research is that only by using these
approaches 'can internal meanings (of people) be examined and reported' (Clarke
2001, p. 155). However, if claims are made for generalisability and replicability,
the research runs into problems of convincing critics of its scientific nature. It is
important, therefore, for qualitative researchers to be mindful of the criteria that
indicate that the research exercise has been carried out rigorously. These criteria
are not to be confused with reliability and validity – that would be to make the
same mistake as to judge a Harley Davidson to be a poor car because it has only
two wheels. Qualitative research of the nature discussed above cannot and should
not be judged by the criteria applied to both quantitative research and qualitative
research of a more positivist turn.

Munhall (1994) provided nine criteria against which phenomenological
research might be judged in terms of rigour, and such criteria might usefully be
applied to any research of a non-positivist turn. For ease of remembrance each
criterion begins with the letter R and they are: resonancy, reasonableness, representativeness, recognisability, raised consciousness, readability, relevance,
revelations, responsibility. Let us look at each one in a little more detail. Resonancy

indicates that the written description/interpretation/analysis resonates with individuals. Reasonableness means that the final product is a reasonable description/interpretation/analysis of the research. Representativeness is a question of whether the research has adequately uncovered aspects of the area to be researched. Recognisability is a question of whether or not people who are not directly involved in the area researched can recognise aspects of it from their own experience. Raised consciousness of something previously unconsidered in the reader shows that the research has been thorough in its exploration. Readability is very important in qualitative research as there is sometimes a tendency to wander into abstract realms of philosophy which are generally of little interest to the reader, who is interested in the results and how they were derived. Relevance indicates that the research is grounded in the needs of nursing and people in care. Revelations, in a similar way to raised consciousness, shows that something previously hidden has been brought to the fore. Finally there is a responsibility to be true to the participants in the research. As can be seen, criteria such as those mentioned are specific to qualitative research and provide grounds for judgement of such research on its own merits.

Ronnie Laing once asserted that:

> It is just possible to have a thorough knowledge of what has been discovered about the hereditary or familial incidence of manic-depressive psychosis or schizophrenia, to have a facility in recognizing schizoid 'ego distortion' and schizophrenic ego defects, plus the various 'disorders' of thought, memory, perceptions, etc., to know, in fact, just about everything that can be known about the psychopathology of schizophrenia or of schizophrenia as a disease without being able to understand one single schizophrenic. Such data are all ways of *not* understanding him.
>
> (Laing 1960, p. 33)

Laing's assertion is a useful reminder to nurses about the role of mental health nursing in the care of people with mental health problems. Nursing is not primarily about understanding the pathology of illnesses such as schizophrenia, it is about understanding the people who suffer from such conditions and helping those people to live with and make sense of the experiences they have. In such a role, qualitative approaches to research have considerable value because they enable the researcher to access aspects of people's life experiences denied to positivist researchers.

In recent years some researchers have moved beyond the qualitative/quantitative debate and concentrated instead on the people who are being researched. The view taken by these researchers is that even though qualitative research accesses the story, experience and/or meaning of those being researched, there is still a power differential between the people being researched and the researcher, with the researcher making the decisions and interpretations (Heron 1996).

The antidote to this is to carry out research *with* people. There is a variety of such research approaches but I will concentrate on two: co-operative inquiry (Heron 1996) and participatory research (Tetley and Hanson 2000).

In co-operative inquiry all of those involved in the research are both co-researchers and co-subjects. Heron (1996) then takes the view that there are different types of knowledge: experiential knowledge, which is that gained through direct encounter; practical knowledge gained through practice of some skill or competence; propositional knowledge, which is knowledge about something that we can explain or expand upon; and presentational knowledge, which is how we first consider our experiences and then present them in terms of our stories. Co-operative inquiry is based on these two ideas: the co-researcher and the different forms of knowledge. In the process of the inquiry the co-researchers cycle through four phases. Phase 1 involves mainly propositional knowledge and is aimed at agreement about the area of the research. Phase 2 involves mainly practical knowledge and is where the co-researchers become co-subjects and note their own and each other's experience. Phase 3 is the stage where the researchers become totally engaged with the experience and, unsurprisingly, mainly involves experiential knowledge. In phase 4 the researchers meet to reconsider their original ideas in the light of their experiences, using mainly propositional knowledge, and at this point the cycle starts again.

Traylen (1994) reported that in interviewing a group of health visitors about their practice she felt that wounds were opened in the process of the interviews that were then left unaddressed. By adopting a co-operative inquiry approach these issues were addressed by the health visitors themselves.

Participatory research is less of a method and more of an ethical approach to the question of researcher and researched. In participatory research, decisions are shared on important questions such as the research question, research design, data collection, analysis, reporting and acting on findings (Tetley and Hanson 2000). Northway (2000) indicated that participatory research provides a way to recognise the disempowerment of people who receive mental health services. In a piece of research carried out with the ForUs organisation in South Wales, participatory research was employed to investigate issues around medication for people receiving mental health care (Northway *et al.* 2001).

## CONCLUSION

In this chapter I have not set out to provide an exhaustive study of qualitative research methods. Such an exercise would be beyond the scope of a single chapter and there are a number of texts which concentrate on qualitative research methods in considerable detail. I have chosen instead to concentrate on methods which can be described as non-positivist in approach. Such methods are sometimes referred to as being at the softer end of the research spectrum, in recognition of their being furthest removed from empirical scientific methods such as randomised controlled trials. In taking this route within this chapter I have indicated the caveats that should be borne in mind by researchers in this area – i.e. that the research does not set out to represent an external reality that can be replicated and generalised. Consequently, attempts to show reliability and validity are neither desirable nor useful. Nevertheless there are criteria by which the rigour of such research may be judged, and I have provided examples of such criteria which should be of value to both researchers in their practice and readers of research in their criticism of research.

I have also discussed the role of participatory approaches in research which facilitate the empowerment of people traditionally seen as the subjects of research.

The value of the research approaches discussed in this chapter to community mental health nursing is that they enable nurses to investigate issues emerging from experience and relationships in ways that more positivist approaches, in their search for generalisable themes, are unable to achieve.

# REFERENCES

Ashworth, P. (1997a) 'The variety of qualitative research. Part one: introduction to the problem', *Nurse Education Today*, 17: 215–218.

Ashworth, P. (1997b) 'The variety of qualitative research. Part two: non-positivist approaches', *Nurse Education Today*, 17: 219–224.

Beech, I. (1997) 'Research as power: a reply to Gournay and Ritter', *Journal of Psychiatric and Mental Health Nursing*, 4: 443–444.

Beech, I. (1999) 'Bracketing in phenomenological research', *Nurse Researcher*, 6 (3): 35–51.

Berg, A. and Hallberg, I. (2000) 'Psychiatric nurses' lived experiences of working in in-patient care on a general team psychiatric ward', *Journal of Psychiatric and Mental Health Nursing*, 7 (4): 323–334.

Burnard, P. and Hannigan, B. (2000) 'Qualitative and quantitative approaches in mental health nursing: moving the debate forward', *Journal of Psychiatric and Mental Health Nursing*, 7: 1–6.

Clarke, L. (2001) *Contemporary nursing: culture, education and practice*, Salisbury: Academic Publishing Services.

Crotty, M. (1996) *Phenomenology and nursing research*, Melbourne: Churchill Livingstone.

Crotty, M. (1998) *The foundations of social research*, London: Sage.

Giorgi, A. (1970) *Psychology as a human science: a phenomenologically based approach*, New York: Harper and Row.

Giorgi, A. (1985) *Phenomenology and psychological research*, Pittsburgh: Duquesne University Press.

Gournay, K. and Ritter, S. (1997) 'What future for research in mental health nursing?', *Journal of Psychiatric and Mental Health Nursing*, 4: 441–442.

Graham, I. (2001) 'Seeking a clarification of meaning: a phenomenological interpretation of the craft of mental health nursing', *Journal of Psychiatric and Mental Health Nursing*, 8 (4): 335–346.

Hagan, T. and Green, J. (1994) *Mental health needs assessment: the user perspective*, Wakefield: Wakefield Healthcare.

Heron, J. (1996) *Co-operative inquiry: research into the human condition*, London: Sage.

Laing, R. (1960) *The divided self*, Harmondsworth: Penguin.

Leonard, V. (1994) 'A Heideggerian concept of person', in Benner, P. (ed.) *Interpretive phenomenology: embodiment, caring and ethics in health and illness*, Thousand Oaks, CA: Sage.

Marrow, C. (1996) 'Using qualitative research methods in nursing', *Nursing Standard*, 11 (7): 43–45.

Morrison, P. (1992) *Professional caring in practice*, Aldershot: Avebury.

Munhall, P. (1994) *Revisioning phenomenology: nursing and health science research*, New York: National League for Nursing.

Northway, R. (2000) 'The relevance of participatory research', *Nurse Researcher*, 7 (4): 40–52.

Northway, R., Parker, M. and Roberts, E. (2001) 'Collaboration in research', *Nurse Researcher*, 9 (2): 75–85.

Paley, J. (1997) 'Husserl, phenomenology and nursing', *Journal of Advanced Nursing*, 26: 187–193.

Pejlert, A., Asplund, K., Gilje, F. and Norberg, A. (1998) 'The meaning of caring for patients in a long-term psychiatric ward as narrated by formal care providers', *Journal of Psychiatric and Mental Health Nursing*, 5 (4): 255–264.

Stevenson, C. and Beech, I. (2001) 'Paradigms lost, paradigms regained: defending nursing against a single reading of postmodernism', *Nursing Philosophy*, 2 (2): 143–150.

Streubert, H. and Carpenter, D. (1995) *Qualitative research in nursing: advancing the humanistic imperative*, Philadelphia: Lippincott.

Tetley, J. and Hanson, E. (2000) 'Participatory research', *Nurse Researcher*, 8 (1): 69–88.

Tilley, S., Pollock, L. and Tait, L. (1999) 'Discourses on empowerment', *Journal of Psychiatric and Mental Health Nursing*, 6 (1): 53–60.

Traylen, H. (1994) 'Co-operative inquiry with health visitors', in Reason, P. (ed.) *Participation in human inquiry*, London: Sage.

van den Berg, J. (1972) *A different existence: principles of phenomenological psychopathology*, Pittsburgh: Duquesne University Press.

van Manen, M. (1990) *Researching lived experience: human science for an action sensitive pedagogy*, London, Ont.: Althouse.

Walters, A. (1995) 'The phenomenological movement: implications for nursing research', *Journal of Advanced Nursing*, 22: 791–799.

# FURTHER READING

Munhall, P. (1994) *Revisioning phenomenology: nursing and health science research*, New York: National League for Nursing.
An accessible introduction to the qualitative approach in general, and phenomenology in particular, with particularly interesting views on rigour, reliability and validity.

Reason, P. (ed.) (1994) *Participation in human inquiry*, London: Sage.
Moving forward from the qualitative–quantitative debate to propose a new approach to human science enquiry that deals with the researcher/researched split.

Streubert, H. and Carpenter, D. (1995) *Qualitative research in nursing: advancing the humanistic imperative*, Philadelphia: Lippincott.
This volume is presented in a thoughtful way with various qualitative approaches presented in a theoretical way, each followed by a chapter on practical application.

# CONCLUSION

## Ben Hannigan and Michael Coffey

As the chapters in this book have attested, community mental health nurses have travelled a long way from their modest beginnings almost half a century ago. CMHNs can now be found in a wide variety of practice areas, employing any of a range of therapeutic approaches. However, CMHNs still struggle to identify and articulate their particular contribution to mental health care. This struggle is reflected, in part, by the use of two different terms to describe nurses who work with people with mental health problems living in the community: 'community mental health nurse' (CMHN), and 'community psychiatric nurse' (CPN). Both terms are used in this book, in – apparently – an entirely interchangeable way.

The expansion of the CMHN workforce and the growth of work in specialist areas mean that, in reality, it is becoming less and less meaningful to think of community mental health nurses as a single, unified group of practitioners. It is not clear how far, if at all, a core set of 'mental health nursing values' finds expression across different areas of practice. On the surface, at least, the nurse working with children with mental health problems appears to differ remarkably from the nurse working with older people with dementia, or from the nurse specialising in the care of adults with substance misuse problems. Knowledge, skills and attitudes vary, as does the context in which work is accomplished, and as do education needs. Universities and nursing's regulatory bodies have been slow to adapt to this reality, and a future challenge for educators will be to offer the kind of educational experience that reflects the particular needs of different groups of practitioners.

Debates over CMHN identity, specialism and education will be taking place against an ever-changing policy and professional backdrop. In the future, it is possible that nurses at pre-registration level may be trained as 'generalists' (UKCC 2001). This would reduce the speciality of mental health nursing to a post-qualification add-on, with mental health nursing in the community as – presumably – an add-on to the add-on. As mental health nurses are pulled towards their non-mental health nursing colleagues by this drift towards generalism, patterns of community mental health care delivery will continue to pull CMHNs towards their non-nursing mental health professional colleagues. There are already considerable overlaps in the work of mental health nurses and mental health social workers; changes in policy and practice may increase this. How far future community mental health nurses will identify and ally themselves with 'nursing' or with 'mental health work' will be interesting to see.

Certain challenges will continue to face community mental health nurses, irrespective of their professional alignment and their mode of education. The move towards more user-responsive services is tempered by the determination of policy-makers to more closely manage the lives of people with mental health problems in the name of public safety. Nurses, in particular, will need to walk the tightrope between these competing agendas, and find the 'space' in which to practise. Other challenges include meeting the differential mental health needs of women and of men, and of people from ethnic minority groups. Community mental health nursing is still largely 'blind' to the importance of gender and ethnicity. There is also room for CMHNs to become more engaged with the 'bigger picture'. This means influencing policy and practice developments at national and local level, and working to ensure that a mental health nursing 'voice' is heard.

Important research agendas lie ahead. Given the size of the CMHN work-force, it is remarkable how little is still known about models of good practice, about 'what works', and about what helps to support practitioners in managing the stresses and strains of doing mental health work. It is appropriate that future research agendas take account of (and engage with) research in the wider, multi-disciplinary, mental health field. However, there remains an important space, too, for unidisciplinary research of the type that other professions enjoy.

Finally, community mental health nursing has to face the problem of declining recruitment and retention, and low morale. Working as a mental health nurse no longer appears an attractive career option for many. The work is stressful, the responsibilities significant, the pay and conditions often poor. These are significant challenges for the future and we hope that this text provides a basis on which to build our contribution to the community mental health of tomorrow.

# REFERENCE

UKCC (2001) *Fitness for practice and purpose: the report of the UKCC's post-commission development group*, London: UKCC.

# PROFESSIONAL ORGANISATIONS

## The Nursing and Midwifery Council

The Nursing and Midwifery Council (NMC) is the statutory body for nursing, midwifery and health visiting in the UK. The NMC:

- maintains a register of qualified nurses, midwives and health visitors;
- sets standards for education, practice and conduct;
- provides advice for nurses, midwives and health visitors;
- considers allegations of misconduct or unfitness to practise due to ill health.

NMC publications include: the *Code of Professional Conduct*, the most recent version of which appeared in June 2002; *Guidelines for Mental Health and Learning Disabilities Nursing*, which appeared in April 1998; and various sets of standards governing pre- and post-registration education courses.

The NMC's website is: http://www.nmc-uk.org

Documents on this site are usually downloadable in portable document format (PDF).

## The Mental Health Nurses' Association (formerly known as the Community Psychiatric Nurses' Association)

The Mental Health Nurses' Association, known until 2003 as the Community Psychiatric Nurses' Association (CPNA) was formed in the mid-1970s, and is now part of the newly-formed public sector trade union Amicus. Membership of the Association is open to all mental health nurses. Members are able to receive professional support, advice, and educational services. The Association also provides a mental health nursing voice at national and local level, and campaigns alone and with other organisations on a range of mental health and professional issues.

Members receive the journal *Mental Health Nursing*, and are able to participate in both national and local activities, including conferences.

## The Royal College of Nursing

The Royal College of Nursing (RCN) is the UK's largest professional nursing organisation. Membership of the RCN is open to all mental health nurses. Like the CPNA, the RCN offers advice, educational services and professional support, and campaigns on a range of health and nursing issues at all levels.

Members can subscribe to the journal *Mental Health Practice*, and can join a number of specific mental health forums: Mental Health Nursing Forum; Forum for the Development of Mental Health Nursing Practice; Forensic Nursing Forum; and the Children and Young People's Mental Health Forum.

The RCN's website is: http://www.rcn.org.uk

The RCN's mental health zone is: http://www.rcn.org.uk/rcn_extranet/mhz/index.htm

# VOLUNTARY ORGANISATIONS

## Hearing Voices Network

91 Oldham Street, Manchester M4 1LW
Tel.: 0161 834 5768
Website: http://www.hearing-voices.org.uk

The Hearing Voices Network is for people who hear voices, and for their families and friends. The Network promotes greater tolerance and understanding of voice hearing, and seeks to raise awareness about the experience in society as a whole.

## Manic Depression Fellowship

Castle Works, 21 St George's Road, London SE1 6ES
Tel.: 020 7793 2600
Website: http://www.mdf.org.uk

The Manic Depression Fellowship works to enable people affected by manic depression to take control of their lives.
    The fellowship aims to fulfil its mission by:

- supporting and developing self-help opportunities for people affected by manic depression;
- expanding and developing the information services about manic depression;
- influencing the improvement of treatments and services to promote recovery;
- decreasing the discrimination against, and promoting the social inclusion and rights of, people affected by manic depression;
- being an effective and efficient organisation with sufficient resources to sustain and develop its activities, thereby ensuring that members receive a unique, high-quality service.

# MIND

5–19 Broadway, London E15 4BQ
Tel.: 020 8519 2122
Website: http://www.mind.org.uk

MIND is the leading mental health charity in England and Wales, and works for a better life for everyone with experience of mental distress.
MIND's activities include:

- advancing the views, needs and ambitions of people with experience of mental distress;
- promoting inclusion by challenging discrimination;
- influencing policy through campaigning and education;
- inspiring the development of quality services, which reflect expressed need and diversity;
- achieving equal civil and legal rights through campaigning and education.

# Mental Health Foundation

7th Floor, 83 Victoria Street, London SW1H 0HW
Tel.: 020 7802 0300
Website: http://www.mentalhealth.org.uk

The Mental Health Foundation is the leading UK charity working in mental health and learning disabilities. With pioneering research and community projects the Mental Health Foundation aims to improve the support available for people with mental health problems and people with learning disabilities.

# SANE

1st Floor, Cityside House, 40 Adler Street, London E1 1EE
Tel.: 020 7375 1002
Website: http://www.sane.org.uk

SANE has three objectives:
- to raise awareness and combat ignorance about mental illness, and to improve mental health services;
- to provide care and support to anyone concerned about mental illness;
- to initiate and fund research into the causes of, and treatments and potential cures for, schizophrenia and depression through its work at the SANE Research Centre in Oxford.

## Rethink Serious Mental Illness

Head Office, 30 Tabernacle Street, London EC2A 4DD
Tel.: 020 7330 9100/01
Website: http://www.nsf.org.uk

Rethink (formerly the National Schizophrenia Fellowship) is the largest severe mental illness charity in the UK. Rethink is dedicated to improving the lives of everyone affected by severe mental illness, whether they have a condition them-selves, care for others who do, or are professionals or volunteers working in the mental health field.

## Revolving Doors

http://www.revolving-doors.co.uk/home.asp

The Revolving Doors Agency is the UK's leading charity concerned with mental health and the criminal justice system. The Agency runs practical schemes in police stations, prisons and courts to support people who have 'fallen through the net' of mainstream services. What the Agency learns enables them to provide project development support to other agencies and to conduct research and policy work at local and national level.

## The Alzheimer's Society

Gordon House, 10 Greencoat Place, London SW1P 1PH
Tel.: 020 7306 0606
Website: http://www.alzheimers.org.uk

The Alzheimer's Society is the UK's leading care and research charity for people with all forms of dementia and their carers.

## The Sainsbury Centre for Mental Health

134 Borough High Street, London SE1 1LB
Tel.: 020 7403 8790
Website: http://www.scmh.org.uk

The Sainsbury Centre for Mental Health's core aim is to improve the quality of life for people with severe mental health problems by enabling the develop-ment of excellent mental health services, which are valued by users, carers and professionals.

The Sainsbury Centre seeks to achieve this by influencing national policy and practice through a co-ordinated programme of research, service development and training.

## Survivors Speak Out

34 Osnaburgh Street, London NW1 3ND
Tel.: 020 7916 5473

Survivors Speak Out is a national campaigning group of survivors of mental health services. They campaign for better treatment for people with mental health problems, and provide advice and information.

## UK Advocacy Network (UKAN)

Volserve House, 14–18 West Bar Green, Sheffield S1 2DA
Tel.: 0114 272 8171

UKAN is a national federation of independent mental health user-run patients' councils, support groups, advocacy projects and user forums. It collects and disseminates information about patients' councils, advocacy projects and user forums, and provides this information in order to facilitate wider development of user involvement and user-led mental health services.

# JOURNALS AND MAGAZINES

Journals are the best way of keeping up to date with current research and opinion in community mental health nursing. Key UK-based mental health nursing, and multidisciplinary, journals are:

*Journal of Psychiatric and Mental Health Nursing*
This journal provides an international forum for the publication of original contributions that lead to the advancement of psychiatric and mental health nursing practice.

Website: http://www.blackwell-science.com/~cgilib/jnlpage.asp?Journal=jpmhn &File=jpmhn

*Mental Health Nursing*
This is the journal of the Community Psychiatric Nurses' Association. Professional research, debate, opinion and care study papers are regularly published.

Website: http://www.cpna.org.uk

*Mental Health Practice*
This is the Royal College of Nursing's mental health journal. Professional research, debate and opinion pieces are regularly published.

Website: http://www.nursing-standard.co.uk/mentalhealth/index.html

*Journal of Mental Health*
This international peer-reviewed journal provides professionals, managers and others with a forum for the latest ideas and evidence in the field of mental health.

Website: http://www.tandf.co.uk/journals/titles/09638237.html

*Mental Health Today*
This multidisciplinary journal publishes research, debate and policy analysis papers.

*Openmind*
This is MIND's magazine, which regularly publishes lively articles by mental health service users and professionals.

Website: http://www.mind.org.uk/openmind/index.asp

*British Journal of Psychiatry*
The monthly peer-reviewed journal of the Royal College of Psychiatrists.

Website: http://bjp.rcpsych.org

# INTERNET SITES AND DISCUSSION LISTS

## INTERNET SITES

Here we provide a selection of the many internet sites that we have encountered and found useful.

*http://www.york.ac.uk/inst/crd*
The NHS Centre for Reviews and Dissemination (CRD) was established in January 1994 to provide the NHS with important information on the effectiveness of treatments and the delivery and organisation of health care.

CRD, by offering rigorous and systematic reviews on selected topics, a database of good-quality reviews, a dissemination service and an information service, helps to promote research-based practice in the NHS.

Within the NHS R&D programme, CRD is a sibling organisation of the UK Cochrane Centre. The UK Cochrane Centre is part of an international network, the Cochrane Collaboration, committed to preparing, maintaining and disseminating systematic reviews of research on the effects of health care. CRD plays an important role in disseminating the contents of Cochrane reviews to the NHS.

*http://www.fnrh.freeserve.co.uk*
A very useful forensic mental health resource page, set and maintained by Dr Phil Woods.

*http://www.snappygraffix.com/npnr*
The Network for Psychiatric Nursing Research (NPNR) was first conceived in 1993, when it became apparent that mental health professionals were finding it difficult to get up-to-date information about the innovative research and development work being carried out by colleagues within mental health. The objective of the NPNR is to disseminate and develop research and practice within the UK.

*http://www.nelmh.org*
The National Electronic Library for Mental Health (NeLMH) is one of the first virtual branch libraries of the National Electronic Library for Health (NeLH), an initiative announced in the government's Information for Health strategy. The NeLMH is also one of the main areas of focus for the Mental Health Information Strategy announced in the National Service Framework for Mental Health.

*http://www.doh.gov.uk/mentalhealth*
This is the Department of Health's mental health site. Policy documents, guidance and reports all appear here, and are usually downloadable in portable document format (PDF).

*http://www.wales.gov.uk/subihealth/index.htm*
This is the National Assembly for Wales's health website, with links to mental health policy and guidance. Again, documents are usually available in PDF.

*http://www.scotland.gov.uk/whatwedo.asp?topic=health&Submit=Go*
This is the Scottish Executive's health website.

*http://www.ni-assembly.gov.uk/io/sitemap.htm*
This is the Northern Ireland Assembly's main website.

# DISCUSSION LISTS

*http://www.jiscmail.ac.uk/lists/psychiatric-nursing.html*
This psychiatric nursing discussion list includes members from around the world, and is a lively forum for the exchange of news and views.

*http://www.jiscmail.ac.uk/lists/cmhn-education-and-practice.html*
This is a discussion list for people interested in community mental health nursing education and practice.

# INDEX

*A first class service* (DOH 1998) 133
ABC model 242
Abdul (vignette) 118–19
accountability: autonomy 49
ACO *see* assertive community outreach
ACT *see* assertive community treatment
Act (1959): voluntary status admission 10
action: needs for 178
Action Zone approach 155, 156
'Acute Solutions' (Sainsbury Centre 1999) 150
adolescents 343–54; action agenda 350–2; burden 346–7; history 344–6; nurse training 352–4; problem size 346; services collaboration 347–8; strategies 349–50; workforce 348
adults: family therapy 217–18
Africa: cultural aspects 113
aging population 319–27
aims: multidisciplinary teams 70–1, 73
alcohol 313
*All Wales strategy* (Welsh Office 1983) 332
Alzheimer's Society 320
AMHPs *see* approved mental health professionals
analysis: CANSAS 182–3, *see also* needs assessment
anti-anxiety drugs: pharmacology 280
anti-oppressive practice 153
antidepressants: pharmacology 278–9
antipsychotic medication 275–8; atypical 277–8; compliance 281; psychosis relapse prevention 253
anxiety states: gender bias 101; medication 280; primary care provision 79–80; risk assessment effects 193–5; suicide risk 201
approved mental health professionals (AMHPs) 38

art therapy 287–97; community movements 294–5; creativity 288–9, 291; definition 289–90; evidence-based practice 292; music 291–4; storytelling 295, 296; writing 296–7
Asia 113, 114
assertive community outreach (ACO) 314
assertive community treatment (ACT) 388
assertive outreach 261–71; critical success factors 265; definition 264; functions 264; integration 267–8; local service management responsibilities 268–9; location 267; management 266–7; research 262–3; staffing 266; style of working 267; targeting 265–6; team approaches 269–71
assessment: cognitive behavioral 240–3; community mental health care needs 175–84; education/training 391; learning disabilities with mental health problems 334–6; *see also* needs assessment
asylum system 7–8, 91
atypical antipsychotics 277–8
audits: CHI/CHAI 33–4
autonomy: ethical aspects 47–9; respect for 44

baseline exaggeration 335–6
behavioral problems 335–6, 338, 339
belief systems: cultural differences 113
beneficence principle 44
'beneficent coercion' 50
Bennett, Rocky 389
benzodiazepines: pharmacology 280
Bernstein family (case study) 229–32
best practice: NICE establishment 33; *see also* good practice

*Better services for the mentally ill* (DHSS 1975): history 14, 23; multidisciplinary community teamwork 67–8
biological model of mental illness 14
bipolar affective disorder: lithium 279–80
boundaries: teamwork 70–2
bracketing technique 399, 400
Bradford 85
*Bringing Britain together: a national strategy for neighbourhood renewal* (Social Exclusion Unit 1998) 158
*British Journal of Psychiatry* 169–70
*Building bridges* (DOH 1995) 32; dementia care 322, 327; mentally disordered offenders 300; primary care for mental illness 85
burden criterion: child referrals 346–7
burnout: nurses 121–31
Buzan, Tony 243–4

Camberwell Assessment of Need Short Appraisal Schedule (CANSAS) 175, 176, 179–84, 390
CAMHS *see* Child and Adolescent Mental Health Services
cannabis 313
CANSAS *see* Camberwell Assessment of Need Short Appraisal Schedule
*Capable practitioner* initiative 71
capacity-based compulsory treatment model 37
care programme approach (CPA) 25–6; change limitations 94; community mental health teams 69; introduction 32, 92–3
carers' needs: dementia patients 319–27; National Service Framework for Mental Health 222–3; psychosocial family interventions 222–33
Carers' and Users' Expectations of Services (CUES) 179
case histories: storytelling 296
case management: 261-71; assertive outreach 264–9; contemporary 263; history 262; team approach 269–71; *see also* care programme approach
case studies: Abdul (racial issues) 118–19; assertive outreach 269–71; ethical reflection 45; Jane (racial issues) 115; John (racial issues) 118; Joseph (racial issues) 115; Mental Health Review Tribunals 118; Michael (racial issues) 115; multidisciplinary teamwork 73–5; psychosocial family interventions 228–32
CBT *see* cognitive behavioral therapy

Centre for Reviews and Dissemination (CRD) 171–2
change: family therapy 214
CHI *see* Commission for Health Improvement
Chief Male Nurses Association: 1964 Annual Conference 8
Child and Adolescent Mental Health Services (CAMHS) 210, 344–5, 348, 349, 350
children 343–54; agenda for action 350–2; burden on adults 346–7; custody 57–8, 59; family therapy 216–17; historical context 344–6; National Service Frameworks 349–50; nurse employment 348, 352–4; service collaboration 347–8; size of problem 346; specialised interventions 350
chlorpromazine 10, 276
chronic disease management model 84–5
circular interviewing 218
citizenship: service users 94, 98
Claybury Hospital (nr London) 8
Claybury stress/burnout study 122, 123, 126
client-centred services 107
client-directed services 107
clinical governance 348
Clinical Standards Advisory Group (CSAG 1999) 80
clinical supervision 132–44; community psychiatric nurses 136–42; coping/stress management 127; managerial supervision confusion 138, 140; peer involvement 141; rudiments 134–5; training needs 138–9
Clunis, Christopher 191, 386
CMHCs *see* community mental health centres
CMHNs *see* community mental health nurses
CMHTs *see* community mental health teams
co-operative enquiry 402–3
Cochrane Schizophrenia Group 171, 228–32
coercive powers 303: *see also* compliance; compulsory treatment
coexisting substance abuse problems: forensic importance 312–13; prevalence 311–12; substances 313–14; treatment 314–15; treatment effectiveness 315–16; UK studies 312
cognitive aspects: biases/deficits in psychosis 236, 237; learning disabilities 335; psychosocial family interventions 228

cognitive behavioral therapy (CBT): context 238–9; engagement 240; engaging patients 245; Mark (case study) 243–7; problem assessment 240–3; psychosis 235–47

collaboration: professionals dealing with children and adolescents 347–8; service users and mental health workers 90–9; *see also* co-operative enquiry

Commission for Health Improvement (CHI) 33–4, 165

commitment: multidisciplinary teams 73

common sense: risk 188, 189, 190

communication: family interventions 226–7, 230

community care: arts movements 294–5; failure 34–5; introduction 10, 11, 12; policy: 1990 onwards 31–3; risks 26–7; services: gender bias 106–8; suicidal patient management 204–6; treatment orders 37

community mental health centres (CMHCs) 314

community mental health nurses (CMHNs): activities 86; 'community psychiatric nurse' nondistinction 406; coping strategies 126–7; ethical aspects of practice 45–52; mentally disordered offenders 305; nurse–patient relationships: ethics 41–53; problems facing 16; psychosis relapse planning 250–7; stress/burnout 121–31; suicidal patients 202

community mental health teams (CMHTs): boundaries and barriers 70–2; chronic disease management model 85; history 68–70; management problems 69; professional integration problems 67–76

Community Psychiatric Nurses' Association (now the Mental Health Nurses' Association) 408

community psychiatric nurses (CPNs): clinical supervision issues 132–42; 'community mental health nurse' nondistinction 406; community mental health teams relationship 69, 70; dementia care 319–27; history 20–7; non-social work role 21; nursing skills 74–5; psychosocial family interventions 232–3; recognition/training 14; reflective practice issues 141–2; role definition 13, 21; stress/coping 126; training criticisms (early 1990s) 15

*Community Psychiatric Nursing Journal* 24

*Community psychiatric nursing* (RCP occasional paper 1997) 323

comorbidity: substance abuse 310–16

competence: ethical assessment 50

complex health interventions 393

compliance: anti-psychotic medication 281; ethical aspects 41, 49–50; MIND Annual Conference (1998) 97

compulsory treatment: capacity-based model 37; coercive powers 303; draft mental health bill (2002) 38

conceptual aspects: conceptualized risk 189; creativity 288, 289; family therapy 213–14; psychosis 236–8

confidence: promoting in patients 60–3

confidentiality 46–7

conflict resolution: families 228

consent: ethical aspects 49–50

constructivism 212

consultation processes 95–6, 107

consumer-led services *see* user-led services

context 167, 193–5, 238–9

controversial evidence 168

coping strategies: community mental health nurses 121, 126–7; paranoia 245–6

core beliefs: psychosis 236

costs/benefits 292, 390–1

counselling: family therapy 211

counsellors: activities 86

couples therapy 217

CPA *see* care programme approach

CPNs *see* community psychiatric nurses

CRD *see* NHS Centre for Reviews and Dissemination

creativity: art forms 289; art therapy 287–97; concept 288, 289; writing 295, 297

credentialism 20, 24

criminal offences 299–306

crisis intervention 22–3

critical policy analysis 31

critical success factors 265

CUES *see* Carers' and Users' Expectations of Services

cultural issues 111–20

Daily Living Programme 388

Dartington Social Research Unit (DSRU) 347

decision-making: risk 191–3; risk management 187–206; service users 90–9

definitions: assertive outreach 264; evidence 168–9; mental health promotion 151–3; need 177–8;

relapse 252; risk 188, 189, 190; suicide 199

dementia care 319–27; demographics 320–1; nursing roles 321–6; policy trends 320–1; practice diversity 326

demographics 320–1

deontology 43–4

depot injections *see* neuroleptic depot injections

depression: gender bias 101; medication 278–9; primary care 79–80, 84–5; stress in women 104; suicide risk 201; termination of employment 57; women 102–5

descriptive qualitative research 399

diagnosis: cultural aspects 117–19; diagnostic groups 81; gender bias 102, 105–6

diagnostic overshadowing phenomenon 336

*Diagnostic and statistical manual of mental disorders* (DSM-IV) 336–7

direct contact services 349

Disability Discrimination Act 1995 62

discourse analysis 400–1

discrimination 54–66; gender-based 100–10; inclusion promotion 60–3; origins 59–60; social exclusion realities 55–9

discussion lists 417

district nurses 80, 86, 124

distrust: evidence-based care 168

Dobson, Frank: 1998 statement 34, 35

domestic violence 108

dopamine 275–6

DSRU *see* Dartington Social Research Unit

dual diagnosis 310–16

duration (interventions) 228

duty-based approach *see* deontology

eating disorders 79, 80, 101

ECAS *see* Epidemiological Catchment Area Study

ECT *see* electro-convulsive therapy

education *see* training

EE *see* expressed emotion

effectiveness: creativity 288; dual diagnosis 315–16

elderly people: dementia care 319–27

electro-convulsive therapy (ECT): women 105

emotionality: women 103

employment 56–9, 103, 104

empowerment *see* patient empowerment

engagement: CBT 240

English National Board for Nurses, Midwives, and Health Visitors 132

Epidemiological Catchment Area Study (ECAS) 311

EPS *see* extrapyramidal symptoms

ERG *see* External Reference Group

ethics: creativity 288; deontology 43–4; issues 41–53; principles 44; reflection (case study) 45; 'should' questions 42; utilitarianism 43

ethnicity 111–20; case studies 115, 118–19; diagnosis/therapy 117; issues 113–15; multicultural practice 116–17; traditional psychiatry 112–13

evaluation *see* assessment; needs assessment

everyday creativity 288, 289

evidence-based practice 164–86; art therapy 292; context 167; definition 165–6; initiatives adoption 172–3; innovative practice developments 173; mentally disordered offenders 301–4; power conflicts 168–9; psychosocial family interventions 228–32; randomised controlled trials 167–8; resources 170–2; systematic reviews 167

exceptional creativity 288

*The experiences of an asylum doctor* (Montagu Lomax) 91

*Experiencing Psychiatry* 93

expressed emotion (EE) 224–5, 232, 253–5

External Reference Group (ERG) 35, 36

extrapyramidal symptoms (EPS) 277

family therapy 210–19; adults 217–18; children 216, 217; genograms 215; psychosocial interventions 222–33; team working 215; training study 387

FCMHNs *see* forensic community mental health nurses

fear states: risk assessment 193–5; *see also* anxiety states

forensic community mental health nurses (FCMHNs) 123

forensic patients 299–306, 312–13

*Forget me not* report (Audit Commission 2000) 321

formulation stage: needs assessment 183

Foucauldian approach 194

four-tier strategic framework 349–51

functional analysis 242

fundholding: GPs 69

funding: quantitative research 392

*Future healthcare workforce* project 71

gamma-aminobutyric acid (GABA) 275

gender issues 100–10; community services 106–8; depression in women 104–5;

diagnosis 102, 105–6; life events
model 104; mental health 104–5;
social role theory 103–4; societal
reaction theory 105
generalism: CPNs' role development 24;
primary care team 78–9; training 406
genetics: psychosis 238
genograms: family therapy 215
Gittins, Diana 91
global mental health promotion 154
goals *see* aims
good and harm: definition 42
good practice: mental health promotion
159–61; National Service Framework
for Mental Health (DOH 1999a) 36;
NICE 'best practice' 33; suicide risk
assessment 203–4
Gospel Oak Depression Study 389
GPs: activities 86; early lack of support
for CPNs 21; fundholding capability
32, 69; prevention practices 83–4;
referrals: 1990s 24, 25; *see also*
primary care system
Gray, Muir 165, 166
Greene, John 11, 12, 13, 21
Guillebaud Report (1956) 9

harm *see* good and harm
HAS (Audit Commission 1999) 344
HAZs *see* Health Action Zones
health: needs for 177–8
Health Action Zones (HAZs) 155, 156
*The health of the nation* (DOH 1992)
152, 155, 199, 204
health visitors 80, 86, 124
Hearing Voices Network (HVN) 96, 412
hermeneutic circle 400
hierarchy of need (Maslow) 177
high-risk individuals: suicide 201–2
history 7–18; case management 262;
children/adolescents 344–6; CPNs
20–7; family therapy 211–12;
multidisciplinary community
teamwork 68–70
*History of mental health nursing* (Peter
Nolan) 91
homes of patients 47
homicides: community care 26–7
hope 60–3, 252
*Hospital Plan* (MOH 1962) 22, 31
hospital-based mental health nurses 124
household roles: stress in women 104
human psyche 112–13
Hutton, John 97
HVN *see* Hearing Voices Network

ideation: suicide risk 203–4
illness timeline 284

in-patient admissions: women 101
individual needs assessment 176–7
informal carers 304–6
information gathering 181, 182
information giving 226, 230
informed consent 49–50
initiatives adoption 172–3
injections 22–3
Institute of Psychiatry 389, 392
institutional racism 116
intellectual distortion: learning disabilities
334–5
International Self Advocacy Alliance and
Survivors Speak Out 251
internet sites 416–17
interpersonal skills: nurses 74–5
interpretation of psychotic events 246–7
interpretive qualitative research 399, 400
interventions *see* psychopharmacology;
psychosocial family interventions
interview process 399, 400
isolation: gender bias 106; nurses 133;
social exclusion 54–66; support for
nurses 133; women 102

Jamison, Kay 59
Jane (case study) 115
JBCNS *see* Joint Board of Clinical Nursing
Studies
job satisfaction 122–5, 127
John (case study) 118
Joint Board of Clinical Nursing Studies
(JBCNS) 14
*Journal of Psychiatric and Mental Health
Nursing* 169–70
journals 169–2, 414–15
justice principle 44

Kettering assertive outreach team (case
study) 270–1
*Keys to engagement* (Sainsbury Centre for
Mental Health 1998) 262
keyworkers: introduction 26

Labour Government (1997 onwards) 31
Labour Party 33–4
language 339, 401
Largactil *see* chlorpromazine
*Late in the Morning* CD album 293
'learned helplessness' 104
learning disabilities 331–9; assessment
334–6; cognitive disintegration 335;
intellectual distortion 334–5;
interventions 338–9; psychosocial
masking 335; risk perceptions 189–90
legal aspects: community mental health
care 30–40; Disability Discrimination
Act 1995 62; Mental Health Act

(1983) 34, 36, 37; NHS and Community Care Act 1990 31–2; professionalisation of CPNs 20, 24; *Reforming the Mental Health Act* (Secretary of State for Health and Home Secretary 2000a, b) 37
life events models 104
literature sources 169–72
lithium 279–80
local mental health promotion 154
local service management 268–9
location: assertive outreach 267
Lomax, Montagu 91
longterm care 26, 284

Macpherson definition 116
magazines 414–15
*Making it happen* (DOH 2001a): broad model 156; definition 152; framework 149; mental health promotion 156, 159; pro formas 159
management: assertive outreach 266–7; 'managerial supervision' 138, 140; medication 280–4, 389; multidisciplinary teams 69, 71, 72–3
Manchester Clinical Supervision Scale 138
Manchester Regional Hospital Board (1956) 9
Manic Depression Fellowship 251, 410
MAOIs *see* monoamine oxidase inhibitors
marijuana 313
Mark (CBT case study) 243, 244, 245, 246, 247
married women: depression 103, 104
Maslow's hierarchy of need 177
mass media: risk awareness 194
Maudsley Hospital (London) 388
measures *see* assessment; needs assessment
Medical Research Council (MRC) 393
medication: learning disabilities with mental health problems 338; management 280–4, 389; *see also* compliance; psychopharmacology
Mental Health Act (1983) 34, 36, 37, 95
Mental Health Act Commission 101
Mental Health Alliance 37
Mental Health Foundation 97, 411
Mental Health National Service Framework (DOH 1999) 55
Mental Health Nurses' Association 408
Mental Health Nursing Review (DOH 1994) 386–7
mental health promotion (MHP) 149–61; 'Acute Solutions' (Sainsbury Centre) 150; anti-oppressive practice 153; benefits 150–1; definitions 151–3; good practice 159–61; key analysis

levels 152; Single Regeneration Budget 150, 158; user-led services 150
Mental Health Review Tribunals 118
mental hospitals: 1960s 9; Manchester Regional Hospital Board report 9; overcrowding 8; reform from within 9–10
Mental Research Institute (MRI) 212
'mentality' 152–3, 159
mentally disordered offenders 299–306; coercive powers 303; evidence bases 301–4; social support 304–6
MHNs *see* mental health nurses
MHP *see* mental health promotion
Michael (case study) 115
Milan Associates 212, 213, 215
MIND: Annual Conference (1998): medication non-compliance 97; details 410–11; Enquiry into social exclusion 60; service provision for women 107–8; Yellow Card survey 93
Mind Maps® 243–4
Mini PAS-ADD questionnaire 337–8
*Modernising mental health services: safe, sound and supportive* (DOH 1998) 35, 36
monitoring 243, 254
monoamine oxidase inhibitors (MAOIs) 275, 276, 278, 279
mood stabilizers 279–80
Moore, Stan 10–11, 21
Moorhaven Hospital (nr Plymouth) 11–12, 14, 20
morale: mental hospital staff 8
MRI *see* Mental Research Institute
multicultural practice 116–17, 118
multidisciplinary teams: community teamwork 67–76; creating 72–3; future developments 75–6; isolation within 392; nurse experiences 73–5
music therapy 291–2
Music Workshop Project 292–3

National Confidential Enquiry into Suicide and Homicide by People with Mental Illness 198, 204
National Health Service and Community Care Act (1990) 175
National Health Service (NHS): inauguration 8; 'New Labour' 33–4; policy aspects 30–40
National Institute for Clinical Excellence (NICE) 33, 165, 390
National Institute for Mental Health 393
National Schizophrenia Fellowship 223
National Self-Harm Network (NSHN) 96
National Service Frameworks (NSFs) 9, 36; carers' needs 222–3; children and

adolescents' services 349–50; cultural issues 111; dementia care 321; establishment 34; multidisciplinary teams 75; needs assessment 167, 175; objectives 30; primary care provision for mental health 78–9, 87; specifications 82–4; women in-patients 101–2

needs assessment 390; community mental health care 175–84; definitions 177–8; measures 178–9; psychometric properties 179; step-by-step guide 181–4

Needs for Care Assessment (NFCAS) 179

needs-led approach 175–6

negotiation: risk 192–3

Neighbourhood Renewal Fund (NRF) 158

nerve impulses 275, 276

neuroleptic depot injections 22, 23

neurotransmission 275, 276

neutrality position: family therapy 214

New Deal for Communities (Neighbourhood Renewal Unit 2002b) 150, 158

'New Labour' 33–4

*The new NHS: modern, dependable* (Secretary of State for Health 1997) 33, 133

NFCAS *see* Needs for Care Assessment

NHS *see* National Health Service

NHS and Community Care Act 1990 25, 31–2

*The NHS Plan* (DOH 2000): multidisciplinary teams 72; primary care trusts establishment 156; women's needs 107

NICE *see* National Institute for Clinical Excellence

nine criteria: qualitative 401–2

Nolan, Peter 91

non-fiction: creative 297

non-maleficence principle 44

non-positivist qualitative research 398–403

Nottingham 106–7

novelty: creativity 288, 289

NRF *see* Neighbourhood Renewal Fund

NSFs *see* National Service Frameworks

NSHN *see* National Self-Harm Network

nurses: autonomy 47–9; creative role 290, 291; critical policy analysis 31; low status in research teams 392; multidisciplinary team experiences 73–5; nurse—patient relationships 41–53; research involvement 169–70, 291, 392; scientific respectability 291; *see also* community mental health

nurses; psychiatric nurses; school nurses

Nursing and Midwifery Council 408

objectivity: positivist research 398–9

occupational therapists 69

offenders: mentally disordered 299–306

Office for National Statistics (ONS) 346

older people: dementia care 319–27

*One flew over the cuckoo's nest* (Ken Kesey) 10

ongoing formulation problem 244

ongoing psychosis monitoring 243

ONS *see* Office for National Statistics

*Organised Chaos* CD album 292–3

outcome-based approach *see* utilitarianism

outcomes: quantitative research 390, 391

outreach: assertive 261–71

overcrowding 8, 20

*Paradox and counterparadox* (Milan Associates 1978) 212

parasuicide 204–5

parenting 57–8

participatory research 402, 403

PAS-ADD *see* Psychiatric Assessment Schedule for Adults with Development Disabilities

paternalism 51

patients *see* service users

PCTs *see* primary care, trusts

Peat, Lena 11

peer involvement 141

*Perceval's narrative* 91

pharmacology *see* psychopharmacology

'phenomenological nod' 400

Pilkington, Francis 11, 12

PIMRA *see* Psychotherapy Inventory for Mentally Retarded Adults

Plymouth Polytechnic 14

PMHWs *see* primary mental health workers

policy aspects: 1990 onwards 31–3; community mental health care 30–40; dementia care trends 320–1; development 155; regeneration 155–8

population needs 176

positivist qualitative research 398

poverty: unemployment 57

Powell, Enoch 31

power conflicts: evidence 168–9

practice: dementia care 326; ethical aspects 45–52; family therapy concepts 213–14; quantitative research contribution 386–9; *see also* evidence-based practice

practice nurses: activities 86

pragmatic verbal disorders 334–5
predictive models: suicide 199–201
prevalence: coexisting problems 311–12, 333
prevention: depression 81; longterm psychotherapeutic 284; preventive psychiatry 22–3; primary care programmes 81, 83; psychosis relapse 250–7
primary care: system 78–87; teams 68–70; trusts (PCTs) 156
primary mental health workers (PMHWs) 352
privacy: ethical aspects 46–7
problem solving: families 227, 231
prodromal changes 254
professional aspects: collaboration over children/adolescents 347–8; CPN autonomy 20, 25; organisations 408–9; reshaping boundaries 70–3
'professionalisation' 19–20, 23–5
prosodic verbal disorders 334–5
psyche: human 112–13
Psychiatric Assessment Schedule for Adults with Development Disabilities (PAS-ADD) 337, 338
psychiatrists 21, 24, 25, 105
Psychnurse Methods of Coping Questionnaire 126
Psychological Therapies Team (PTT) 71–2, 73, 75
psychometric properties 179
psychopharmacology 274–85; anti-anxiety drugs 280; antidepressants 278–9; antipsychotics 275–8; mood stabilizers 279–80; sedative-hypnotic drugs 280
psychosis: carer's needs 223–4, 228; cognitive behavioral therapy 235–47; event interpretation 246–7; Mark (CBT case study) 244, 245, 246, 247; relapse prevention 250–7
psychosis relapse: antipsychotic medication 253; definition 252; management strategies 257; monitoring 254; prevention 250–7; recovery concept 255–6; 'relapse signatures' 254; stress-vulnerability approach 253–5
psychosocial family interventions 222–33; cognitive restructuring 228; communication 226–7; education 226; evidence base 228–32; home interventions 225; problem solving 227
psychosocial masking 335
psychosocial model of mental illness 14
psychosocial nursing 22, 23

psychosocial suicide risk factors 200, 205
Psychotherapy Inventory for Mentally Retarded Adults (PIMRA) 337
psychotherapy training 211
psychotic experience 243–4
PTT see Psychological Therapies Team
public interest 46–7, 49
public panics 194–5
publications 171–2, 414–15
purchasing power 32, 69

qualitative research: CMHN studies 397–405; co-operative enquiry 402–3; discourse analysis 400–1; hermeneutic circle 400; nine criteria 401–2; non-positivist types 399–403; participatory studies 403; positivism/non-positivism 398
quality 133, 348
quantitative research: CMHN studies 385–96; contribution to current CMHN practice 386–9; costs/benefits 390–1; funding 392; justifications for 390–4; outcomes 390
questionnaires 122, 123, 126, 337

racial discrimination 113–19
randomised controlled trials (RCTs) 167–8
RCP see Royal College of Psychiatrists
RCTs see randomised controlled trials
recovery concept 255–6
Reed Report (DOH/HO 1992) 300, 301
Rees, T.P. (Percy) 9, 10
referrals 85, 86
Reflecting Team Process (Andersen 1987) 216
reflective practice 132–44; issues for community psychiatric nurses 141–2; principles 135; storytelling 295
Reform of the Mental Health Act 1983: proposals for consultation (Secretary of State for Health 1999) 37
Reforming the Mental Health Act (Secretary of State for Health and Home Secretary 2000a, b) 37
reforms: mental hospitals 9–10
refusal: ethical aspects 49–50
regeneration policies 155–8
rejection see social exclusion
relapse see psychosis relapse
'relapse signatures' 254
research: assertive outreach 262–3; case management 262–3; nurse involvement 169–70; qualitative approaches 397–405; quantitative approaches 385–96; see also evidence-based practice

Research Assessment Exercise 392
resources 51–2, 170–2
Rethink Serious Mental Illness 223, 411
Review of Mental Health Nursing (DOH 1994) 386–7
Revolving Doors (organisation) 412
Richardson, Prof. Genevra 35, 36, 37
risk: assessment 191–5; community care 26–7; community nursing environment 188–91; creativity 288, 289; decision-making 187–208; defining 188, 189, 190; suicide 199–201, 204–6
Ritchie Enquiry (1994) 191
roles: community psychiatric nurse 13, 21; dementia care nursing 321–6; nursing skills 74–5; primary care liaison nurses 85; primary care team members 80, 86; social role theory 103–4
Royal College of General Practitioners (RCGP) 83
Royal College of Nursing 409
Royal College of Psychiatrists (RCP) 323, 333

Sainsbury Centre for Mental Health 412; assertive outreach 262, 265; mental health promotion 150, 159, 160; stress survey 125
Sainsbury Mental Health Initiative 125
SANE 411
*Saving lives: our healthier nation* (DOH 1992) 155
schema theory 236
schizophrenia: case study 115; cognitive deficits/bias 237; dopamine hypothesis 276; Hearing Voices Network 96, 412; primary care provision 79; psychosocial family interventions 223–4, 229–32; 'serious mental illness' 322; substance abuse 313–14; suicide risk 201; understanding 402
school nurses: activities 80
scientific respectability: nursing 291
SCM *see* standard case management
secondary prevention: depression 81
sedative-hypnotic drugs 280
selective serotonin reuptake inhibitors (SSRIs) 278
self-esteem: employment 56–60
serious mental illnesses classification 322
service users: asylum system 91; autonomy 47–9; collaboration with mental health workers 90–9; empowerment 94, 97–8; nurse–patient relationships 91, 92
sexual harassment 101; *see also* gender issues

Shaftsbury, Lord 7
shared formulations 243–4
Short Report (DHSS 1985) 25
'should' questions 42
Single Regeneration Budget (SRB) 150, 158
skills requirements 74–5, 191–3
social context 193–5
social domains (CANSAS) 180–1
social exclusion 54–66, 102, 106
social inclusion 60–3
social models 332
social role theory 103–4
social support 304–6
social work: avoidance by CPNs 21
social workers 69, 86
socialisation 103–4
societal reaction theory 105
Somerset 71–2, 73, 75
SRB *see* Single Regeneration Budget
stakeholders 31
standard case management (SCM) treatment 314
standards 34, 36, 82–4, 222–3
status: nurses in multidisciplinary teams 392
stigma *see* social exclusion
storytelling 295, 296
*Strategies for living* initiative (Mental Health Foundation) 97
stress: community mental health nurses 121–31; depression in women 104; questionnaire 122, 123
stress-vulnerability 238–9, 253–5
style of working 267
substance abuse 310–16
success factors 265
suicide: definition 199; high-risk individuals 201–2; patients causing CMHN stress/burnout 122, 123; predictive models 199–201; prevention 198–206; psychosocial risk factors 200; rates 198–9; risk assessment 203–4; risk management 204–6
supervision *see* clinical supervision
Survivors Speak Out 413
systemic family therapy 210–19; clinical areas 216–17; concepts informing practice 213–14; history 211–12; ideas in practice 214–15; Milan team 212; parallels in mental health nursing 212–13; teamworking 215; therapy sessions 215–16; working with adults 217–18
systematic reviews 167

targeting: assertive outreach 265–6

TCPS *see* Transcultural Psychiatry Society (UK)
team approaches: assertive outreach 269–71; children/adolescents 350; multidisciplinary 67–76
tertiary prevention: depression 81
therapeutic creativity 287–97
therapy *see* treatment
Thorn Programme 387
Thornicroft, Professor Graham 35
Thresholds Bridge programme (Chicago) 262
time span (interventions) 228
*Together we stand* HAS report 344
tokenism: service user consultation 95
Townsend, Peter 8
traditional psychiatry 112–13
training: 1960s 14; 1990s 15; CAMHS nurses 352–4; clinical supervisors' needs 138–9; evaluation 391; family interventions 387; generalist 406; medication management skills 389; psychosocial family interventions 226, 230; psychotherapy 211; service user involvement 96
transcultural psychiatry 113–16
Transcultural Psychiatry Society (UK) (TCPS) 114
treatment: cultural aspects 117–19; gender bias 105–6; service user collaboration 90–9; *see also* family therapy; interventions; psychopharmacology
*Treatment choice in psychological therapies and counselling* (DOH 2001) 211
tricyclic antidepressants (TCAs) 278

UK Advocacy Network (UKAN) 413
UKAN *see* UK Advocacy Network

unemployment 56–60
urban policy tradition 157
*Urban regeneration and mental health* (Hoggett *et al.* 1999) 157–8
US influence on UK mental health practices 22–3, 24, 25
User Focused Monitoring 93, 160–1
user-led services 90–9, 150
utilitarianism 43

value for money 292, 390–1
voluntary organisations 410–13
voluntary status admission 10
vulnerability 238–9, 253–5, 333–4

Warlingham Park Hospital (nr Croydon) 10–11, 20, 21
wars: public mood 195
WAT *see* Workforce Action Team
websites 416–17
Welsh strategy *see* child and adolescent mental health services
*Who cares?* (HEA 1997) 323
women: depression 102–5; ECT 105; emotionality 103; in-patient admissions 101; isolation 102; issues 100–10; needs 107; service provision 107–8
Workforce Action Team (WAT) 71, 75, 96
workforce development plans 348
*Working in partnership* (DOH 1994) 15, 91, 132–3, 327
World Health Organisation (WHO) 151, 154, 332
worldviews: cultural differences 113
writing 296

Yellow Card survey (MIND) 93

Zito, Jonathan 386

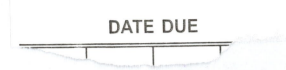

DATE DUE